REGULATING PESTICIDES IN FOOD

THE DELANEY PARADOX

Committee on Scientific and Regulatory Issues
Underlying Pesticide Use Patterns and Agricultural Innovation

Board on Agriculture

National Research Council

NATIONAL ACADEMY PRESS
Washington, D.C. 1987

NATIONAL ACADEMY PRESS • 2101 Constitution Avenue, NW • Washington, DC 20418

This project was supported by the U.S. Environmental Protection Agency. Although the research described in this document has been funded wholly or in part by the U.S. Environmental Protection Agency under assistance agreement CR-812181-01 to the National Academy of Sciences, it has not been subjected to the agency's peer and administrative review and therefore may not necessarily reflect the views of the agency, and no official endorsement should be inferred.

Preparation of this publication was supported by funds from the W. K. Kellogg Foundation; Dow Chemical U.S.A.; CIBA-GEIGY Corp., Agricultural Division; General Foods Corp.; ICI Americas Inc., Agricultural Chemicals Division; Lilly Research Laboratories; Mobay Chemical Corp., Agricultural Chemicals Division; Rhone-Poulenc, Inc., Agrochemical Division; Rohm and Haas Co.; and Shell Companies Foundation.

Library of Congress Catalog Card Number 87-61095

ISBN 0-309-03746-8

Committee on Scientific and Regulatory Issues Underlying Pesticide Use Patterns and Agricultural Innovation

RAY THORNTON, *Chairman*, University of Arkansas
DARRYL BANKS, New York State Department of
  Environmental Conservation
DONALD BISSING, FMC Corporation
GERALD A. CARLSON, North Carolina State University
FERGUS CLYDESDALE, University of Massachusetts
T. ROY FUKUTO, University of California, Riverside
GEORGE KENNEDY, North Carolina State University
RICHARD A. MERRILL, University of Virginia
WARREN R. MUIR, Hampshire Research Associates, Inc.
GAIL M. PESYNA, E. I. du Pont de Nemours & Co., Inc.
DEXTER SHARP, Monsanto Co. (retired)
EARL SWANSON, University of Illinois
MICHAEL R. TAYLOR, King & Spalding
FRED H. TSCHIRLEY, Michigan State University (retired)
ARTHUR C. UPTON, New York University
EILEEN VAN RAVENSWAAY, Michigan State University
PAUL WAGGONER, Connecticut Agricultural Experiment Station

Staff

RICHARD WILES, *Project Officer*
*CONNIE MUSGROVE, *Project Officer*
JOHN WARGO, *Consultant*
DELORES CARTER, *Senior Secretary*
ROMA DECOTEAU, *Senior Secretary*

---

*Through January 1987

iii

Board on Agriculture

iv

Preface

In February 1985, the U.S. Environmental Protection Agency (EPA) asked the Board on Agriculture of the National Research Council to study the EPA's methods for setting tolerances for pesticide residues in food. Specifically, the EPA asked the board to examine the current and likely future impacts of the Delaney Clause on the tolerance-setting process. The Delaney Clause is a provision of the Federal Food, Drug and Cosmetic (FDC) Act, which is the law that governs the setting of pesticide tolerances. The clause purports to bar the EPA from granting any tolerance for a pesticide residue that has been found to induce cancer in animals and that concentrates in processed food. The board was asked to consider the impact of this prohibition on the availability of agricultural pesticides and the protection of the public health.

To conduct the study, the board formed the Committee on Scientific and Regulatory Issues Underlying Pesticide Use Patterns and Agricultural Innovation. The committee includes experts in agricultural pest control, pesticide development, agricultural economics, cancer risk assessment, public health, food science, regulatory decision making, and law.

The committee undertook three principal tasks in preparing this report. First, it examined the statutory framework for setting tolerances for pesticide residues in food and the operation of the tolerance-setting process at the EPA. Second, it developed a computerized data base for estimating the impacts of the current standards for setting tolerances on dietary cancer risk as well as on pesticide use and development. Third, it analyzed the impacts of different standards for establishing pesticide tolerances on dietary cancer risk and pesticide use and development.

The report is organized into six chapters preceded by an Executive Summary that contains the committee's findings, conclusions, and recommendations. Chapter 1 introduces the problem. Chapter 2 describes the current law and administrative system for setting pesticide tolerances, with special attention to the sometimes divergent mandates of the FDC Act and the Federal Insecticide, Fungicide and Rodenticide Act (FIFRA). Chapter 3 presents a profile of potential cancer risk from tolerances currently associated with pesticide residues in food. It helps to illuminate the scope of the problem confronting the EPA. Chapters 4 and 5 describe four alternative scenarios for establishing or adjusting tolerances for oncogenic pesticide residues and compare the change in potential cancer risks and pesticide use patterns likely to be achieved under each scenario. Chapter 6 shows the prospects for developing new chemical pesticides and other innovative approaches to pest control and summarizes potential implications of the current regulatory framework for these innovations.

The committee is impressed by the challenges facing the EPA in its efforts to regulate pesticide residues in food. The law is textually complex and difficult to implement. Relevant scientific knowledge is expanding rapidly, presenting new issues and problems daily. Public demands and expectations are unrelenting. The committee hopes this report will assist the EPA's effort in this important area of regulation.

RAY THORNTON
Chairman

Acknowledgments

The complexity of this report posed unusual challenges to the committee. Many people deserve special thanks for their contributions to this task.

The committee's analysis—and this report—would not have been possible without support and cooperation from Environmental Protection Agency officials and scientists: Douglas Campt, Reto Engler, John A. Moore, Steven Schatzow, and Richard Schmidt. These and other individuals facilitated the committee's use of the agency's Tolerance Assessment System and provided other essential data and guidance needed to understand current EPA policy and practice.

The committee expresses its appreciation to John P. Wargo, Yale University, for designing the data base and responding to requests for additional analyses. It also thanks Bruce S. Wilson, U.S. Court of Appeals for the Eighth Circuit, for providing the legal history of the Delaney Clause.

The committee is grateful for the diligence and creativity of the Board on Agriculture staff, particularly that of project officers Connie Musgrove and Richard Wiles. The substantive contribution of Richard Wiles is especially noteworthy. The committee also appreciates the dedication of Delores Carter and Roma DeCoteau as they worked on the manuscript through many drafts. And it thanks the editors, Carla Carlson and Grace Jones Robbins.

Contents

EXECUTIVE SUMMARY 1

1 INTRODUCTION 17
FIFRA and the FDC Act, 18
The Delaney Clause and the Purpose of This Report, 20
The Committee's Tasks, 21

2 THE CURRENT SYSTEM: THEORY AND PRACTICE . . 23
Registration of Pesticides Under FIFRA, 23
Tolerance Setting Under the FDC Act, 24
The Data Call-In Program, 36
The Delaney Clause—A Closer Examination, 37
Summary of Problems and Issues Posed by the
    Delaney Clause, 40

3 ESTIMATES OF DIETARY ONCOGENIC RISKS 45
Introduction, 45
Description of the Data Base and the Analytical Method, 50
Estimation of Oncogenic Risk, 63
EPA's Interpretation of the Delaney Clause to Date, 83
Case Studies of Potential Policy Precedents, 91
Projecting Past Actions into the Future, 96
The Short-Term Potential Impact of the Delaney Clause, 97

ix

4 THE SCENARIOS AND THE RESULTS. 100
Introduction, 100
Analytical Methods, 102
Description of the Scenarios and Results, 103

5 COMPARING THE IMPACT OF THE SCENARIOS. . . . 118
The Impacts of the Scenarios on Herbicides, Insecticides,
    and Fungicides, 118
The Impacts of the Scenarios on Individual Active
    Ingredient Risk, 120
A Crop-Level Analysis: The Impacts of the Scenarios on
    Benefits and Risks, 123
Alternatives to the Scenarios, 129

**6 PESTICIDE INNOVATION AND THE ECONOMIC
EFFECTS OF IMPLEMENTING THE
DELANEY CLAUSE** 136
The Innovation Process and the Pesticide Industry, 137
Review of Industry R&D and Studies to Date, 139
Future Prospects in Chemical Pest Control, 145
Chemical Pesticide Prospects Relative to Dietary Risks, 148
Innovation Prospects in Pest Control, 150
Special Challenges to Innovation, 155

APPENDIXES

A. Legislative History of the Pesticide Residues Amendment
of 1954 and the Delaney Clause of the Food Additives
Amendment of 1958 *Bruce S. Wilson* 161
B. Analytical Methodology for Estimating Oncogenic Risks
of Human Exposure to Agricultural Chemicals in Food
Crops *John P. Wargo* 174
C. Case Studies of the EPA's Application of the Delaney Clause
in the Tolerance-Setting Process *Richard Wiles* 196
    Fosetyl Al, 196
    Benomyl, 198
    Captan, 201
    Chlorobenzilate, 204
    Dicamba, 206
    EBDCs, 208
    Metalaxyl, 214
    Permethrin, 217
    Thiodicarb, 220

D. Pesticide Innovation 226
   Trends in Innovation *Earl R. Swanson* 226
   Weed Control *Fred H. Tschirley* 228
   Insect Control *T. Roy Fukuto* 234

E. Survey of Pesticide R&D Directors: How Do Current
   Laws Affect Agricultural Pesticide Research Productivity? . . . 249

INDEX 257

Tables and Figures

TABLES

1-1   Section 408 and 409 Food Tolerances Listed in the CFR, 19

2-1   Food Tolerances in the CFR, 35

2-2   Food Tolerances in the CFR for 53 Oncogens, 36

3-1   Agricultural Use Information for Selected Oncogenic Herbicides, 47

3-2   Fungicide Use for 10 Major U.S. Food Commodities, 48

3-3   Potentially Oncogenic Pesticides Identified by the EPA, 52

3-4   Number of Pesticides Identified as Oncogens by the EPA, 56

3-5   Comparative Consumption of Selected Crop Groups, 58

3-6   Comparative Consumption of Selected Raw and Processed Crops, 58

3-7   Presumed Oncogenic Pesticides with Section 409 Tolerances, 63

3-8   Processed Foods in the Tolerance Assessment System (TAS) Compared with Section 409 Tolerances, 64

3-9   Estimated Oncogenic Risk from Dietary Exposure to 28 Pesticides, 68

3-10   Estimated Oncogenic Risk Distribution by Pesticide Type on Fresh and Processed Foods, 69

3-11   Crop Requirements for Processing Studies Under Current EPA Guidelines, 70

3-12   Worst-Case Impact of the Delaney Clause, 71

3-13   Industry Recommendations of Processed By-products Requiring Tolerances, 72

3-14   Animal Feeds Not Subject to Feed-Additive Regulations, 73

3-15   Estimated Oncogenic Risk from Meat, Milk, Dairy, and Poultry Products, 74

3-16   Distribution of Estimated Oncogenic Risk by Pesticide Type, 74

3-17 Estimated Oncogenic Risk from Dietary Exposure to Selected Herbicides, 76

3-18 Estimated Oncogenic Risk from Dietary Exposure to Selected Insecticides, 77

3-19 Estimated Oncogenic Risk from Dietary Exposure to Selected Fungicides, 77

3-20 Fifteen Foods with the Greatest Estimated Oncogenic Risk, 78

3-21 Estimated Oncogenic Risk from Herbicides in Major Foods, 79

3-22 Estimated Oncogenic Risk from Insecticides in Major Foods, 80

3-23 Estimated Oncogenic Risk from Fungicides in Major Foods, 80

3-24 Estimated Oncogenic Risk from All Active Ingredients Used on Selected Foods, 83

3-25 Foods with the Greatest Estimated Oncogenic Risk from Herbicides, 84

3-26 Foods with the Greatest Estimated Oncogenic Risk from Insecticides, 84

3-27 Foods with the Greatest Estimated Oncogenic Risk from Fungicides, 85

3-28 Estimated Oncogenic Risk from Tolerances over Time, 86

3-29 Tolerance Actions for Which the Delaney Clause Was Cited, 88

3-30 Pesticide Active Ingredients Under Review for Which the Delaney Clause Has Been a Concern, 89

3-31 Pesticides with Retracted or Unpursued Tolerance Applications, 90

3-32 Number of Cancer Studies Due for Pesticide Active Ingredients, 1986–1990, 96

3-33 Potential Short-Term Impact of the Delaney Clause on Selected Fungicides, 97

3-34 Potential Short-Term Impact of the Delaney Clause on Selected Herbicides, 98

4-1 Key Features of the Four Scenarios Examined by the Committee, 104

4-2 Scenario 1—Reduction in Estimated Risk, 105

4-3 Scenario 1—Effect on Active Ingredients, Tolerances, and Crops, 106

4-4 Impacts of Scenario 1 on Major Crop Uses for Registered Pesticides, 107

4-5 Scenario 2—Reduction in Estimated Risk, 108

4-6 Scenario 2—Effect on Active Ingredients, Tolerances, and Crops, 109

4-7 Impacts of Scenario 2 on Major Crop Uses for Registered Pesticides, 111

4-8 Scenario 3—Reduction in Estimated Risk, 112

4-9 Scenario 3—Effect on Active Ingredients, Tolerances, and Crops, 113

4-10 Impacts of Scenario 3 on Major Crop Uses for Registered Pesticides, 114

4-11 Scenario 4—Reduction in Estimated Risk, 115

4-12 Scenario 4—Effect on Active Ingredients, Tolerances, and Crops, 116

4-13 Impacts of Scenario 4 on Major Crop Uses for Registered Pesticides, 116

5-1 Estimated Risk Reduction for Each Type of Pesticide by Scenario, 119

5-2 Impact of Scenarios on Different Pesticide Active Ingredients, 121

5-3 Risk, Acre Treatment, and Expenditure Reductions for Selected Crop-Pesticide Combinations, 122

5-4 Potential Short-Term Impact of the Delaney Clause on Selected Fungicides, 132

5-5   Estimated Change in Dietary Oncogenic Risk in Some Crops from Revoking Benomyl Tolerances, 133
5-6   Estimated Change in Dietary Oncogenic Risk in Some Crops from Revoking EBDC Tolerances, 134
6-1   Pesticide Industry Total R&D Expenditures, 141
6-2   Number of Chemicals Registered for the First Time as Pesticides Under FIFRA (1967–1984), 143
6-3   Evaluation of Experimental and Unregistered Citrus Insecticides, 146
6-4   Number of Herbicides in Field Tests, 147
6-5   Evaluation of Experimental and Unregistered Fungicides, 148
6-6   Current Status of Pesticides and Available Alternatives, 149

FIGURES

3-1   Percentage of theoretical maximum residue contribution for oncogenic pesticides by pesticide type, 60
3-2   Percentage of estimated dietary oncogenic risk from fungicides, herbicides, and insecticides, 75
3-3   Concentration of total estimated dietary oncogenic risk in selected foods, 78
3-4   Risk from tolerances granted before and after 1978, 87
6-1   Pesticide development from production to commercialization, 138
6-2   Estimated dietary oncogenic risk and R&D expenditures by pesticide type, 150

REGULATING
PESTICIDES
IN FOOD

Executive Summary

In February 1985, the Environmental Protection Agency (EPA) asked the Board on Agriculture of the National Research Council to study the EPA's methods for setting tolerances for pesticide residues in food. Specifically, the EPA asked the board to examine the impact of the Delaney Clause on the tolerance-setting process. Although the Delaney Clause appears on its face to be a minor feature of the complex statutory scheme governing the regulation of pesticides and pesticide residues in food, its potential impact on the EPA's future decision making is great.

The EPA establishes tolerances for pesticide residues on raw commodities under section 408 of the Federal Food, Drug and Cosmetic (FDC) Act. Enacted in 1954, this law stipulates that tolerances are to be set at levels deemed necessary to protect the public health, while taking into account the need for "an adequate, wholesome, and economical food supply." Section 408 thus explicitly recognizes that pesticides confer benefits and risks and that both should be taken into account in setting raw commodity tolerances.

Pesticide residues that concentrate in processed food above the level authorized to be present in or on their parent raw commodities are governed by the FDC Act's section 409, the law governing food additives. Under section 409, such residues must be proven safe, which is defined as a "reasonable certainty" that "no harm" to consumers will result when the additive is put to its intended use. Consideration of benefits is not authorized. Moreover, section 409 contains the Delaney Clause. This clause prohibits the approval of a food additive that has been found to

1

"induce cancer" (or, under the EPA's interpretation, to induce either benign or malignant tumors—i.e., is oncogenic) in humans or animals.

The dichotomous statutory standards applicable to tolerance setting inspired this study. A pesticide regulated on a risk/benefit basis at the time of registration and in the setting of tolerances for residues in or on raw agricultural commodities becomes, solely because it concentrates in processed food, subject to the Delaney Clause's ostensible zero-risk standard. This shift in criteria has potentially far-reaching effects. If any portion of a crop to which an oncogenic pesticide has been applied is processed in a way that will concentrate residues, the EPA's current policy is to deny not only a section 409 tolerance for the processed food but also a section 408 tolerance for residues of the pesticide in or on the raw commodity. Further, if required section 408 tolerances cannot be granted for a food-use pesticide, the EPA must also deny registration of the pesticide under the Federal Insecticide, Fungicide and Rodenticide Act (FIFRA).

The EPA's policy concerning application of the Delaney Clause to new pesticides and new uses is fairly clear. The EPA's policies are currently less settled regarding the large number of already-registered pesticides, however, and are expected to come under intense pressure in coming years. The sources of this pressure are the following:

• The EPA has instituted programs to expand substantially the data on the toxicological properties of pesticides and the tendency of individual pesticides to concentrate in processed foods.

• Once tested in accordance with contemporary standards, many older pesticides are likely to be identified as oncogenic or potentially oncogenic, inviting regulatory action by the EPA.

• As more data on the tendency of pesticides to concentrate in processed food become available, many more currently registered pesticides will be shown to need section 409 tolerances and thus will become subject to the Delaney Clause.

It is unlikely that the EPA will be able to avoid applying the Delaney Clause to registered pesticides. Thus, as the agency proceeds through the reregistration process, it must determine how to apply the zero-risk standard of the Delaney Clause to a significant number of currently registered, commercially important pesticides. Because of the potential magnitude and complexity of this task, the EPA asked the Board on Agriculture to undertake this study.

The committee undertook three principal tasks. First, it examined the statutory basis of tolerance setting for pesticide residues in food and the operation of the tolerance-setting process at the EPA. Second, it developed a computerized data base to estimate the potential dietary oncogenic risk associated with pesticides determined or suspected by the EPA to be oncogenic. Third, using the data base it had developed, the committee analyzed the impact of alternative approaches to tolerance setting on estimated cancer risks and pesticide use and development.

THE COMMITTEE'S ESTIMATES OF ONCOGENIC RISK

The analytical methods involved in estimating oncogenic risks from pesticide residues in food contain many areas of scientific and technical uncertainty. The assumptions made to account for these uncertainties can have profound implications for the resulting risk estimates. For example, the calculation of exposure to pesticide residues in a given foodstuff can yield risk estimates that vary by an order of magnitude. The committee assumes all residues are at the tolerance level, although actual residues may be different. Likewise, assumptions regarding how and when to aggregate risks from a pesticide used on a variety of crops can significantly alter risk estimates. The quantification of a pesticide's oncogenicity potency, called a Q star or Q^*, can also vary by orders of magnitude, depending on such factors as whether a surface area or body weight correction is made in extrapolating risks from rodents to humans, the choice of extrapolation model, or whether malignant and benign tumors are combined when calculating the response to a given dose. The Q^*'s used by the committee were calculated by EPA scientists and have not been formally peer reviewed.

The EPA generally follows a conservative policy in estimating risk. Whenever assumptions must be made, the agency attempts to make them in a way that minimizes the chance of underestimating risks. The cumulative result of these assumptions is an upper-bound estimate of additional oncogenic risk above the background cancer risk of 1 in 4 or 0.25 (2.5×10^{-1}). For perspective, it is worth noting that an additional dietary oncogenic risk of 1 in 1 million or 1×10^{-6} would raise this background risk of 0.25 to 0.250001. In developing the risk estimates contained in this report, the committee adopted what it understood to be the EPA's current methodology for quantitative risk assessment, recognizing that many key elements of the agency's risk assessment procedures are under review. This report only notes the importance of these assumptions and underlying issues; it does not offer resolutions.

In arriving at a regulatory position on an oncogenic pesticide, the EPA considers the relative significance of all the evidence of oncogenicity for a compound. This "weight-of-the-evidence" approach involves considering many qualitative factors such as the tumor type, results of mutagenicity bioassays for the compound, and negative oncogenicity test results. In calculating the distribution of dietary oncogenic risk and the consequences of regulatory scenarios examined in this report, the committee did not use weight-of-the-evidence techniques. Instead, it relied entirely on the quantitative risk assessment methods that the EPA uses. Risk estimates are generally shown with the EPA's oncogenic classification for the compound, however. This classification system is designed to characterize a pesticide's oncogenicity in humans (see Chapter 3).

The reader should understand that a wide margin of uncertainty surrounds nearly all of these numbers. With this in mind, the reader should focus on general patterns of risk distribution and how key parameters change when policy alternatives are assessed, not on specific point estimates of risk.

The committee further emphasizes that all risk estimates in this report are limited to oncogenic risk from pesticide residues in food. This does not imply, however, that other risks presented by pesticides or other routes of exposure are less important. Indeed, the regulation of pesticides involves a consideration of many health and environmental risks, only one of which involves residues of oncogenic pesticides in food.

ESTIMATED ONCOGENIC RISK AND ITS DISTRIBUTION IN THE FOOD SUPPLY

To characterize the universe of oncogenic pesticides, the committee adopted the list of 53 suspected oncogenic compounds that the EPA transmitted to Congressman Henry Waxman (D-Calif.) in October 1985. Of these compounds, the committee limited its analysis to three types of pesticides—herbicides, fungicides, and insecticides. The risk estimates discussed in this report are derived from only 28 of these 53 active ingredients (see Chapter 3). To roughly characterize the benefits associated with the use of these oncogenic compounds, the committee assembled crop use and farm-level expenditure estimates averaged over three years on all 53 compounds.

Findings

The committee's analysis indicates that the Delaney Clause will be central to the EPA's decision making in future years.

First, the EPA considers a substantial fraction of all herbicides, fungicides, and insecticides to be oncogenic or potentially oncogenic in animal studies. On the basis of pounds of pesticide applied, 60 percent of all herbicides are oncogenic or potentially oncogenic. (This number includes two compounds not on the "Waxman list" that have since been found to be suspect oncogens, raising the percentage from around 40 percent to just over 60 percent.) By volume, 90 percent of all fungicides fall into this category, as do about 30 percent of all insecticides.

Second, for the 53 oncogenic compounds, the committee has identified 31 processed foods with approved section 409 tolerances. All of these appear to conflict with the Delaney Clause. Moreover, the committee has identified an additional 778 processed foods *with no 409 tolerances* for which oncogenic pesticides are registered. Residues of these pesticides are expected to concentrate in many of these processed foods. Hence, over the next few years, the EPA will face bringing several hundred additional pesticide uses into compliance with section 409 of the FDC Act and the Delaney Clause.

Third, over the next five years, the EPA is scheduled to complete regulatory actions that will force decisions on compliance with the Delaney Clause for 10 currently registered oncogenic pesticides. These pesticides account for between 80 and 90 percent of the total estimated dietary oncogenic risk from residues of the 28 compounds that comprise the committee's risk estimate (see Chapter 3).

Fourth, the committee explored the distribution of dietary oncogenic risk from residues of these 28 pesticides. Fungicides account for about 60 percent of all currently estimated dietary oncogenic risk from these 28 compounds. Of the remaining risk, 27 percent stems from crop uses of herbicides and 13 percent from insecticides. Fungicides, however, account for only about 7 percent of all pesticide sales and less than 10 percent of all pounds applied. Further insights derived from the committee's analyses of these 28 pesticides include the following:

• About 55 percent of the total estimated dietary oncogenic risk stems from residues on crops that have raw and processed food forms.
• About 20 percent is associated with consumption of the processed forms of these crops. Approximately 35 percent is from consumption of the raw form of the same crops.
• About 45 percent of estimated dietary oncogenic risk is from foods that the EPA considers to have no processed form. These foods include many fruits and vegetables and *all* meat, milk, and poultry products.

These figures lead to several observations:

• At most, the Delaney Clause could apply to processed-food residues responsible for only one-fifth of the estimated dietary oncogenic risk from pesticides. However, its implementation could eliminate another 35 percent of the estimated risk from residues on the raw forms of these processed foods because it is the EPA's policy to deny section 408 raw food tolerances when section 409 tolerances cannot be established for the processed forms of the same crop.

- Foods accounting for nearly one-half of the total estimated dietary risk (all meat, milk, poultry, and pork products and many fruits and vegetables) are ostensibly beyond the scope of the Delaney Clause, because under current EPA guidelines they have no processed form.

Fifth, dietary oncogenic risk appears to be concentrated in a relatively small number of pesticides and crops. Nearly 80 percent of the estimated dietary oncogenic risk (from all 178 food uses of the 28 compounds that comprise the committee's risk estimate) is from residues of 10 pesticides on only 15 different foods.

IMPACTS OF FOUR ALTERNATIVE WAYS TO REGULATE ONCOGENIC RESIDUES

The committee studied the implications of four theoretical policy scenarios, or frameworks, for regulating residues of oncogenic pesticides in food. The committee emphasizes that these scenarios are artificial constructs chosen not because they reflect any current regulatory approach but rather because they represent a plausible range of approaches. Further, the committee does not offer a legal opinion on the compatability of any of these scenarios with current law or interpretation. These tasks were not in the committee's charge.

Scenario 1 applies a zero-risk standard for oncogenic risk to all pesticide residues on both raw and processed foods. If the EPA determined that a pesticide was oncogenic, all food tolerances for that pesticide would be revoked.

Scenario 2 applies a zero-risk standard for oncogenic risk to all pesticide residues in *processed* foods: any residue of an oncogenic pesticide in a processed food would be disallowed. This scenario further assumes that when residues of an oncogenic pesticide are present in the processed portion of a crop, tolerances for both raw and processed forms would be revoked.

Scenario 3 would revoke all tolerances for a pesticide on a crop when the combined estimated cancer risk from the residues of that pesticide on both the raw and processed forms of a crop exceeds 1 in 1 million or 1×10^{-6}.

Scenario 4 would revoke all tolerances for a pesticide on a crop when the total risk from residues of a pesticide on all *processed* forms of a crop exceeds 1×10^{-6}. As under scenario 2, when residues on the processed form of the crop trigger revocation, both raw and processed food tolerances would be revoked.

Results of the Scenarios

Scenario 1 would revoke all tolerances for all oncogenic pesticides and eliminate all estimated dietary oncogenic risk.

Scenario 2 would revoke tolerances that would reduce dietary oncogenic risk (from the 28 pesticides that constitute the committee's estimate of dietary oncogenic risk) by 55 percent, ignoring about 45 percent of total estimated dietary risk from foods with no processed form.

Scenario 3 would reduce total estimated risk from these 28 compounds by 98 percent, while revoking only 32 percent of all tolerances for the 28 oncogenic pesticides.

Scenario 4 would eliminate just 35 percent of the estimated dietary oncogenic risk, while revoking the smallest percentage of all tolerances.

The most significant finding from the committee's crop level analyses is that under a "negligible risk" standard applicable to residues on both raw and processed food—illustrated by scenario 3—a high percentage of total risk is eliminated while a low percentage of "benefits" (as measured here by acre treatments and expenditures) are lost. For certain crops, scenario 4 would also eliminate a high percentage of total risk while affecting a low percentage of benefits. Scenario 4 would be less effective at reducing overall risk, however, by not addressing tolerances on three of eight crops.

Scenarios 1 and 2 have the same effect on all crop-pesticide combinations examined except peanut fungicides; all oncogenic risk from residues on these crops would be eliminated. In most cases, tolerances associated with a significant percentage of current pesticide expenditures and acre treatments on these crops would be lost. For certain crops in certain regions, the loss of all oncogenic compounds—particularly fungicides—would cause severe short-term adjustments in pest control practices because of the lack of economically viable alternatives.

Findings

The four scenario analyses suggest that progress toward risk reduction could be the greatest and most uniform when raw and processed foods are subject to a consistent risk standard. The potential advantages of a negligible risk standard, with no consideration of benefits, are also highlighted. Such a standard, consistently applied, could eliminate most existing dietary oncogenic risk while allowing continued use of—and benefits from—certain low-risk compounds.

AN ANALYSIS OF THE FUNGICIDES: A SPECIAL CASE

Fungicides present a unique problem. The EPA needs to establish hundreds of new processed-food tolerances for these compounds, but about 90 percent by weight of all fungicides now applied are considered potential oncogens. All but 1 of the 14 oncogenic fungicides were registered more than 15 years ago. These older pesticides are relatively inexpensive, remain effective in various applications, and provide significant benefits to agricultural producers and consumers. These fungicides are important in the production of many high-value fruit and vegetable crops, particularly in the eastern and southeastern regions of the country. The eleven fungicides in the committee's total risk estimate represent less than 10 percent of all acre treatments with pesticides, but are responsible for about 60 percent of the total estimated dietary oncogenic risk.

The mode of action of fungicides makes it difficult to develop compounds that are nontoxic to genetic material. As a result, few effective non-oncogenic new fungicides are being developed. Only four fungicides registered since 1972 have gained greater than 5 percent of the market share for any food crop. Data on several of these compounds indicate oncogenicity and other chronic effects, however.

The combination of the above factors makes the regulation of oncogenic risk from fungicide residues extremely complex. It is the committee's view that literal application of the Delaney Clause will significantly complicate the EPA's efforts to reduce dietary oncogenic risks from fungicides. The committee performed several simple analyses (see Chapter 5) showing that sequential tolerance revocations or denials for one active ingredient at a time could in some cases actually *increase* human dietary oncogenic risk and in many other cases only lower it slightly. These results would occur when the use of a fungicide presenting an equal or greater risk *increased* after tolerances for a less-hazardous compound were revoked.

In response to this dilemma, the committee examined the effect of cropwide tolerance reductions as a means for reducing estimated dietary risk from fungicides. Even a cursory analysis suggests that this and other new regulatory strategies warrant detailed study in terms of their potential to bring about significant reduction in dietary oncogenic risk while preserving beneficial fungicide uses. Cropwide tolerance reductions could reduce the total estimated dietary oncogenic risk from fungicides by up to 50 percent with only modest enforcement effort and minor adjustments in the agricultural sector.

PESTICIDE INNOVATION AND ALTERNATIVE PEST-CONTROL METHODS

Despite the development of pest resistance to chemical pesticides, environmental damage, applicator risk, and fears of cancer associated with pesticide use, most farmers believe that pesticides are a critical part of a reliable and cost-effective pest control strategy. If a large number of tolerances for oncogenic pesticides are revoked over the next five years, adequate replacement pesticides, particularly fungicides, probably would not be available for several major fruit and vegetable crops. For herbicides, however, the prospects are more optimistic. Considering all alternatives being developed, it appears that the loss of several major oncogenic herbicides would not pose a serious threat to agriculture. The outlook for insecticides lies somewhere between that for herbicides and fungicides.

The simultaneous loss of several oncogenic fungicides as described above could present serious disease control problems in certain crops in major production regions. Further, the rate of successful new product development within the three major categories of pesticides is almost inversely proportional to dietary risk; innovation has not been occurring to address the problem of oncogenicity.

Alternative Technologies

Advances in classical plant breeding, innovation in biological and cultural pest control systems, and progress in genetic engineering offer some promise for nonchemical pest control in the future. Nonchemical approaches will be encouraged by tolerance revocations if more profitable chemical controls are not available. For many crops, especially fruits and vegetables, there are few equally effective technologic alternatives to chemical pest control. More important, as with synthetic chemical pesticides, R&D efforts in alternative technologies do not appear directed toward the pest problems most likely to be affected by Delaney Clause–driven tolerance revocations; breeding for disease resistance is an important exception.

Because of the time needed to further develop plant genetic engineering techniques, new technologies involving or derived from biotechnology will not be available to reduce the impact of the next five years of regulatory actions. Although plant breeding offers the promise of more pest-resistant crop varieties, these new varieties will probably lower rather than eliminate the need for pesticides. The objective of biocontrol techniques is to establish a more stable pest control situation in the long run, but these methods are often complex and do not always provide the certainty that chemical pesticides provide. The problems with these alternative technologies will delay the adoption of nonchemical techniques in the absence of incentives.

The Effect of the Delaney Clause on R&D

In the long term, a rigorous application of the Delaney Clause to both existing and new pesticides is likely to shift the focus of public and private

R&D away from oncogenic compounds and reduce the total investment in chemical pesticides. This shift and reduction of investments will depend on factors that the committee was not able to examine quantitatively, including the structure of the industry (corporate mergers), regulatory developments, and scientific breakthroughs. If gross sales of agricultural chemical companies are reduced or if net returns become more variable as a result of tolerance revocations, however, revenues available for these R&D activities will decline and overall innovation is likely to fall. These declines in R&D investments are more likely if revocations lead to increased use of nonchemical controls—developments that provide no profit for pesticide companies.

The Minor Use Issue

All fruit and vegetable crops grown in the United States are considered "minor" crops in terms of pesticide use. Most minor crops have no recognized processed forms under EPA regulations. Most minor crops also present relatively small oncogenic risks. The important issue with these crops is whether pesticides currently vital to their production will remain available when the tolerances for oncogenic pesticides on other crops are revoked pursuant to the Delaney Clause.

Certain minor crops with processed forms *do* present potentially significant risk, however. Apples, tomatoes, grapes, potatoes, and citrus are directly vulnerable to tolerance revocations under any version of the Delaney Clause. In contrast to most minor crops, these crops represent intermediate markets for pesticide producers and therefore provide an incentive for product development. In this fashion, the continued availability of pesticides for small minor crops is linked to the continued availability of pesticides on "minor" crops representing larger markets.

Liability for crop failures or crop injury is another potential obstacle to future pesticide availability for small minor crops. This results from the limited acreage of these minor crops and hence the limited pesticide market they provide, relative to potential liability for control failures. Liability is high because these crops have high per acre value and must meet high-quality standards.

The Delaney Clause and Pest Resistance

A distinct value of many widely applied, suspect oncogenic fungicides is that even after years of use, pests show little if any resistance to them. In contrast, a number of pests have developed some degree of resistance to many of the new, non-oncogenic or more weakly oncogenic fungicides and insecticides. The viability of many of these newer compounds is often linked to their simultaneous use with the older oncogenic compounds. Given the large number of tolerances for older fungicides that may be revoked under the Delaney Clause, there is a critical need to develop non-oncogenic fungicides as well as resistance management programs for these fungicides in the next five years.

MAJOR CONCLUSIONS AND RECOMMENDATIONS

The committee's analysis and findings support four basic conclusions. The first deals with the legal and institutional base for regulating oncogenic pesticide residues in food. The second addresses the possible roles of other than zero oncogenic risk criteria in targeting regulation on pesticide uses that pose potentially significant human health hazards. The third involves the need for and structure of an overall strategy for the EPA as it moves ahead with the task of bringing all existing pesticide registrations and tolerances into compliance with the law, including the Delaney Clause. The fourth describes the adoption of an analytical framework to facilitate a more systematic examination of the risks and benefits associated with pesticides.

Legal Basis for Regulation

Pesticide residues in food, whether marketed in raw or processed form or governed by old or new tolerances, should be regulated on the basis of consistent standards. Current law and regulations governing residues in raw and processed food are inconsistent with this goal.

First, the committee can discover no scientific reason for the law's different treatment of raw and processed food tolerances. Because the committee could find no scientific reason for this disparity, it recommends the consistency and simplification of treating them alike.

Second, residues stemming from the use of older pesticides should be subject to the same scrutiny and standards as those applied to residues from new pesticides. Although concentrating on new pesticides that might present new dangers was a reasonable policy when the regulation of pesticides began, new analyses, data, and criteria provide compelling reasons for uniform treatment of old and new compounds. Neither the FDC Act nor FIFRA provides a clear basis for treating residues of new pesticides differently from those of old pesticides. Subjecting old tolerances to contemporary safety criteria is essential.

The committee's analysis demonstrates that about 90 percent of estimated dietary oncogenic risks from pesticides stems from uses sanctioned by tolerances granted before 1978. The only way for the EPA to reduce dietary risk substantially is to subject old pesticides to the same regulatory scrutiny it applies to new agents. Doing so in the context of reregistration will provide the EPA with an opportunity to reduce public exposure to at least some of the oncogenic pesticides that now are routinely present in food.

Third, the two agencies charged with implementing and interpreting the Delaney Clause—the EPA and the Food and Drug Administration (FDA)—should continue to work to achieve consistent legal interpretations of their common statute and compatible regulatory policies based on the best contemporary science. As long as the Delaney Clause is a part of the FDC Act, better cooperation and communication between EPA and FDA scientists and policy-level officials will be increasingly important as the two agencies work to develop policies for implementing this provision. The effective functioning of both agencies depends on the development of consistent policies for achieving the widely supported goal of eliminating added carcinogens from the food supply whenever feasible and prudent.

A Nonzero Standard for Oncogenic Risk

A negligible risk standard for carcinogens in food, applied consistently to all pesticides and to all forms of food, could dramatically reduce total dietary exposure to oncogenic pesticides with modest reduction of benefits.

The committee believes that the elimination of oncogenic pesticide residues from human food is an appropriate aspiration of regulation. The committee recognizes, however, that residues of several dozen oncogenic pesticides may be found in hundreds of different foods. Many such residues pose little risk to humans, whereas some clearly warrant attention and, quite probably, regulatory action. The problem of implementing action against many pesticides with limited personnel and resources should be minimized. Moreover, the challenge for regulators grows increasingly complex as science and technology advance. Improvements in analytical chemistry and residue detection capabilities, new toxicological data, changing pesticide use practices, and the development of new pesticides and foods establish an urgency *and* the feasibility to devise a strategy for attaining a safer food supply.

One option for regulators is to adopt a negligible risk standard in setting and revising tolerances for all oncogenic pesticides found in food. The committee sees merit in such a standard if its adoption can speed up progress toward risk reduction and help the EPA focus its limited resources on pesticides and crops that pose significant oncogenic risks.

The committee notes with concern that current EPA policy has allowed continued use of pesticides that pose estimated dietary oncogenic risks as high as 1 in 10,000 (1×10^{-4}). The adoption of a negligible-risk standard would provide added justification for the agency to reduce relatively high risks while deferring actions on relatively low or perhaps even zero risks. The committee would not endorse the adoption of such a standard if it were not consistently applied to all pesticides and all forms of human food.

The committee is aware that a zero-risk standard applied to pesticide residues in all foods would eliminate that source of oncogenic risk in the diet. The committee believes, however, that in certain regions and on certain crops, the implementation of such a policy would cause severe adjustments in agricultural practices, particularly in control of plant diseases. This policy could impede agency discretion necessary to achieve significant risk reduction over the next 5 to 10 years while maintaining viable disease control alternatives.

The committee's analysis highlights several advantages of a consistently applied negligible-risk standard over even strict adherence to the traditional zero-risk interpretation of the Delaney Clause, which applies a zero-risk standard only to processed foods and their parent raw commodities:

- The committee found that, if consistently applied, a negligible-risk standard applied to raw and processed foods (assuming no consideration of benefits) could lead to the elimination of 98 percent of existing dietary risk from exposure to the 28 pesticides comprising the committee's estimate of dietary oncogenic risk. In contrast, a zero-risk standard applied only to oncogenic residues in processed foods and their parent raw commodities would reduce estimated risk by just 55 percent. In reality, however, benefits must be considered, and not all residues will concentrate. Also, the risk reduction achieved under both scenarios will probably be less than suggested. Nonetheless, the committee believes that the relative effectiveness of these two scenarios will remain constant and that any plausible negligible-risk standard that treats section 408 and 409 tolerances consistently will lead to greater risk reduction than a zero-risk standard applied only to section 409 tolerances.

- A uniform negligible-risk standard could give the EPA the flexibility needed to reduce dietary oncogenic risks over time. One important option would be the ability to grant tolerances for new chemicals that might pose a slight oncogenic risk (currently prohibited by the Delaney Clause), if use of such pesticides would displace more hazardous products now routinely used. In the past, the EPA has applied the Delaney Clause to deny tolerances for weak oncogens on certain crops. To date, the agency has not invoked the clause to revoke any existing tolerances (in most cases citing lack of acceptable data on oncogenicity and residue concentration). This application of the Delaney Clause has had the effect of preserving the market share for, and continuous dietary exposure to, pesticides that present relatively greater dietary oncogenic risks.

• A negligible-risk standard for tolerance setting would aid the EPA in focusing regulatory resources on the crop and pesticide combinations presenting the greatest oncogenic risk. On the other hand, a zero-risk standard does not encourage and may not allow the EPA to discriminate between relatively significant and relatively insignificant oncogenic risks. Indeed, the Delaney Clause has focused considerable agency resources on protracted scientific assessments designed to determine whether a pesticide is an "oncogen" per se and whether the risk associated with a particular use of that pesticide is zero, or some very small level that is well beyond the predictive power of currently available toxicological tests and risk assessment methods.

The advantages of a consistently applied negligible-risk standard will depend on how fast the EPA will reregister old chemicals, the sequence that will be followed, and perhaps most important, how the benefits will be taken into account. Risk reductions of the magnitude that the committee's analyses suggest are not guaranteed because the analyses did not incorporate benefit considerations. The benefits of some pesticide uses may justify greater risks. The level of risk reduction achieved through the adoption of such a negligible-risk standard will depend on the importance the EPA places on the benefits of specific pesticide uses.

Targeting High-Risk Pesticide and Crop Uses

The committee's analysis (described on pages 50–66) suggests that about 80 percent of oncogenic risk from the 28 pesticides that constitute the committee's risk estimates is associated with the residues of 10 compounds in 15 foods. Logic argues that the EPA should focus its energies on reducing risk from the most worrisome pesticides on the most-consumed crops, and compelling reasons support such a strategy.

First, if the EPA developed a regulatory position on all oncogenic pesticides used on a given crop, the agency would have a realistic chance of dealing with the special problems that arise when there is more than one oncogenic pesticide used on a particular crop. As a class, the fungicides present special difficulties because nine oncogenic compounds account for about 90 percent of all fungicide sales. Further, these nine compounds present comparable risks and generally are viable substitutes for one another. In this situation the agency's historical approach—regulating one pesticide at a time across all of its uses—is not well suited to ensuring real risk reductions. This approach could even *increase* oncogenic risk when revocation of one agent allows a more potent oncogen to gain wider use.

The recommended strategy would also help preserve the benefits of pesticide uses that pose very low, but possibly not zero, risks. For example, most suspect oncogenic pesticides used on corn, soybeans, and cotton present very low dietary oncogenic risks. Further, the committee's analysis indicates that when estimated dietary oncogenic risks from herbicides or insecticides on these crops are deemed high, they can generally be substantially reduced through actions affecting one or two compounds. Most pesticides used on these crops would probably be passed over if a policy were in effect that targeted pesticide uses presenting relatively high dietary oncogenic risk. Such pesticide uses could come under scrutiny for other reasons, however, such as other health effects, ecological problems, or groundwater contamination.

The Adoption of an Analytical Framework

The EPA should develop improved tools and methods to more systematically estimate the overall impact of prospective regulatory actions on health, the environment, and food production. Rapid advances in computer technology, as well as the EPA's successful efforts to computerize major data sets like the Tolerance Assessment System (TAS) make such progress readily attainable.

The EPA's current approach to pesticide regulation focuses on the risks and benefits of one active ingredient at a time across all its uses. Much of the committee's analysis rested on new analytical manipulations of EPA data sets. Insights gained on the distribution and relative magnitude of risks and benefits associated with pesticide use are the foundation of the committee's recommendations. The analytical framework and data base that the committee developed on a prototype basis are described in detail in Chapters 3–5 and Appendix B. The framework the EPA might develop and utilize could be more thorough and precise. The committee's preliminary work provided intriguing new insights, however. The data base that the committee developed is extremely valuable in comparing the effectiveness of different regulatory policies that reduce dietary oncogenic risks from pesticides.

Use of new analytical tools and data bases could help the EPA get ahead of its growing work load. The refinement of such a system would allow the EPA to project with increased confidence a wide range of impacts associated with its regulatory actions. For example, the committee's rudimentary analysis demonstrates that certain strategies for implementing the Delaney Clause could increase dietary risk, and vigorous application of the Delaney Clause to tolerances for residues in processed foods may not be the most effective strategy for minimizing dietary exposure to oncogenic pesticides.

It is important to note that this study's preoccupation with oncogenic hazards simplifies the challenges that the EPA actually faces. In developing regulatory decisions, the EPA must take into account trade-offs between oncogenic risks and other sorts of health and environmental hazards among all pesticides registered for a particular use. Nonetheless, this more complicated task would be aided by the analytical tools discussed in this report.

1

Introduction

The modern increase in pesticide use demonstrates how technological advancements can be beneficial and harmful at the same time. Effectively used, pesticides can kill or control pests, including weeds, insects, fungi, bacteria, and rodents. As a result, chemical pest control has won a central place in modern agriculture, contributing to the dramatic increases in crop yields achieved in recent decades for most major field, fruit, and vegetable crops. The production systems for most crops in most regions of the United States are dependent on at least one pesticide, and often several—some for weed control, some to control insect pests, and others for the control of a variety of plant diseases. The amount of pesticide use varies by region, however. Oats in the northern plains require little or no pesticide use, whereas vegetables in humid regions of the South may require 20 or more pesticide applications in a single growing season.

The focus of this study is limited to pesticide use on food crops. Although pesticides help protect food crops from insect pests, weeds, and diseases, most are potentially dangerous substances whose use requires careful control. They work because they are toxic to target organisms or otherwise disrupt natural processes necessary for the organisms' survival. Some are toxic only to target pests and pose little threat to other life forms, including humans. Many, however, are capable of harming nontarget species.

Pesticides are dispersed widely to treat crops, pastureland, and harvested fruits and vegetables. Consequently, most pesticide applications result in some contact with nontarget crops and organisms as well as

17

applicators (persons who apply pesticides), farm workers, food handlers, and ultimately food consumers. Drinking water is also an increasingly significant source of human exposure to pesticides. All of these routes of exposure present concerns, but this study is limited to dietary exposure from oncogenic residues in food and to the process designed to control this route of exposure.

FIFRA AND THE FDC ACT

The societal response to the dual nature of pesticides has been the development of a comprehensive regulatory system that seeks to make possible the beneficial use of pesticides while minimizing their public health and environmental risks. The current system originated with enactment of the 1947 Federal Insecticide, Fungicide and Rodenticide Act (FIFRA). The system now is defined by a comprehensively amended FIFRA and—for pesticides likely to appear on human foods—by various provisions of the Federal Food, Drug and Cosmetic (FDC) Act. The basic goals of these statutes are to allow only those pesticide uses that (1) do not have "unreasonable adverse effects" on human health or the environment and (2) have benefits outweighing whatever risks might exist. These goals are easy to state but difficult to implement. Complex issues and scientific uncertainties arise in estimating risks and benefits of pesticide uses. There is no simple, widely accepted method for balancing risks and benefits. Moreover, the avoidance of unsafe residues requires not only an operational definition of safety but a costly and complex system for monitoring and enforcement. The responsibility for deciding which pesticides may be used and what residues can be tolerated lies with the Environmental Protection Agency (EPA).

The EPA performs two main tasks. First, under FIFRA, the EPA decides what pesticide uses can be registered or approved in the United States. A single pesticide may have many potential uses. For example, the insecticide dimethoate is used to control a variety of pests on nearly 30 different crops, including cotton, tomatoes, and corn. In this report, a pesticide use refers to the application of a pesticide on a particular crop. The EPA registers each use under a statutory standard that requires balancing of benefits of a pesticide use against its potential risks to human health and the environment.

The EPA's second main task—and the focus of this study—is the establishment of legal limits (tolerances) specifying the amount of pesticide residue that can be present in or on foods sold in interstate commerce. The EPA performs this function under the authority of the FDC Act. It is a huge administrative task. A single pesticide intended for use on a single crop is likely to leave residues on the raw agricultural

TABLE 1-1 Section 408 and 409 Food Tolerances
Listed in the CFR

Type of Pesticide	Number	
	Section 408	Section 409
Insecticides	3,654	63
Herbicides	2,462	39
Fungicides	1,256	20
Total	7,372	122

NOTE: This table does not include feed-additive tolerances listed in the CFR.

commodity. It can also find its way into numerous processed food and animal products. Moreover, most pesticides are used on several crops.

On the basis of field testing to measure residue levels, the EPA establishes tolerances to cover all expected residues on food. Over 8,500 food tolerances for all pesticides are currently listed in the *Code of Federal Regulations* (CFR). Approximately 8,350 of these tolerances are for residues on raw commodities (promulgated under section 408) and about 150 for residues known to concentrate in processed foods (promulgated under section 409). Table 1-1 shows the number of tolerances issued for insecticides, herbicides, and fungicides, which are the major classes of pesticides.

The EPA's tolerance-setting task is made complicated by divergences between FIFRA and the FDC Act. Most notably, some legal standards within the FDC Act apply to pesticide residues present in or on raw commodities and some apply to pesticide residues in processed foods. In deciding whether to establish a raw agricultural commodity tolerance for a fresh food such as tomatoes, the EPA is authorized to balance the benefits of using the pesticide to produce a crop against the potential human health effects of any residue that would result—a process similar to that undertaken when the pesticide is considered for registration under FIFRA.[1]

Some processed foods contain higher levels of residues than allowed by the raw commodity tolerance because residues concentrate during processing. An example is the fungicide benomyl, which concentrates in processed tomato products. This phenomenon can have important regulatory implications because the FDC Act does not allow the EPA to consider the benefits of a pesticide's use in setting tolerances for residues that concentrate in processed foods. Tolerances for such residues are instead set under the same risk-only standard that governs intentional food additives: a residue must be proven safe.[2]

THE DELANEY CLAUSE AND THE PURPOSE OF THIS REPORT

The regulatory consequences of residue concentration in processed food are profound if a pesticide has been found to induce cancer in experiments on animals. Such a residue, or food additive for legal purposes, is subject to the FDC Act's most famous provision—the Delaney Clause. The EPA has interpreted the Delaney Clause as generally prohibiting the establishment of *any* processed-food tolerances for an oncogenic pesticide (a pesticide capable of inducing tumors), regardless of whether or to what extent its residue is judged to pose a hazard to human health. It is this policy that has occasioned the current study.

The objectives of this study are to describe and, to the greatest extent possible, estimate the consequences for public health and agricultural innovation of these dichotomous standards for setting pesticide tolerances. The EPA's request for this study followed its recognition that the procedures necessary to implement the two standards had grown exceedingly complex and sometimes produced results that were difficult to reconcile scientifically. Moreover, the agency realized that an increasing number of regulatory decisions would hinge on its policies for dealing with oncogenic residues in processed foods as the results of new residue chemistry and chronic toxicity studies became available as part of its ongoing pesticide reregistration process.

In describing the need for the study, EPA officials anticipated that application of the Delaney Clause could have a major impact on pesticide availability. Agricultural producers could face high costs if they were forced to adjust cropping patterns and pest control methods. In addition, the agency emphasized a potential paradox. Adherence to the strict standard of the Delaney Clause in establishing *new* tolerances could preclude commercial introduction of potentially lower-risk pesticides. These lower-risk pesticides would then be stopped from replacing older, potentially more hazardous compounds that have not been fully tested or, if tested, have not been brought into compliance with all current statutory requirements. The EPA was also concerned that actions dictated by the law's preoccupation with oncogenicity might make it more difficult to address other health and environmental hazards.

The EPA asked the National Research Council's Board on Agriculture to study the current system for tolerance setting, especially as affected by the Delaney Clause. The agency also asked the board to evaluate the clause's impact on the EPA's ability to accomplish the central goals of pesticide regulation enunciated by Congress: permitting beneficial uses of pesticides while minimizing public health and environmental risks. The board appointed the Committee on Scientific and Regulatory Issues Underlying Pesticide Use Patterns and Agricultural Innovation to respond to these questions.

THE COMMITTEE'S TASKS

The committee began by developing an analytical framework and a data base to assess the impact of the current system (and possible alternatives) on the future availability of pesticides and on human exposure to oncogenic pesticide residues. As explained in Appendix B, the committee, with the EPA's cooperation, assembled an extensive data base. This data base covers 289 registered pesticide active ingredients currently used on food crops by

- Tolerance levels,
- Crop use,
- The likely need for processed food tolerances (because residues tend to concentrate),
- Potential human exposure based on average dietary consumption patterns,
- Regulatory status and history, and
- Toxicological properties.

The committee carried out a series of analyses using the data base. From the results, the committee estimated the effects of different regulatory strategies across all registered pesticides. Based on risk assessment and other analytic methods routinely used by the EPA, this data base analysis has yielded approximate answers to such general questions as—

- How large is the potential human oncogenic risk from pesticides in the diet?
- What pesticides pose the most significant risks?
- What crops account for the greatest exposure and largest risks?
- What general conclusions can be drawn regarding the characteristics of the most hazardous and least hazardous pesticides?

The committee's report of data responsive to these questions, primarily in Chapter 3, must be interpreted with great caution. It is especially important to note that only estimated cancer risks and no other human health risks were assessed. Further, estimates of oncogenic risks are derived using methods designed to identify conservative upper bounds on potential human risk. The estimates presumably overstate true human risk. But with these caveats the analysis provides some important insights, which are described below.

The potential impact of the Delaney Clause on the availability of pesticides and human exposure to oncogenic pesticides is explored in Chapters 4 and 5. In these chapters, four scenarios, or theoretical policy constructs, were evaluated to determine which approach or approaches to tolerance setting will maximize the availability of useful pesticides while minimizing public health and environmental risks.

Throughout the study, the committee has been impressed by the complexity of the tasks that Congress has delegated to the EPA. The committee has come to appreciate the sometimes perplexing scientific and administrative issues posed by each regulatory decision. Before the agency can sanction a new chemical use or restrict or eliminate an old risk, it must assemble and evaluate large amounts of scientific and economic data. It must deal with an array of sometimes competing considerations. It must pay attention to consistency among decisions, especially when far-reaching impacts on the public health, environment, and economy are potentially at stake. It must regularly incorporate scientific advances in risk assessments. In spite of scientific advances and an exponential increase in data that must be evaluated in estimating risks and benefits of pesticide use, the EPA shoulders these complex tasks with budget constraints and limited resources that have shrunk considerably since 1980.

A major part of the EPA's difficulty in reaching and defending regulatory decisions is caused by the law itself rather than the amount or complexity of data. By statute, the propensity of a pesticide residue to concentrate in processed food has been made the linchpin for determining which of two quite different statutory standards applies to the tolerance-setting decision. For oncogenic pesticides that do concentrate, the agency's exercise of scientific judgment is curtailed because the Delaney Clause purports to demand not only zero risk but zero exposure. As a result, agency resources have been diverted toward inquiries regarding the fact and extent of concentration, which may often be insignificant in terms of public health protection, but of great consequence in practice. The committee began the study with the understanding that the Delaney Clause could have substantial impacts on the pesticide program, but was unsure of how to characterize or measure the impacts. The report's analyses shed new light on these impacts.

The committee hopes that this study will provide a framework for policymakers in the EPA, the Congress, and elsewhere to make informed judgments about whether the current system for tolerance setting should be changed. The committee offers some general conclusions concerning the desirability of change and suggests how the prospective consequences of alternative policies should be analyzed. If further refined, the analytical framework and data base used herein may help clarify whether strict adherence to the Delaney Clause contributes to or detracts from achievement of Congress' goals.

NOTES

1. "In establishing any such regulation [raw agricultural commodity tolerance] the Administrator shall give appropriate consideration . . . (1) to the necessity for the production of an adequate, wholesome, and economical food supply." 21 USC § 346(b).
2. "No such regulation [food additive tolerance] shall issue if a fair evaluation of the data before the Secretary fails to establish that the proposed use of the food additive under the conditions of use to be specified in the regulation, will be safe." 21 USC § 348(C)(3)(A).

2

The Current System:
Theory and Practice

The issues this report addresses arise from the interaction between two different statutes, the EPA's administrative practices and the growth in new information about pesticide toxicity and prevalence. The questions posed by the Delaney Clause can be understood only in the context of the system under which the EPA regulates pesticides. This chapter describes that system and identifies the developments that give rise to questions about the Delaney Clause. It concludes by summarizing the major issues the current study is intended to help resolve.

REGISTRATION OF PESTICIDES UNDER FIFRA

The central event in the regulation of a pesticide is registration, which is EPA approval of one or more of its uses under the Federal Insecticide, Fungicide and Rodenticide Act (FIFRA). EPA registration of a pesticide use is required before the pesticide can be lawfully sold in the United States. The use of a pesticide in a manner inconsistent with the terms and conditions of its registration is unlawful.

The registration process is linked with the tolerance-setting process. Pesticides that are to be registered for use on food crops must be granted tolerances under the Food, Drug and Cosmetic (FDC) Act. Tolerances authorize and place legal limits on the presence of pesticide residues in or on raw agricultural commodities and, in appropriate cases, processed foods. The EPA will not register the use of a pesticide on food crops unless tolerances have first been granted to cover any residues expected to remain in or on food. Registration is nevertheless the logical starting point for a discussion of pesticide regulation because registration governs the uses of pesticides that result in food-borne residues.

Section 3 of FIFRA sets forth the standards for registration. The basic requirements are that the pesticide use must be able to accomplish its intended effect without causing "unreasonable adverse effects on the environment," which the law defines as "any unreasonable risk to man or the environment, taking into account the economic, social, and environmental costs and benefits of the use of any pesticide."[1] In proceedings to cancel or suspend the registration for use of a pesticide, the law further directs the EPA to consider the impact of the proposed action "on production and prices of agricultural commodities, retail food prices, and otherwise on the agricultural economy."[2]

Thus, FIFRA is a "balancing" statute. Congress recognized that pesticide uses can yield both risks and benefits and directed the EPA to consider both in deciding whether to permit particular uses of a pesticide. To grant registration, the EPA must conclude that the food production benefits of a pesticide outweigh any risks.

Under FIFRA the burden rests on the manufacturer or other would-be registrant to provide the data needed to support registration. The EPA regulations spell out in detail the data required in 40 CFR Parts 158 and 162.[3] Required data include substantiation of the product's usefulness and disclosure of its chemical and toxicological properties, likely distribution in the environment, and possible effects on wildlife, plants, and other elements in the environment. If the applicant's data fail to prove that the product's use poses "no unreasonable adverse effects on the environment," registration is denied. In theory, the registrant continues to bear this burden even after registration and may be called on to prove its case again if new scientific data cast doubt on the EPA's original assessment of risk or balancing of benefits.

The conclusion of a successful registration process is the approval of a label for the product. This label sets forth detailed and legally binding instructions for use of the pesticide on certain crops, including any limitations or conditions on how or when the pesticide must be applied or not applied. Label specifications are generally designed to avoid adverse effects on the environment or on adjacent or future crops, to ensure efficacy, and to minimize applicator exposure.

TOLERANCE SETTING UNDER THE FDC ACT

Pesticides that are to be registered for use on food crops must have been granted tolerances covering expected residues of the pesticide in raw and processed foods. Two different sections of the FDC Act, enacted four years apart, apply to the setting of tolerances. One, section 408, governs tolerances for pesticide residues on raw commodities. The other, section 409, governs tolerances for pesticide residues that concentrate in processed foods.

Section 408—The Statutory Standard

Congress enacted section 408 of the FDC Act in 1954 to enhance regulatory control over pesticide residues in food. It authorizes the establishment of tolerances for pesticide residues in or on raw agricultural commodities before they leave the farm gate. These tolerances are to be set at levels deemed necessary to protect the public health, while considering the need for "an adequate, wholesome, and economical food supply." Like the FIFRA standard for registration, section 408 of the FDC Act explicitly recognizes that pesticide uses confer benefits and risks and that both should be taken into account. The inquiry authorized by section 408 may not be as broad as that under FIFRA, yet section 408 clearly allows although does not compel the EPA to consider factors other than risks to human health.[4]

Residues of a pesticide on a raw agricultural commodity that exceed a section 408 tolerance or for which no tolerance has been established are deemed unsafe. The commodity itself is characterized as adulterated (and thus unlawful) under the FDC Act.[5]

Section 409

Section 409 of the FDC Act is the source of the Food and Drug Administration's (FDA) general authority to regulate the purposeful addition of substances to food. This provision empowers the FDA to require premarket approval for a varied universe of food additives, including artificial sweeteners, preservatives, chemical processing aids, animal drug residues, and packaging materials. Precisely how section 409 affects the EPA's regulation of pesticides requires some explanation.

Section 201(s) of the FDC Act initially defines the term "food additive" broadly to include "any substance the intended use of which results or may reasonably be expected to result . . . in its becoming a component of food."[6] But it then expressly excludes from the definition pesticide residues in or on raw agricultural commodities, presumably because they are already covered by section 408. By necessary implication, however, pesticide residues in processed foods remain food additives and thus subject to the premarket approval requirement of section 409.[7] The FDA has primary responsibility for implementing section 409, but the EPA has been delegated responsibility for regulating pesticide residues that are food additives.

Like section 408, section 409 establishes a procedure to secure approval for the uses of food additives. However, the standard for granting approvals under section 409 differs fundamentally from the risk-benefit standard of section 408. Section 409 requires the sponsor of a food additive to prove with reasonable certainty that no harm to consumers will result when the additive is put to its intended use.[8] This so-called "general safety standard" for food additives is strictly risk based. It allows consideration of an additive's potential health risks and, by negative implication, seems to preclude consideration of any economic or other benefits.

In section 409, Congress also created a special rule for food additives that have been found to induce cancer in humans or animals. Under the famous Delaney Clause—enacted as a proviso to the general safety standard—no such additive can be approved (in the case of a pesticide this means "granted a tolerance") under section 409.[9]

A food additive that has not been approved under section 409 or that is present in food at a level exceeding a section 409 tolerance is deemed unsafe. Unsafe food additives, as well as the foodstuffs containing them, are adulterated and subject to the same enforcement procedures and penalties applicable to raw agricultural commodities.

If Congress had stopped here, pesticide residues in raw commodities and those in processed foods would be subject to different standards, but the distinction would be clear. The former would be regulated under the balancing criteria of section 408; the latter would be regulated under the risk-only standard of section 409, reinforced by the Delaney Clause. But Congress did not stop here, and it is Congress' further effort to integrate sections 408 and 409 that contributes much of the complexity in pesticide tolerance setting. In brief, not all pesticide residues in processed foods are regulated as food additives.

When it adopted section 409 in 1958, Congress realized that many, if not most, processed foods would contain at least some of the residues of pesticides lawfully present (under section 408) on the raw agricultural commodity used in their production. To facilitate regulation of pesticide residues falling within the definition of food additive—and hence requiring approval under both section 408 and section 409—Congress in effect exempted from "food additive" regulation residues that are present in a processed food at levels no higher than *sanctioned on the raw agricultural commodity*. Section 402(a)(2)(C) of the FDC Act provides

that where a pesticide chemical has been used in or on a raw agricultural commodity in conformity with an exemption granted or a tolerance prescribed under section 408 and such raw agricultural commodity has been subjected to processing such as canning, cooking, freezing, dehydrating, or milling, the residue of such pesticide chemical remaining in or on such processed food shall, notwithstanding the provisions of sections 406 and 409, not be deemed unsafe if such residue in or on the raw agricultural commodity has been removed to the extent possible in good manufacturing practice and the concentration of such residue in the processed food when ready to eat is not greater than the tolerance prescribed for the raw agricultural commodity. . . .[10]

As a general rule, this proviso allows EPA approval of a residue under section 408 to suffice, as long as any residues in food processed from the raw agricultural commodity do not exceed the level authorized under section 408 (see the boxed article "Concentrating Residues"). Such residues remain subject to the balancing standard of section 408, and they escape the Delaney Clause.

Under this statutory framework, the concentration of a pesticide's residues in processed food has profound implications. To expose them, the committee first summarizes the procedural and analytical steps the EPA follows in setting tolerances under sections 408 and 409 and describes the universe of tolerances promulgated to date. Then the committee examines more fully the significance of discovering that pesticide residues concentrate in processed food.

The Tolerance-Setting Process Under Sections 408 and 409

OVERVIEW OF THE PROCESS

Most tolerance-setting proceedings are initiated when a pesticide manufacturer files a petition with the EPA requesting establishment of a tolerance. The petition must be accompanied by or make reference to scientific data and technical information that the manufacturer believes satisfy the agency's data requirements. This information also must support a judgment that the tolerance can be established in compliance with statutory standards. The formal procedures for handling completed petitions under sections 408 and 409 differ slightly, but the same basic supporting data are mandated.

After reviewing a petition for completeness, the EPA publishes a notice in the *Federal Register* inviting comment on the proposed tolerance. At this point the underlying safety and residue data generally are not subject to examination by members of the public.[11] After analyzing all the available data and considering any comments submitted in response to the proposal, the EPA either denies the petition or establishes a final tolerance. A notice announcing the EPA's action, including a brief summary of reasons, is published in the *Federal Register*. The tolerance is eventually codified in the *Code of Federal Regulations* (CFR). Both

Concentrating Residues: What Are They and When Does Delaney Apply?

The FDC Act dispenses with the need for a food or feed additive tolerance for any pesticide residue in processed food or feed when "the concentration of such residue in the processed food . . . is not greater than the tolerance prescribed for the raw agricultural commodity. . . . " Concentrating residues requiring food or feed additive tolerances must meet the act's safety standard. Under the Delaney Clause, the pesticide presumably cannot be approved if found to induce cancer in man or animal. Thus, the EPA's interpretation of the language relating to concentration can be critical. The central issue is whether the law makes the *fact* or the *level* of concentration the determining factor. Although there has been some confusion on the matter, the EPA's current position is clear. It is the *fact* of concentration that necessitates section 409 tolerances and thus potentially triggers the application of the Delaney Clause.

Raw agricultural commodity tolerances are based on the results of field trials designed to achieve the highest residue levels likely under normal agricultural practice. These studies include such methods as using the highest recommended application rates under weather and climatic conditions that prolong and in some cases exacerbate residues. Because of this, the tolerance is often higher than the actual residues found at harvest on crops grown in regions where application rates are lower and where residues dissipate more rapidly. In these cases a residue theoretically could concentrate during processing yet not exceed the level allowed on the raw agricultural commodity, which is the section 408 tolerance.

On occasion, tolerance petitioners have asked the EPA to set section 408 tolerances high enough to allow concentration of residues during processing to levels below these tolerances. The EPA reports it has denied all such requests and has relied on 40 CFR § 180.4 (1986), which states: "The tolerance established ordinarily will not exceed that figure which the Administrator of the Environmental Protection Agency states, in his opinion, reasonably reflects the amounts of residue likely to result."

When seeking a section 408 tolerance for a specific crop, the petitioner must address the need for section 409 tolerances by showing whether the residues concentrate as a result of specific processes such as drying, milling, or juicing. In determining whether a section 409 tolerance is required, the EPA focuses on whether residues in any processed product exceed those found on the unprocessed crop, not whether residues concentrate above some hypothetical section 408 tolerance. If residues concentrate, an average concentration factor is determined. The section 409 tolerance is set at a level equal to the section 408 tolerance multiplied by this concentration factor.

The logic of the EPA's practice is clear. A section 408 tolerance represents a residue level that *may* in some cases be realized. A section 409 tolerance must reflect the possible residue levels in processed foods derived from that raw commodity. (Source: 40 CFR § 180.4 (1986).)

statutes permit opponents of a tolerance to object, request a hearing, and ultimately challenge the EPA's final decision in court, but these formal procedures are almost never invoked. Indeed, relatively few tolerance petitions evoke written comment from members of the public other than those affiliated with the pesticide industry.

SPECIFIC DATA REQUIREMENTS

Data requirements for tolerance petitions are spelled out in EPA regulations and guidelines. Much of the required information duplicates that needed to support registration under FIFRA, and is already available. Key elements of the data package include a description of the chemistry of the pesticide itself; identity and quantity of residues expected to be present in food; analytical procedures used in obtaining the residue data, which must be complete enough to permit replication by a competent analyst; residues in animal feed derived from crop by-products or from forages and resulting residues, if any, in meat, milk, poultry, fish, and eggs; and toxicity tests on the parent compound and any major impurities, degradation products, or metabolites.

The gathering and interpretation of residue chemistry data are some of the most difficult technical challenges that the registrant and the EPA face. The objective is to estimate and fully track the principal food residues, including metabolites and degradation products, that are likely to result from the commercial use of a pesticide under varying climatic and soil conditions. This generally requires extrapolation from data on a limited number of field trials in different parts of the country where the pesticide would possibly be used. In considering the level at which to set a tolerance, the EPA will generally select the highest residue levels reported in such tests.

The toxicity data required for each active ingredient and for major impurities or metabolites typically include the results of the following studies and reflect the need for data on all risks as well as those posed by residues in food:

- Acute oral, dermal, and inhalation studies;
- Two-generation reproduction study;
- Chronic feeding studies on rodents and nonrodents;
- Oncogenicity studies on mice and rats;
- Mutagenicity studies on gene mutation, structural chromosomal aberration, and other effects toxic to genetic material;
- Teratogenicity studies on rats and rabbits;
- Delayed neuropathy studies on chickens; and
- Plant and animal metabolism studies.

The agency may grant exemptions from one or more of these requirements when the petitioner can show it is scientifically appropriate to do so.

ONCOGENICITY AND CARCINOGENICITY

Throughout its work, the committee encountered disparate usages of the terms oncogen, oncogenicity, carcinogen, and carcinogenicity. In conventional scientific terminology, oncogen means a substance capable of producing benign *or* malignant tumors. The EPA has adopted this definition.[12] The term carcinogen is generally reserved for substances capable of producing malignant tumors. The committee will follow these usages in this report.

Confusion can arise when these terms are used in a regulatory context. For example, the FDA apparently interprets the Delaney Clause as prohibiting approval of carcinogens, whereas the EPA apparently treats it as prohibiting oncogens—theoretically a broader interpretation. It is unclear to the committee how significant this difference is in actual practice. It seems likely, though, that there are more oncogenic pesticides than carcinogenic ones; chronic feeding studies will sometimes reveal oncogenicity even when a pesticide's capacity to cause malignant tumors is uncertain. Thus, the EPA's more conservative approach generally expands the universe of pesticides to which the Delaney Clause applies.

The description of a substance that is merely a suspect oncogen or carcinogen also may be confusing. A substance may be characterized as an oncogen or carcinogen even though the evidence on which the statement is based may be incomplete (for example, it consists of results from a single test in one species or sex), weak (for example, a trend was seen in a chronic bioassay but not at a statistically significant level), or otherwise flawed (for example, a statisically significant effect was observed in a study of flawed design or execution). In such cases, the EPA may evaluate the potential human risk of such substances as suspect or possible oncogens or carcinogens. The criteria the EPA uses in judging whether a compound is an oncogen for the purposes of the Delaney Clause constitute a critical regulatory variable. The implications will be considered later in this report.

Finally, the important scientific distinction between substances found to be oncogenic or carcinogenic in animals and those found to have the same effects in humans is often obscured or overlooked. Because of the limits of epidemiological data, regulatory agencies typically rely solely upon animal studies in evaluating the safety of compounds for humans. In the absence of convincing data documenting causality between pesticide exposure and cancer in humans, however, it is inaccurate to refer to such substances as human oncogens or carcinogens. Rather, such chemicals are animal oncogens or carcinogens. (It should be noted, however, that the Delaney Clause does not require proof of carcinogenicity in humans.) In its scheme for categorizing evidence of carcinogenicity, the EPA properly reserves the term "human carcinogen" for substances where available human data are sufficient to support that finding. In other cases, the EPA uses the terms "probable human carcinogen" and "possible human carcinogen," depending on the strength of available animal evidence, short-term in-vitro mutagenicity assays, and any other relevant data.[13]

Appreciation of these distinctions and possible differences in the approaches of the EPA and the FDA is important to complete understanding of the impact of the Delaney Clause. One set of issues lies within the gray areas of the sciences of toxicology, pathology, and risk assessment. Another set clusters around the regulatory consequences of a given scientific judgment. In recent years, the EPA and the FDA have agreed in their regulatory judgments on chemicals with clear, strong indications of carcinogenic potential and on chemicals with very weak or equivocal evidence of oncogenicity. But chemicals that fall between these extremes are vexing.

In this study, the committee follows the EPA's criteria and terminology. The term oncogen will be used in cases when the EPA would judge the animal evidence sufficient to trigger the Delaney Clause. The committee will attempt to clarify its terms throughout the report and cautions readers to remember that tables and text generally depict only *potential* human risk, usually under worst-case scenarios.

TOLERANCE SETTING FOR NON-ONCOGENIC PESTICIDES UNDER SECTION 408

The core of the typical tolerance-setting process under section 408 is the effort by the EPA to compare the quantity of residues to which humans might be exposed through consumption of pesticide-treated food with the level it judges, based on the available toxicological data, as safe. If the EPA finds that the pesticide (or its expected impurities, metabolites, and degradation products) does not cause a statistically significant increase in the incidence of tumors in animals, it concludes the Delaney Clause is not applicable. Then, the EPA calculates a safe level of exposure, following the conventional analysis of calculating an Acceptable Daily Intake (ADI) for the substance in question.

The first step in calculating an ADI is determining from the battery of toxicity studies the "no observable effect level" (NOEL) for the most sensitive toxic response that is considered to be of potential human health concern. In any study, the NOEL is the highest dose level of pesticide (consumed in the daily diet per unit of body weight) at which no adverse effect was observed. It is the dose level nearest to but less than the lowest dose producing observable indications of toxicity. The study displaying the lowest NOEL is generally selected to establish the ADI. This is calculated by dividing the NOEL by a safety factor (typically 100) to yield the ADI, which is also expressed in milligrams of pesticide per kilogram of body weight per day. (The safety factor of 100, an accepted convention in toxicology, is derived by assuming that [1] humans are 10 times as sensitive as the most sensitive animal tested, and [2] some humans are 10 times as sensitive as the least susceptible human.) Regulatory scientists regard the ADI arrived at in this fashion as a level of dietary exposure that virtually all individuals could consume on a daily basis and even exceed on occasion without experiencing adverse effects.

The next step in evaluating whether a proposed tolerance is toxicologically supportable is calculation of the theoretical maximum residue contribution (TMRC) for each food form in which the pesticide could occur. The sum of the TMRCs for all food forms represents the cumulative TMRC for the pesticide. If the TMRC for a proposed use combined with the TMRC for all other already-approved uses is less than the ADI, the proposed new tolerance that has met other requirements is generally approved. If the TMRC exceeds the ADI, the EPA either denies the tolerance or explores with the petitioner ways to lower the TMRC from the proposed or other uses.

In calculating the TMRC, the EPA seeks to avoid underestimating food consumption and exposure to residues by assuming that (1) each pesticide is used on *all* harvested crop acres for which a tolerance exists or is proposed and (2) pesticide residues are present at the full tolerance level in every food consumed. Together these assumptions generally exaggerate estimates of dietary exposure to residues. Very few pesticides are used on anywhere near 100 percent of the total acreage of a crop grown in the United States, and measured residues are usually below the tolerance. However, the EPA routinely uses these conservative assumptions to account for gaps in information about actual exposure and uncertainties about health effects.

Although the EPA is empowered by law to consider the benefits of pesticide use in establishing section 408 tolerances, it rarely does so. Residues that pass the foregoing ADI/TMRC analyses are regarded as safe. (Indeed, given the 100-fold safety factor and the conservative assumptions about exposure built into the TMRC, there is thought to be a wide margin of safety.) The petition is then said to be toxicologically supportable and is generally approved without examination of benefits. If the TMRC exceeds a pesticide's ADI, the agency may examine the benefits or, as noted above, explore with registrants possible ways to reduce the TMRC by changing the timing, rate, method, or diversity of crop uses for the given pesticide. Before the pesticide use is registered, however, other important potential environmental effects of the pesticide's use and other routes of human exposure must be evaluated. These include the pesticide's effects on birds, fish, and wildlife; ground-water contamination; and hazards to applicators.

TOLERANCE SETTING FOR ONCOGENIC COMPOUNDS UNDER SECTION 408

The EPA's analysis proceeds somewhat differently if the pesticide is a suspected oncogen. In this case, the agency does not seek to identify a NOEL or calculate an ADI. Its approach is based on quantitative risk assessment models developed specifically to provide upper-bound esti-mates of human cancer risks, based on animal bioassay data, assuming a lifetime of exposure to the pesticide. On the basis of such risk assess-ments, the EPA makes a judgment about whether a given tolerance for a specific pesticide use poses an unreasonable risk to humans.

The use of quantitative risk assessment in this context raises questions that go beyond the scope of this report.[14] However, a basic understanding of the methodology and limitations of risk assessment is essential to the analysis presented in subsequent chapters.

In brief, risk assessment is a complex extrapolation process. It involves first extrapolating from the effects seen at the generally high doses used in animal studies to the much lower dosages ordinarily consumed by humans in the diet. Then, one predicts from the animal test model results that might occur in humans under actual exposure conditions. The assessment of the oncogenic risk posed by any given substance thus reflects both the potency of the substance and human exposure to it. Once potency is determined, the level of risk to food consumers from a particular pesticide use is a function of exposure to residues in food: the higher the residue levels in foods (or frequency of consumption), the higher the risk.

The risk assessment process is beset by uncertainty and by gaps in knowledge, even on such basic points as the relevance of particular animal test models to humans and the true qualitative and quantitative relationships between effects seen at high doses and those likely to occur at low doses. To compensate for such gaps in knowledge, the EPA and other agencies that use quantitative risk assessment typically adopt conservative assumptions that are designed to avoid understating the potential human risk. For example, results from the most sensitive animal species are used in extrapolating from high doses to low doses, mathe-matical models are selected that are thought to avoid understating potential human risk, and assumptions are made concerning potential human exposure to the substance that almost certainly overstate true human exposure. Most experts believe that these conservative assumptions together produce risk estimates that represent the likely upper bound of potential human risk. It is generally accepted that the true human risk is probably less than the reported risk estimate.

Risk estimates are typically expressed in terms of the probability that an individual member of a population will experience cancer from exposure to the substance in question over his or her lifetime. Thus, a risk estimate of 1 in 1 million or (1×10^{-6}) from a specified level of exposure is a statement that at the 95 percent upper-bound confidence limit, there is no greater than a 1 in 1 million chance that an exposed individual, or that 1 person out of 1 million exposed individuals, will experience cancer from daily lifetime exposure to the substance in question. To keep these risk estimates in perspective, all individuals now face about a 1 in 4 chance of contracting cancer. Heavy smokers face far worse odds.

In setting tolerances for oncogenic pesticides under section 408, the EPA performs the risk assessment described above and decides whether the risk posed is acceptable—that is, whether the risk is negligible enough to justify a tolerance. To the committee's knowledge, the EPA has not formally adopted any numerical cutoff for oncogenic risks it views as negligible. Without question, however, the EPA has approved many section 408 tolerances for oncogenic pesticides. (See the case studies in Appendix C.)

The committee's review of EPA tolerance actions in recent years suggests that when the estimated upper-bound risk is less than 1 in 1 million (1×10^{-6}), the agency rarely disapproves a tolerance. Tolerances likely to pose greater risk than 1 in 10,000 (1×10^{-4}) are rarely granted. Decisions to approve tolerances carrying an upper-bound risk between 1 in 1 million and 1 in 10,000 are generally, but not always, made after taking steps to reduce dietary exposure and confirming that risks from other routes of exposure are also small.

In reaching decisions on dietary risks that fall between 1×10^{-4} and 1×10^{-6}, the EPA enlarges its inquiry. Under section 408, the agency may consider the benefits of a pesticide's use. The agency generally evaluates benefits in relation to all risks, when data are available, in deciding whether to grant a tolerance for a pesticide for which the upper-bound oncogenic risk estimate falls between 10^{-4} and 10^{-6}. On occasion the EPA's consideration of benefits has been relatively thorough and its judgment has proved central to the ultimate decision. (See the case studies in Appendix C.) In most cases, however, whether dealing with an oncogen or non-oncogen the EPA rests its tolerance decision on a judgment about the safety of the pesticide residue without regard to benefits.

TOLERANCE SETTING UNDER SECTION 409

As noted, section 408 of the FDC Act allows the EPA to consider the benefits of pesticide use and does not forbid approval of oncogenic residues. Section 409, which applies to concentrated residues in processed food, differs in both respects. It does not expressly allow the EPA (or the FDA in its consideration of direct food additives) to consider the benefits of a pesticide's use.[15] In the Delaney Clause, it forbids the approval as safe of any food additive shown to "induce cancer in man or animal."

In the case of non-oncogens, these differences in statutory language have little practical importance. The EPA evaluates the human risk associated with a proposed section 409 tolerance for a non-oncogen using the same ADI/TMRC analysis it follows under section 408. If the TMRC is less than the ADI, the residue is judged safe, and a 409 tolerance is granted.

In regulating oncogens, however, the EPA immediately confronts the Delaney Clause. When a pesticide that requires a section 409 tolerance (because its residues concentrate in some processed foods) has also been found to be oncogenic in animals, the EPA simply declines to grant a tolerance. There is no consideration of whether the residue poses a risk to humans or whether the risk might be judged acceptable. Tolerances in the CFR as of June 1986 are shown in Table 2-1.[16]

It is obvious how the fact of concentration can decisively affect the regulatory fate of a pesticide use. If residues of an oncogenic pesticide occur *but do not concentrate* in processed food, the EPA can estimate risk, make a safety judgment, and then balance risks with the pesticide's benefits. In these cases, a food additive tolerance is not required; the raw agricultural commodity tolerance suffices. If the oncogenic pesticide concentrates in the processed food, the EPA automatically denies a tolerance without further analysis.

Although the impacts of the Delaney Clause on petitions to establish

TABLE 2-1 Food Tolerances in the CFR

Type of Pesticide	Number
Insecticides	3,806
Herbicides	2,543
Fungicides	1,305
Other	823
Total	8,477

TABLE 2-2   Food Tolerances in the CFR for 53 Oncogens

Type of Pesticide	Number	
	Section 408	Section 409
Herbicides	915	9
Insecticides	843	3
Fungicides	712	12
Other	55	7
Total	2,525	31

new section 409 tolerances for oncogenic pesticides are clear-cut, its impact on already-established tolerances has been very different. New information demonstrating that a pesticide has oncogenic potential and concentrates in processed food would seem to necessitate the Delaney Clause prohibition. Yet, the EPA has not invoked this provision to revoke a single such tolerance.

As shown in Table 2-2, 31 section 409 tolerances and 2,525 section 408 tolerances exist for pesticides shown to be oncogenic in animal tests.

THE DATA CALL-IN PROGRAM

A driving force that will compel the EPA to confront the implications of the Delaney Clause is FIFRA's requirement that all registered pesticides be reregistered on the basis of contemporary scientific standards and data, with priority given to pesticides used on food. To implement this long-standing mandate, the EPA in 1981 instituted the Data Call-In Program, which was designed to elicit the toxicity information needed to make reregistration decisions. The agency also requests a wider range of data in their registration standards program. The toxicity and residue chemistry data generated by these programs in the future will substantially enlarge the number of pesticides that, under current law and policy, seem to require section 409 tolerances and thus could be affected by the Delaney Clause.

By 1990, the agency should have received updated oncogenicity data for nearly all pesticides registered for use on foods. It is impossible to predict which or how many active pesticide ingredients will be found to be oncogenic once all are adequately tested. But, based on past experience (53 out of 289 pesticides used on foods are determined by the EPA to be oncogenic) and assuming continuity in the EPA's interpretation of oncogenicity studies, about 20 percent of the registered pesticides for which data are submitted may be found to be oncogenic.

The EPA determines whether a pesticide residue concentrates in processed food and thus requires a section 409 or food additive tolerance on the basis of residue chemistry data. The EPA currently has complete residue chemistry data on less than 25 percent of pesticides used on foods. The agency is working to complete this segment of its data base although residue data are coming in at a slower pace than toxicity data.

The EPA confronts some difficult issues in this area. EPA scientists acknowledge that the agency's current requirements for food-processing studies do not cover all foods in which residues are likely to concentrate. Concerned food-processing companies have asked the EPA to review the need for evaluating residue concentration in 20 additional crops. The agency must decide how far to pursue metabolites, degradation products, and impurities to determine whether there is concentration. And the EPA is debating how and when to test for concentration in certain dried foods, animal feeds, animal products, and complex mixtures in highly processed foods.

It would be an enormous task to reliably determine whether residues of all pesticides now covered by section 408 tolerances concentrate in processed foods. For those pesticides with scores of raw food tolerances, it would require more time and money to satisfy residue chemistry data requirements than to develop a complete new set of chronic toxicity data. (See Appendix E for a discussion by industrial research directors.) One outcome seems clear. Completion of the data base on pesticide residues in processed foods will substantially enlarge the number of pesticide uses for which section 409 tolerances will be required. The Delaney Clause will halt many of the required tolerances because the pesticides will be found to be oncogenic in animal tests. Residue chemistry data, required to elicit information to assess dietary exposure to pesticide residues in raw and processed foods, will reveal many concentrating residues for which no 409 tolerances are now approved.

THE DELANEY CLAUSE—A CLOSER EXAMINATION

The foregoing discussion explains the role that the Delaney Clause plays in pesticide tolerance setting and suggests why the provision will loom larger in future EPA decisions. This impending collision between law and practice triggered the current study and independently inspired a closer examination of the history and current interpretation of this noteworthy provision. The FDA, the agency principally responsible for implementing the Delaney Clause, has examined these issues for many years.

In the early 1970s the FDA first suggested the possibility of using quantitative risk assessment to evaluate the safety of substances found oncogenic or carcinogenic in animal studies. The FDA proposed this method of evaluation when it implemented the DES Proviso, which was added to the Delaney Clause in 1962.[17] As part of the Drug Amendments in 1962, Congress provided that the Delaney Clause would not bar approval of carcinogenic drugs and feed additives administered to food-producing animals if upon examination by methods acceptable to FDA no residue of the material could be found in the edible tissues of the animals.[18] Convinced that the use of any animal drug would leave some residue, the FDA in 1979 interpreted this proviso to mean no residue above a level posing no significant increased risk of cancer in humans, that is, a level judged by the FDA to be safe. The agency proposed to use quantitative risk assessment to determine the residue level corresponding to an increased lifetime risk of no more than 1×10^{-6} for an individual. It termed this the sensitivity-of-the-method (SOM) approach and continues to use it in regulating residues of carcinogenic animal drugs and feed additives in human food.

Throughout the 1970s, the FDA continued to grapple with developments in science (paralleling those now confronting the EPA) that put great pressure on the traditional understanding of the Delaney Clause. Increased and more sensitive chronic toxicity testing and advances in analytical methods identified many more natural and man-made carcinogens in human food. Many of these were residual reactants, trace constituents of direct food additives, or components of packaging materials that migrated into food in minute amounts.

One source of authority for the exercise of judgment is found in the language of the clause itself. The Delaney Clause applies only if the FDA (or the EPA) finds that a substance "induces cancer when ingested by man or animal." The legislative history makes clear that Congress intended the agencies to exercise sound scientific judgment in deciding whether a substance induces cancer. The clause seems to preclude the agency from ignoring the results of an animal ingestion study solely on the basis of the conclusion that such results are irrelevant to humans. Yet, the agency is surely allowed, perhaps even required, to evaluate whether the study was properly designed and conducted. The statute also leaves open the questions of whether cancer induction must be demonstrated by more than a single well-conducted study or how to weigh conflicting results from two or more studies. In practice, a single, properly conducted, positive test has been adequate, in the EPA's judgment, to trigger a finding of oncogenicity.

The statute is also silent on exactly what "induce cancer" means. Is it sufficient that an additive or pesticide increases the incidence of benign tumors in the test animals? Or must there be convincing—or at least some—evidence of malignancy? How should benign and malignant tumors seen in the same study be interpreted? The FDA has not chosen a rigid position, but generally it has looked for evidence of malignancy before taking action solely on the basis of the Delaney Clause. EPA scientists have been more conservative. In several cases they found that a substance meets the "induce cancer" criterion where there has been no indication of malignancy (see Appendix C).

In addition to the SOM approach, the FDA has used other interpretations of the Delaney Clause intended to limit application. Two of these—the constituents policy and the de minimis interpretation—deserve discussion here.

The constituents policy rests on an interpretation of the phrase "no additive shall be deemed to be safe if it is found to induce cancer. . . ." The FDA now interprets the term "additive" to refer to the added substance as a whole and not to each of its individual constituents. Thus, if a constituent of a food additive or color additive has been found to induce cancer, but the parent additive has not, the FDA will not invoke the Delaney Clause. Instead it will evaluate the safety of the additive under the general safety standard. The carcinogenicity of the trace constituent will be taken into account by performing a quantitative risk assessment. The parent additive will be approved as safe under the general safety standard if the assessed risk from the carcinogenic constituent is insignificant. The FDA's benchmark for judging safety in this context is a lifetime upper-bound risk estimate of 1×10^{-6}.

The FDA has applied its constituents policy in evaluating several residual reactants in color additives and some migrating components of packaging materials. One reviewing court upheld this interpretation of the Delaney Clause. A significant example of the application of the constituents policy to pesticide tolerance setting is discussed later in this report.

The FDA's latest and potentially most far-reaching effort to expand its discretion under the Delaney Clause is its de minimis interpretation. The FDA first used this interpretation in evaluating certain color additives that induced cancer in animals. The levels of human exposure to the colors were extremely small. Risks posed were estimated to be extremely low—in some cases orders of magnitude below 1×10^{-6}. The FDA announced in June 1985 that it interpreted the Delaney Clause as not prohibiting such extremely small risks. Six months later, the agency used the de minimis concept to approve the use of methylene chloride to decaffeinate coffee, based on the conclusion that the risks posed by permitted residues were no greater than 1×10^{-6}.[19]

The FDA's de minimis interpretation of the Delaney Clause has been more controversial than the agency's constituents policy. The de minimis interpretation recently has been challenged in a petition for judicial review of the FDA's decision to permanently list two color additives.[20]

Because the de minimis interpretation departs from the FDA's traditional interpretation of the Delaney Clause, the policy's legality will remain uncertain until there is a definitive court ruling.

From a policy standpoint, the FDA's de minimis interpretation is an important development. If upheld, it would replace the zero-risk interpretation of the Delaney Clause with a no-significant-risk standard. For carcinogens, the requirements of the general safety clause and the Delaney Clause would have become congruent. Even if the FDA's statutory interpretation is overruled, its policy judgment that cancer risks of less than 1×10^{-6} may be considered safe when derived by methods using a clearly defined set of conservative assumptions could have important implications for pesticide tolerance setting.

SUMMARY OF PROBLEMS AND ISSUES POSED BY THE DELANEY CLAUSE

The committee identified four different risk standards in the current law which could apply to residues of an *oncogenic* pesticide on the food and feed forms of a single crop.

- For residues on raw agricultural commodities consumed as food, tolerances may reflect a weighing of risks and benefits.
- When residues concentrate in processed food, the Delaney Clause would bar any tolerances for that crop.
- For concentrated residues in processed animal feeds such as soybean hulls, tolerances may be denied under the Delaney Clause unless approvable under the SOM approach discussed above.
- For most hays, fodders, and other nonprocessed livestock feeds, tolerances would be granted under section 408 regardless of whether residues concentrate, based on an assessment of the cancer risks associated with dietary exposure to residues in the animal products ultimately consumed by humans.

This diversity dramatizes the problems presented by the current framework for setting tolerances for pesticide residues on agricultural commodities.

Inconsistency

The current system treats pesticide residues inconsistently in two ways. One is exemplified by the dichotomous risk standards in sections 408 and 409. From the outset of its deliberations, the committee has been unable to identify any sound scientific or policy reason for regulating pesticides present in or on raw commodities differently than those present on processed foods. From the standpoint of consumer protection, the source of exposure—raw commodity versus processed food—seems irrelevant.

The other inconsistency is the system's disparate treatment of old and new pesticides. Old pesticides, especially those first registered before 1972, generally were not tested adequately for oncogenicity. They were approved on the basis of limited residue chemistry data, particularly concerning metabolites. Consequently, there was very limited knowledge of the pesticides' capacity to concentrate in processed food. Many of these pesticides are widely used today even though some are suspected oncogens and usually lack section 409 tolerances that would almost surely be required if complete residue chemistry data were available. Pesticides recently registered for use on foods, on the other hand, have generally been tested rigorously. With more complete residue chemistry data, the EPA is more likely to recognize the need for section 409 tolerances which, if a pesticide proves even weakly oncogenic, cannot be granted.

This inconsistency in treatment of old and new pesticides is very important. If the standards applied to new chemicals are justified to protect the public, the same standards should be applied to older pesticides. If older pesticides are judged to not pose a public health problem, then contemporary requirements restricting new, less oncogenic pesticides may be overly protective and may impede introduction of useful new pesticides.

The Issue of Concentration in Processed Foods

Another major problem derives from the current law's emphasis on whether a pesticide residue concentrates in processed food. For an oncogenic pesticide, this fact can prove crucial. If it is found to concentrate, it will be denied a section 409 tolerance under the current system. Consequently, the pesticide will lose the underlying section 408 tolerance and FIFRA registration for that use. If a crop has no *recognized* processed form (see the boxed article "Subsection O"), then tolerances for an oncogen can be granted if the risks are deemed acceptable. If a crop has a processed form but residues do not concentrate, an oncogen can be granted a tolerance under the general safety clause of section 409. Such differences based on the fact of concentration in certain processed foods make no discernible sense in terms of public health protection.

Paradoxical Regulatory Results

The committee can envision situations in which the current system would compel results that, at least in the short term, actually increase the human cancer risks from pesticides. For example, suppose a registered

---

Subsection O

The Delaney Clause prohibits a food or feed additive tolerance for any pesticide that is found to cause cancer in humans or animals when the residues of that pesticide *concentrate in a processed food or feed* above the level allowed in the raw agricultural commodity. The Delaney Clause does not directly govern residues of these pesticides in raw foods. The clause can have a significant effect on raw food tolerances, however. The EPA has successfully used the Delaney Clause to deny tolerances for an oncogenic pesticide *on an entire crop* when residues are found to concentrate in the processed portion of that crop.

As a result, the definition of a processed food is critical to the scope and impact of the Delaney Clause. The criteria that the EPA uses to define processed foods and feeds are in a nonregulatory companion to 40 CFR 158, Subpart K, entitled "Pesticide Assessment Guidelines Subdivision O: Residue Chemistry." These criteria are guidelines, not regulations. Yet, they represent the EPA's current thinking on processed versus raw foods and feeds. The EPA is currently reviewing and revising the criteria. When the criteria emerge in final form they could have a significant effect on which crops and pesticides might be most affected by the Delaney Clause. Currently, however, *most* pesticides lack residue studies on a range of processed foods.

---

pesticide X with known oncogenic effects and an existing substitute Y which is a weaker oncogen are under review. Both agents produce roughly equal benefits for comparable uses. X does not concentrate in any processed apple products, but Y concentrates marginally. The EPA could be forced by the Delaney Clause to deny a section 409 tolerance for Y and also would be compelled to cancel its section 408 tolerance and registration. Pesticide X would claim a larger share of the market. Human cancer risk would rise, not fall.

Another example involves a registration application and tolerance petition for a new pesticide with data that show weak indications of oncogenicity. The new pesticide is destined for a crop use for which there are two registered, relatively potent oncogenic pesticides. Registration of the new product is delayed by a prolonged dispute over whether a metabolite causes the potential oncogenicity and whether it concentrates in processed foods. Even though approving the new chemical may reduce dietary cancer risk because it would displace more potent, approved oncogens, the EPA probably would maintain the status quo under current policy. Examples of this scenario can also be found in actions now pending before the EPA.

Another twist of the old standards versus the new creates other paradoxes. Suppose the EPA is deciding whether to cancel an old compound that poses clear oncogenic hazards. The availability of effective registered substitute chemicals is important in estimating the material's benefits and, hence, in balancing its risks and benefits. The agency's inability under current law and policy to register a new, weakly oncogenic substitute chemical when residues concentrate in processed food exaggerates the perceived benefits of the older products. Registrations and tolerances may be denied even though EPA scientists are convinced that the new chemical would pose less risk and provide essentially equal food-production benefits.

The following chapters explore the likelihood that the current system will often produce such paradoxical, indefensible results. Alternative policy constructs are explored that might help the agency more efficiently reduce public health hazards while ensuring an adequate inventory of pesticides.

NOTES

1. 7 USC § 136(a) (1978).
2. *Ibid.*
3. 40 CFR Parts 158 and 162 (1986).
4. 21 USC § 346(b) (1984).
5. 21 USC §§ 342(a)(2)(B) and 348(a) (1984).
6. 21 USC § 321(s) (1984).
7. H.R. 2284. 84th Cong., 2d sess. (1958).
8. 21 CFR § 170.3(i) (1986).
9. 21 USC § 348(c)(3)(A) (1984).
10. 21 USC § 342(a)(2)(C) (1984).
11. This is because previously unpublished data are the registrant's confidential proprietary information. The EPA sometimes will press a petitioner to allow public access to its safety data. This occurs when the agency regards the tolerance decision as difficult or potentially controversial, such as when significant safety questions are posed.
12. 40 CFR § 162.3(bb) (1986).
13. U.S. Environmental Protection Agency. 1986. Guidelines for Carcinogenic Risk Assessment. *Federal Register* 51(185): 33,992–34,003.
14. National Research Council. 1983. Risk Assessment in the Federal Government: Managing the Process. Washington, D.C.: National Academy Press.
15. There is disagreement whether section 409 allows the EPA or the FDA to consider the benefits of individual food additives in deciding whether they are safe. The FDA has consistently taken the view that it does not. In the past, the FDA weighed a pesticide's benefits in deciding whether to approve a 409 tolerance. This interpretation seems difficult to reconcile with the section's language and history. It also conflicts with the view of the FDA, the agency primarily responsible for interpreting and administering this section of the FDC Act. No court squarely holds that the EPA's view is untenable.
16. 21 CFR Parts 193 and 561 (1986); 40 CFR Part 180 (1986).
17. 21 USC § 348(c)(3)(A) (1984).
18. *Ibid.*

19. In August 1986 the FDA applied the de minimis interpretation to approve two color additives, D&C Orange No. 17 and D&C Red No. 19. This approval inspired the interpretation's development. U.S. Food and Drug Administration. 1986. *Federal Register* 51(August 7): 28,331–28,346.

20. *Ibid.* The colors are D&C Orange No. 17 and D&C Red No. 19. The petition for review was filed by Public Citizen in the U.S. Court of Appeals for the District of Columbia Circuit. *Public Citizen* v. *Young*, No. 86-1548 (D.C. Cir. filed Oct. 9, 1986) (a decision could be rendered later this year).

3

Estimates of Dietary Oncogenic Risks

INTRODUCTION

To provide some perspective on the potential impact of alternative policies for setting tolerances, this chapter assesses the estimated dietary oncogenic risks associated with 28 out of 53 pesticides that the EPA has identified as oncogenic or potentially oncogenic. The purposes of this exercise are to gain a sense of the magnitude and distribution of current dietary risks and crops associated with oncogenic pesticides and to establish an estimate from which to measure the direction and magnitude of changes in dietary risk and pesticide use that could result from different policies for setting tolerances for oncogenic pesticide residues in food.

All risk estimates in this report are limited to oncogenic risks from residues of currently registered pesticides in or on food. The study focuses on the potential impact of the Delaney Clause on agricultural innovation and the public's dietary oncogenic risk. Oncogenic risks associated with exposure to residues in drinking water or other sources are not included. The risks of other chronic health effects are not examined. The committee has confined its review to risks from herbicides, insecticides, and fungicides that the EPA has found to be oncogenic. Plant growth regulators, rodenticides, and other types of pesticides are not considered.

A number of analyses were performed on the selected pesticides. The most important analyses are examinations of the distribution of dietary risks by (1) the type of pesticide (insecticide, herbicide, or fungicide), (2)

45

type of tolerance (processed versus raw food), (3) crop, and (4) the year in which a tolerance was granted. Each analysis is presented as part of the characterization of estimated oncogenic risk. The committee wishes to make clear that emphasis should not be placed on specific risk estimates associated with particular pesticides, groups of tolerances, or food types. The analysis is subject to a wide range of uncertainty, even though based on state-of-the-art data.

In developing these estimates, the committee used data that the EPA provided and followed the agency's risk assessment procedures as closely as possible. Basic questions addressed include

• How many and what percentage of all pesticides used on food are currently thought by the EPA to be oncogens?
• How is the risk from these pesticides distributed across crops and among types of pesticides?
• How is the risk distributed by age of tolerance?
• What portion of risk is associated with section 408 raw agricultural commodity tolerances in contrast to section 409 processed-food tolerances?

Pesticide Use Patterns in the United States

The benefits of pesticide use are not examined in rigorous fashion in this report, nor are they considered in the process of making most decisions on tolerances. The committee lacked the time and resources to perform detailed benefit assessments for all oncogenic pesticides. Instead of benefit analyses, use and sales data are given for various pesticides and crops. This information is presented in terms of the number of acres treated with a pesticide, the pounds applied and annual expenditures. The portion of herbicide and fungicide use accounted for by oncogens is described in Tables 3–1 and 3–2. A more detailed analysis of the benefits associated with oncogenic pesticides used on eight selected crops is presented in the next chapter.

To appreciate the potential impact of the Delaney Clause, one should note the percentage of all pesticide use that is accounted for by oncogenic herbicides, insecticides, and fungicides. Approximately 480 million pounds of herbicides are used annually in the United States. Of these, about 300 million pounds are agents that the EPA presumes to be oncogenic or for which positive oncogenicity data are currently under review by the agency (see Table 3-1). These agents account for about 50 to 60 percent of all expenditures on herbicides in U.S. agriculture. In 1985, these expenditures added up to about $1.4 billion of the $2.7 billion spent on all herbicide products.[1] (Not all oncogenic herbicides are

TABLE 3-1 Agricultural Use Information for Selected Oncogenic Herbicides

Herbicide[a]	Pounds Applied (millions)	All Herbicide Pounds Applied (%)
Alachlor (Lasso)	85	18
Trifluralin (Treflan)	39	8
Metolachlor (Dual)	38	8
Glyphosate (Roundup)	8	8
Linuron (Lorox)	7	1.5
Paraquat (Gramoxone)	2.8	1.5
Oryzalin (Surflan)	1.7	0.6
Acifluorfen (Blazer)	1.4	0.3
Subtotal	182.9	38.2
Atrazine[b]	79	17
2,4-D[b]	39	8
Total	300.9	63.3

[a]The names of the biggest-selling pesticide brands are listed next to the appropriate chemical compounds to serve as examples in this table and in those following.

[b]These compounds are not on the list of oncogens the EPA made available to the committee (see the discussion of the Waxman list on pp. 50–51). After this correspondence, however, the EPA received data that show positive results for oncogenicity. The EPA has not officially characterized these compounds as oncogenic, but it is significant for the purposes of this report that they induced tumors when tested on animals. Also, the EPA may classify these compounds as oncogenic in the future. These compounds are not included in any risk estimates contained in this report.

SOURCE: U.S. Department of Agriculture, 1984, Inputs: Outlook and Situation Report, No. IOS-6, Washington, D.C.: U.S. Government Printing Office; Gianessi, L. P., 1986, A National Pesticide Usage Data Base, Washington, D.C.: Resources for the Future, photocopy; and unpublished data from the EPA for the years 1981 through 1985.

considered in the analyses presented in this report. Specifically, data indicating oncogenicity for the herbicides atrazine and 2,4-D were received by the EPA after the committee's analysis. These pesticides are included here and in Table 3-1 to indicate the potential impact of the Delaney Clause. Atrazine and 2,4-D are not treated as oncogens for any subsequent analysis presented in this study.)

In terms of pounds applied, the percentage of oncogenic insecticides is relatively small. This is primarily because two oncogenic synthetic pyrethroid insecticides, permethrin and cypermethrin, are applied at very low rates per acre. The percentage of all acre treatments by oncogenic insecticides is higher, however. (One acre treatment is defined as one acre to which one pesticide has been applied one time.) Presumed oncogens

TABLE 3-2 Fungicide Use for 10 Major U.S. Food Commodities

	Fungicide Use Level[a]				
Crop	Oncogenic Expenditures[b] (%)	Oncogenic Acre Treatments[c] (%)	Planted Acres Treated with Fungicides[a] (%)	Total Treated Acres[a] (million)	Total Fungicide Expenditures[a] (million)
Potatoes	91	80	55	3.2	16.4
Peanuts	83	85	81	6.6	38.3
Apples	53	59	78	3.2	23.5
Tomatoes	52	49	60	2.6	14.6
Plums, prunes	50	49	48	0.1	1.8
Cherries	49	47	80	0.4	3.8
Peaches	38	37	79	1.0	8.2
Almonds	27	26	78	0.7	11.5
All citrus	17	8	72	2.9	29.0

[a]This includes organic and inorganic compounds.

[b]This is the sales value of oncogenic compounds as a percent of total fungicide sales on that crop. It includes expenditures on inorganic compounds such as copper and sulfur.

[c]This is expressed as the percentage of total fungicide acre treatments on that crop. It includes acre treatments with inorganic compounds.

SOURCE: Webb, S.E.H., 1981, Preliminary Data: Pesticide Use on Selected Deciduous Fruits in the United States, 1978, Economic Research Service Staff Report No. AGES810626, Washington, D.C.: U.S. Department of Agriculture; Parks, J. R., 1983, Pesticide Use on Fall Potatoes in the United States, 1979, Economic Research Service Staff Report No. AGES830113, Washington, D.C.: U.S. Department of Agriculture; Ferguson, W. L., 1984, 1979 Pesticide Use on Vegetables in Five Regions, Springfield, Va.: National Technical Information Service; and unpublished data from the EPA for the years 1981 through 1985.

make up between 35 and 50 percent of all insecticide acre treatments and expenditures.[2]

In comparison, fungicides include the highest percentage of oncogenic compounds. Table 3-2 describes fungicide use on 10 major crops. About 90 percent of all agricultural fungicides show positive results in oncogenicity bioassays. These oncogenic fungicides represent from 70 million to 75 million of the 80 million pounds of all fungicides applied annually in the United States.[3]

Pesticide Use Data

Pesticide use patterns in U.S. agriculture—and thus pesticide residues in food—are changeable. In any growing season, economic factors can alter which pesticides are used on a given crop in a given area. The price of the crop might be up or down, affecting how much growers are willing to spend for a certain amount of pest control. Weather and soil conditions can preclude or command certain treatments. The presence or absence of a given pest affects pesticide use. The emergence of pest resistance to previously applied pesticides can lead to rapid shifts in pesticide use patterns. Government acreage reduction programs and other policies alter crop- and land-use patterns, which thereby affect pesticide use.

Pesticide use patterns also vary widely across major crops. Nearly all cultivated cropland in the United States is treated annually with at least one herbicide. About 15 percent of these acres receive a treatment with a fungicide. Some crops do not depend greatly on any pesticide. This is particularly true of improved pasture and hay, small grains, and some orchard crops. Virtually all perishable fresh fruits and vegetables, on the other hand, depend heavily on pesticides. Some are treated a dozen or more times each year with six or more different active ingredients.

Farmers spent about $5 billion on pesticides in 1984. These costs represent a little more than 21 percent of farm expenditures for manufactured products such as seed, fertilizer, electricity, fuels, and oils. Pesticides accounted for only 4 percent of all production costs, however. Hired-labor costs were twice as much as pesticide costs; interest on debt and depreciation costs were five times as much.[4]

Problems in Estimating Current Risk

The analytical methods involved in estimating oncogenic risks from pesticide residues in food presume resolution of complex technical and policy issues. The risk assessment methodology currently used by the EPA is guided by a set of standard procedures. These procedures are modified on an ad hoc basis when the situation warrants. In each analysis, the committee adopted what it understood to be the EPA's current methodology. The committee recognizes, however, that many key elements of the agency's risk assessment procedures are under review.[5]

Choosing one set of assumptions can have profound implications for the resulting estimates. For example, depending on how the agency establishes average expected residue levels in food, the calculation of exposure to pesticide residues in a given foodstuff can yield risk estimates that vary by orders of magnitude. Assumptions of how and when to aggregate risks from a pesticide used on a variety of crops will also influence risk estimates. A pesticide's oncogenicity potency factor, called a Q star or Q* (see the boxed article "The 'Q Star' " on pp. 54–55), can also vary by orders of magnitude. This variation depends on such factors as whether a surface area or body weight correction is made in extrapolating risks from rodents to humans, whether malignant and benign tumors are combined, and what extrapolation model is used.

The EPA generally follows a conservative policy in estimating risk. The agency tries to make necessary assumptions in a way that minimizes the chance of underestimating risks. The result is that these risk estimates probably overstate true oncogenic risk. The substitution of more refined information on exposure to residues, or the potency of the oncogen at low doses, could alter risk estimates substantially. This report only notes the importance of these assumptions and underlying issues; it does not offer guidance on how to solve the problems associated with them.

The EPA provided all the data used to establish the committee's estimates of current dietary risk. The committee made no adjustments in the EPA's data. In certain cases, the committee used the data in new analyses to understand the theoretical impact of different regulatory standards and methods of calculating risks and benefits.

Although estimated oncogenic risks generally are presented in a quantitative fashion, a wide margin of uncertainty surrounds nearly all of the numbers. With this in mind, the reader should focus on general patterns of risk distribution and how key parameters change when policy alternatives are assessed in Chapter 4, not on specific point estimates of risk.

DESCRIPTION OF THE DATA BASE AND THE ANALYTICAL METHOD

An estimate of a chemical's oncogenic potential generally is derived from the results of chronic feeding bioassays, which typically involve rats or mice. The committee was not charged with the task, nor did it have the expertise or resources, to review the EPA's toxicological data for the purpose of making case-by-case determinations of oncogenic potential. For this analysis, the committee adopted the list of 53 pesticides that the EPA preliminarily has determined to have oncogenic potential. The EPA transmitted this list to Congressman Henry Waxman on October 21, 1985. The pesticides on the list are presented in Table 3-3. As the EPA receives and analyzes additional oncogenicity data, some active ingredients on the list may be removed and others added. The committee did not guess how many currently untested pesticides will be oncogenic. Although more oncogenic pesticides will be found, the committee cannot say which ones or how many.

In this report, pesticides that the EPA has characterized as suspect oncogens are treated as oncogens, even though a final judgment on oncogenicity may not have been reached on the basis of available data. This approach parallels EPA policy. Once the EPA determines that a pesticide has oncogenic potential, even on a preliminary basis, the pesticide is treated as an oncogen for regulatory purposes.[6] For consistency in the following chapters, the committee treats all chemicals on the Waxman list as oncogenic compounds. In such cases the EPA usually does not approve new food tolerances for these pesticides until a thorough risk/benefit assessment of all current uses is complete.[7]

The Universe of Oncogenic Pesticides

In Chapter 2, the committee discussed some of the uncertainties surrounding the determination of a pesticide's potential to induce cancer. Of the 289 pesticides identified for this study as the universe of pesticides used on foods, the EPA found 53 active ingredients oncogenic or potentially oncogenic. This figure represents about 18 percent of all pesticides used on foods. Unfortunately, the data supporting many of these pesticides are incomplete. For some, particularly certain insecticides, most registered uses on foods have been canceled.

The committee did not assess the quality or completeness of the oncogenicity data supporting these 289 pesticides. The EPA's registration standards program is designed for this purpose, however. Data supporting 115 pesticides registered for use on foods, most of which were registered before 1980, have been assessed under the program. (New active ingredient registrations generally require two valid oncogenicity studies and are rarely subject to a registration standard.) Of the 115 older pesticides, only 23 percent fully satisfied the oncogenicity data requirement; 41 percent had some oncogenicity data on file but did not fully satisfy the EPA's current oncogenicity data requirements; and 36 percent had no adequate oncogenicity data on file.

Oncogenic *risk* is estimated by multiplying human exposure to pesticides by the Q*. The agency supplied the committee with potency factors for 30 of the 53 oncogenic pesticides currently used on food. The committee used 28 of these potency factors in generating the estimates of oncogenic risk. The number and percentage of oncogenic pesticides with available potency factors are shown in Table 3-4. Two chemicals for which the EPA has calculated potency factors, daminozide and asulam, are excluded from the committee's analysis. Daminozide, a plant growth regulator, is not characterized as a herbicide, insecticide, or fungicide; asulam has no food tolerances. The Q*'s and the food consumption and tolerance information in the EPA's Tolerance Assessment System (TAS) form the principal components of the risk calculations in this report.

Table 3-4 illustrates that the committee derived its risk estimates from a roughly equivalent percentage of currently used oncogenic insecticides, fungicides, and herbicides. The portion of oncogenic active ingredients analyzed ranges from 63 percent for insecticides to 79 percent for

TABLE 3-3 Potentially Oncogenic Pesticides Identified by the EPA

Active Ingredient (common/trade name)	Year First Tolerance Granted	Type	Volume of Use (pounds active ingredient/year)[a]	Major Crop Uses
Acephate[b] (Orthene)	1972	Insecticide	1,900,000	Citrus
Acifluorfen (Blazer)	1980	Herbicide	1,400,000	Soybeans
Alachlor[b] (Lasso)	1969	Herbicide	85,000,000	Corn, soybeans
Amitraz (Baam)	1968	Insecticide	50,000	Cattle
Arsenic acid	NA	Herbicide	NA	Cotton
Asulam	1975	Herbicide	NA	Sugar cane
Azinphos-methyl[b] (Guthion)	1956	Insecticide	2,500,000	Peaches, pome fruits
Benomyl[b] (Benlate)	1972	Fungicide	2,000,000	Citrus, rice, soybeans, stone fruits
Calcium arsenate	NA	Insecticide	NA	Stone fruits
Captafol[b] (Difolatan)	1959	Fungicide	6,000,000	Apples, cherries, tomatoes
Captan[b]	1955	Fungicide	10,000,000	Almonds, apples, peaches, seeds
Chlordimeform[b] (Galecron)	1968	Insecticide	NA	Cotton
Chlorobenzilate	1956	Insecticide/ acaricide	1,500,000	Citrus
Chlorothalonil[b] (Bravo)	1961	Fungicide	6,000,000	Fruits, peanuts, vegetables
Copper arsenate	1971	Insecticide	NA	Vegetable crops
Cypermethrin[b] (Ammo, Cymbush)	1984	Insecticide	600,000	Cotton
Cyromazine[b] (Larvadex)	1984	Insecticide	NA	Poultry
Daminozide (Alar)	1967	Growth regulator	875,000	Apples, peanuts
Diallate	1969	Herbicide	500,000	Sugar beets
Diclofop methyl[b] (Hoelon)	1980	Herbicide	1,200,000	Soybeans
Dicofol (Kelthane)	1955	Insecticide/ acaricide	2,500,000	Citrus, cotton
Ethalfluralin[b] (Sonalan)	1982	Herbicide	NA	Soybeans
Ethylene oxide	NA	Bactericide	NA	Spices, walnuts
Folpet[b]	1955	Fungicide	1,500,000	Cherries, fruits, vegetables
Fosetyl Al[b] (Aliette)	1983	Fungicide	NA	Pineapples
Glyphosate[b] (Roundup)	1976	Herbicide	8,000,000	Hays, orchard crops
Lead arsenate	1955	Insecticide	NA	Apples, orchard crops
Lindane	1955	Insecticide	200,000	Avocados, pecans
Linuron[b] (Lorox)	1966	Herbicide	7,000,000	Soybeans
Maleic hydrazide	1955	Growth regulator	300,000	Onions, potatoes
Mancozeb[b] (Dithane M-45)	1962	Fungicide	16,000,000	Fruits, small grains, vegetables

TABLE 3-3 *Continued*

Active Ingredient (common/trade name)	Year First Tolerance Granted	Type	Volume of Use (pounds active ingredient/year)[a]	Major Crop Uses
Maneb[b]	1957	Fungicide	10,000,000	Fruits, small grains, vegetables
Methanearsonic acid	NA	Herbicide	4,000,000	Cotton
Methomyl (Lannate)	1963	Insecticide	4,500,000	Citrus, cotton, vegetables
Metiram[b]	1967	Fungicide	1,000,000	Fruits, small grains, vegetables
Metolachlor[b] (Dual)	1976	Herbicide	38,100,000	Corn, soybeans
O-Phenylphenol[b]	1955	Fungicide	200,000	Citrus, orchard crops
Oryzalin[b] (Surflan)	1974	Herbicide	1,700,000	Soybeans, vineyards
Oxadiazon[b] (Ronstar)	1977	Herbicide	NA	Rice
Paraquat (Gramoxone)	1961	Herbicide	2,800,000	Rice, soybeans
Parathion[b]	1955	Insecticide	7,000,000	Citrus, cotton
PCNB	1955	Fungicide	2,500,000	Cotton, peanuts, vegetables
Permethrin[b] (Ambush, Pounce)	1978	Insecticide	500,000	Vegetables
Pronamide[b] (Kerb)	1972	Herbicide	100,000	Lettuce
Sodium arsenate	NA	Insecticide	NA	Pears
Sodium arsenite	NA	Fungicide, herbicide, insecticide	NA	Grapes
Terbutryn[b]	1959	Herbicide	600,000	Barley, wheat
Tetrachlorvinphos	1969	Insecticide	NA	Cattle, poultry
Thiodicarb (Larvin)	1985	Insecticide	NA	Cotton, soybeans
Thiophanate-methyl	1972	Fungicide	30,000	Fruits, nuts, vegetables
Toxaphene	1955	Insecticide	NA	Cattle
Trifluralin (Treflan)	1963	Herbicide	39,000,000	Soybeans
Zineb[b]	1955	Fungicide	3,500,000	Fruits, small grains, vegetables

[a]Webb, S.E.H., 1981, Preliminary Data: Pesticide Use on Selected Deciduous Fruits in the United States, 1978, Economic Research Service Staff Report No. AGES810626, Washington, D.C.: U.S. Department of Agriculture; Parks, J. R., 1983, Pesticide Use on Fall Potatoes in the United States, 1979, Economic Research Service Staff Report No. AGES830113, Washington, D.C.: U.S. Department of Agriculture; Ferguson, W. L., 1984, 1979 Pesticide Use on Vegetables in Five Regions, Springfield, Va.: National Technical Information Service; Gianessi, L. P., 1986, A National Pesticide Usage Data Base, Resources for the Future, Washington, D.C., photocopy; and unpublished data from the EPA for the years 1981 through 1985, excluding 1983, for crops affected by PIK.

[b]These are compounds for which risk estimates were performed.

The "Q Star"

A pesticide's oncogenic potency is expressed quantitatively as a "Q star" or Q*. The Q* is the slope of the dose response curve from animal tests yielding a positive oncogenic response. The slope represents the change in tumor incidence *(Y)* over the change in dose *(X)*. The units of the potency factor are tumors/mg of pesticide/kg of body weight/day. The Q* represents the estimated tumor incidence expected to occur at the relatively low doses of pesticides in the human diet. It is based on a purely mathematical extrapolation of tumor incidence observed at the high doses used in animal tests. The potency factor does not consider the type, site, or diversity of tumors observed in animal tests. In most cases, however, the potency factors used by the EPA express a combination of malignant and benign tumors. A high Q* indicates a strong oncogenic response (more tumors) to the administered dose; a low number indicates a weak response. Most Q*'s that the committee obtained from the EPA are average Q* calculations derived from several positive oncogenicity studies. These Q*'s were calculated by EPA scientists and have not been formally peer reviewed.

The Q* is considered a conservative or risk-averse model for quantifying oncogenic potency. As such, it represents the 95 percent upper-bound confidence limit (UCL) of tumor induction likely to occur from a given dose. On the other hand, the maximum likelihood estimate (MLE) represents the average probability for tumor induction from a given dose. Oncogenic potency factors derived by the two methods are similar in many cases. In some cases, however, the factors differ by several orders of magnitude, with the Q* calculation generally characterizing a compound as more potent. The EPA relies on the Q* at the 95 percent UCL in risk assessment to provide a margin of safety for uncertainties in characterizing the oncogenic response, for the existence of more sensitive individuals in the exposed population, and for possible synergism of pesticides and metabolites.

The committee relied solely on the Q* in estimating oncogenic potential. Therefore, the estimated oncogenic risks for certain pesticides may appear overstated. More sophisticated judgments of the human risk from dietary exposure to oncogenic agents consider qualitative evidence. This evidence includes the type of tumors produced and whether they are malignant or benign, have metastasized, or are evident in more than one sex and animal species. Such a judgment would entail a "weight-of-the-evidence" approach to risk assessment, which the EPA relies upon in regulatory decision making. The EPA's weight-of-the-evidence classification system for carcinogens is explained in the boxed article "The EPA's

Classification System for Carcinogens," on p. 67. In Tables 3-9 and 3-17 through 3-19, risk estimates are presented with the EPA's classification of the qualitative weight of the evidence.

Quantitative Oncogenic Potency Factors (Q*) for Each Active Ingredient Designated by the EPA as Oncogenic

Active Ingredient (trade name)	Q*
Chlordimeform (Fundal, Galecron)	9.4×10^{-1}
Linuron (Lorox)	3.28×10^{-1}
Oxadiazon (Ronstar)	1.3×10^{-1}
Ethalfluralin (Sonalan)	8.7×10^{-2}
Alachlor (Lasso)	5.95×10^{-2}
Oryzalin (Surflan)	3.4×10^{-2}
Permethrin (Ambush, Pounce)	3.0×10^{-2}
Captafol (Difolatan)	2.50×10^{-2}
Chlorothalonil (Bravo)	2.4×10^{-2}
Asulam	2.0×10^{-2}
Cypermethrin (Ammo, Cymbush)	1.9×10^{-2}
Mancozeb (Dithane M-45)	1.76×10^{-2}
Maneb	1.76×10^{-2}
Metiram	1.76×10^{-2}
Zineb	1.76×10^{-2}
Pronamide (Kerb)	1.6×10^{-2}
Diclofop methyl (Hoelon)	1.1×10^{-2}
Acephate (Orthene)	6.9×10^{-3}
Fosetyl Al (Aliette)	4.3×10^{-3}
Folpet	3.5×10^{-3}
Cyromazine (Larvadex)	2.4×10^{-3}
Captan	2.30×10^{-3}
Metolachlor (Dual)	2.10×10^{-3}
Benomyl (Benlate)	2.065×10^{-3}
Terbutryn	1.87×10^{-3}
Parathion	1.80×10^{-3}
O-Phenylphenol	1.57×10^{-3}
Glyphosate (Roundup)	5.9×10^{-5}
Azinphos-methyl (Guthion)	1.5×10^{-7}

fungicides. The committee received Q*'s for only 7 of 19 oncogenic insecticides. Therefore, it initially appears that the committee examined a disproportionately small number of insecticides. Conclusions regarding relative risk distribution would thus appear to be significantly influenced by the unevenness of the sample. When the sample is adjusted to account for compounds with significant use cancellation, however, the results appear more even.

The situation with insecticides is unique because many oncogenic

TABLE 3-4   Number of Pesticides Identified as Oncogens by the EPA

Active Ingredients	Herbicides	Insecticides	Fungicides	Other	Total
Number identified as oncogens	17	19	14	3	53
With Q*'s[a] (number/%)	11/64	7/37	11/79	1/33	30/57
No Q*'s[a]; major uses canceled[b] (number/%)	0/0	5/26	0/0	0/0	NA
Total (number/%)	11/64	12/63	11/79	0/0	NA
Currently used oncogenic ingredients not considered in committee's analysis of risk (number/%)	6/36	7/37	3/21	NA	NA

[a]Quantitative calculation of oncogenic potency.
[b]These chemicals are toxaphene, lindane, sodium arsenite, copper arsenate, and ethylene oxide.

insecticides with no Q*'s have suffered widespread or total use cancellations. This is not the case with oncogenic herbicides or fungicides. Of the 12 insecticides with no Q*'s, 4 have had most or all uses canceled; one has tolerances for three crops and no available data on use. The risk from these compounds will not increase in the future. The committee did not consider the remaining seven insecticides in its risk analyses. Those insecticides account for only 37.3 percent of the 19 insecticides identified by the EPA as oncogenic or potentially oncogenic. The committee lacked potency estimates for a similar percentage of the fungicides and herbicides.

Pesticide use and the impacts of certain regulatory scenarios on current patterns of use were characterized for all 53 oncogenic active ingredients when data were available and relevant to the analysis. However, this information was used primarily in the crop-level analyses in Chapters 4 and 5.

Estimating Dietary Exposure to Pesticide Residues

The average consumer is exposed to pesticide residues, although in minute quantities, in nearly every food, including meat, dairy products, fruits, vegetables, sugar, coffee, oils, dried goods, and most processed foods. Because pesticide residues are ubiquitous, there is great need for a scientifically rigorous method for estimating dietary exposure to and risk from these residues.

Many assumptions are necessary to estimate dietary exposure to pesticides. Simply, exposure to pesticide residues in food is a function of the quantity and type of foods one eats and the amount of residues on or in those foods.

Food Consumption Data

Estimates of dietary exposure to pesticide residues are based on food consumption estimates. These can vary widely, depending on the methods and data sources used. For example, the recently completed EPA TAS replaced an older EPA data base that rested upon a less sophisticated set of food consumption data developed in the 1960s. The TAS made possible the analyses presented in this report, and will substantially advance the EPA's capacity to assess pesticide residues in the diet. Some of the key improvements and limitations in the TAS are described below.

Until 1985 the EPA used the Food Factor system, which was based on a 1966 (USDA) food consumption survey. As developed by the EPA, the Food Factor system made no distinction between the differing dietary patterns of various segments of the population. The TAS, on the other hand, is derived from the USDA's 1977–1978 food consumption survey, a nationwide study of food consumption patterns. The study contains dietary consumption estimates for 376 food types, which can be broken down by population subgroups according to sex, race, age, and region. Most significantly as far as this study is concerned, the TAS incorporates specific consumption estimates for raw and processed food forms for most crops consumed in the United States. For example, where the Food Factor system estimated consumption of raw and processed apples, TAS estimates consumption of a greater variety of raw and processed forms, such as whole apples, applesauce, apple juice, and dried apples. Tables 3-5 and 3-6 compare selected Food Factor system and TAS consumption estimates. (The TAS is described in more detail in Appendix B.)

Some changes in consumption patterns are evident from these tables. Table 3-5 shows that TAS consumption estimates for milk and dairy products, citrus, tomatoes, peppers, apples, and pears are higher than those in the Food Factor system. Consumption of root vegetables, leafy vegetables, red meat, and grains has declined.

The TAS ratios of raw to processed food forms of a given crop are significantly different from Food Factor ratios. Table 3-6 shows great differences between TAS and Food Factor estimates of the percentage of selected crops consumed in processed form. For three of the crops analyzed (apples, grapes, and oranges), the percentage of the crop

TABLE 3-5 Comparative Consumption of Selected Crop Groups (grams/day)

Crop	TAS	Food Factor System
Citrus[a]	85	57
Fruits, pome[b]	47	41
Grains[c]	118	206
Meat, red[d]	132	162
Milk and dairy[e]	635[i]	429
Vegetables, fruiting[f]	49	44
Vegetables, leafy[g]	33	41
Vegetables, root[h]	106	165

[a]Citrus fruits include grapefruit, lemons, limes, oranges, and other fruits.

[b]Pome fruits include apples and pears.

[c]Grains include corn, oats, rice, rye, and wheat.

[d]Red meat includes cattle, hogs, and sheep.

[e]Milk and dairy products include fresh fluid milk, processed milk, cream, frozen milk desserts, cheese, butter, and other products.

[f]Fruiting vegetables include peppers and tomatoes.

[g]Leafy vegetables include broccoli, cabbage, cauliflower, celery, collards, kale, lettuce, mustard greens, rhubarb, and spinach.

[h]Root vegetables include beets, carrots, onions, potatoes, sugar beets, sweet potatoes, and turnips.

[i]This consumption level was calculated with a TAS conversion factor to estimate consumption of whole fluid milk. This conversion was necessary to make TAS milk consumption, otherwise expressed as milk solids, compatible with the Food Factor consumption figures for whole milk. The committee's risk estimates for milk and dairy products do *not* use this conversion factor. Because of this, the risk from pesticide residues in whole milk may be underestimated.

TABLE 3-6 Comparative Consumption of Selected Raw and Processed Crops (in percent)

Crop	TAS		Food Factor System	
	Fresh	Processed	Fresh	Processed
Apples	67	33	79	21
Grapes	29	71	60	40
Oranges	12	88	62	38
Potatoes	99	1	87	13
Tomatoes	61	39	49	51

assumed to be consumed in processed form in TAS rose 57 to 131 percent over Food Factor estimates. For two others (tomatoes and potatoes), it fell by 30 and 90 percent, respectively.

Although the TAS permits analyses of estimated food consumption patterns for specific population subgroups, all analyses in this report are based on U.S. mean consumption estimates. Current food consumption patterns may be different from those during 1977–1978; therefore, the estimates used may not reflect the contemporary diet accurately.

METHOD FOR ESTIMATING RESIDUES IN FOOD

The committee had to use estimates for all pesticide residues in food because of very limited actual data. The estimates used are based on current food tolerances in the *Code of Federal Regulations* (CFR). Tolerances are typically expressed as parts per million (ppm) of pesticide X on food Y. Because pesticide residues are generally below the tolerance and only occasionally above it, the estimates used may overestimate actual exposure. Dietary exposure to residues of a given pesticide on a given food is estimated by converting the tolerance from parts per million into milligrams in the daily diet. The conversion of an individual tolerance into a dietary intake estimate is performed by multiplying the tolerance by the consumption estimate. This number is then divided by 1,000 to attain comparable units because tolerances are expressed in parts per million and consumption estimates are expressed in kilograms. Estimated exposure levels, expressed in milligrams of pesticide in the daily diet, generally are aggregated for all foodstuffs in which a pesticide *could* be found.

The TAS greatly facilitates analysis of dietary exposure patterns. It incorporates all tolerances published in the CFR and additional estimates of pesticide residues not covered by a published tolerance in processed and raw foods. (These residues are discussed further in the next subsections and in Appendix B.) Although consumption estimates for drinking water and for water added or used during processing or cooking are included in the TAS, these estimates are not considered here.

METHOD FOR ESTIMATING EXPOSURE TO RESIDUES

The EPA traditonally has estimated dietary exposure conservatively by incorporating worst-case assumptions. Pesticide residues are assumed to be present in foods at the published tolerance level. The agency also generally assumes that 100 percent of the acreage of a crop that could be treated with a pesticide will be treated. Estimating exposure in this way nearly always produces an overestimate of actual dietary exposure across

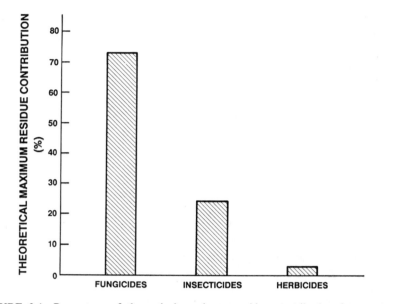

FIGURE 3-1 Percentage of theoretical maximum residue contribution for oncogenic pesticides by pesticide type.

the whole population, assuming pesticides are applied at the prescribed application rate. This conservative bias is reflected in the term the EPA uses for this calculation, the Theoretical Maximum Residue Contribution (TMRC). The agency has acknowledged for a long time the shortcomings of this method. The EPA contends, however, that the two assumptions together introduce a prudent safety factor in its overall assessment of pesticide risks. Figure 3-1 presents the distribution of TMRC for oncogenic fungicides, insecticides, and herbicides. Fourteen oncogenic fungicides account for 73 percent of the TMRC, 19 insecticides for 24 percent, and 17 herbicides for 3 percent.

To estimate current oncogenic risk, the committee considered several ways to develop more realistic calculations of current dietary exposure. One method would be to adjust exposure calculations by taking into account the percentage of each crop treated with a pesticide. To carry out this adjustment, data would be needed on the percentage of acres of all crops treated with all pesticides. It would bias the results if the adjustment were made only for crops and pesticides for which accurate use data are available.

The committee was able to compile such data for the pesticides used on some crops—a step necessary in carrying out the crop analyses in the next chapter. For the risk-estimate tables in this chapter, however, lack of data on use precluded this adjustment. Moreover, the validity of adjusting estimated average exposure on the basis of percentage of acres treated rests on the unlikely assumption that the residue from any given pesticide is evenly distributed throughout the population. Although the committee did not study this issue in depth, it is aware that many foods are grown and consumed within one or a few regions of the country. This is particularly true with fresh milk, and vegetables and fruits in season. Consumers in the Southeast are likely to consume a different mix and different levels of pesticide residues than consumers in California. In Chapter 5, the committee discusses some regional pesticide use problems in more detail.

Other complications in estimating the level of residues in or on a food following application of a pesticide need to be considered in assessing the TMRC concept and in choosing a method to estimate exposure. First, residues found in *most* foods are consistently below the legal limit or tolerance, but this is not always the case. Recent General Accounting Office (GAO) and FDA reports concluded that about 3 to 4 percent of all samples checked contained unlawful residues.[8] These residues were either above the tolerance level or appeared on a food for which there was no tolerance. Moreover, many foods contain residues of several pesticides. There is no way to know how or whether these interact. Pesticides are sometimes misused. Unexpected and undetectable residues can find their way into the food supply.

For these reasons, the committee found no defensible basis or method to adjust tolerances or residue estimates systematically in the TAS.

METHOD FOR ESTIMATING RESIDUES IN PROCESSED FOODS

One of the committee's most important tasks was to compare the oncogenic risks to humans in *raw* versus *processed* foods. The distinction is the key to assessing the regulatory impact of the Delaney Clause.

Most pesticides registered on food crops before 1978 lack tolerances and data for residues in *processed* foods, even though the EPA suspects that such residues are often present at concentrated levels. Dietary exposure to these pesticides will be underestimated without considering the expected residue levels in these processed foods separately from the residue levels and consumption estimates for fresh foods.

To deal with such cases, the EPA built an operating assumption into the TAS: residues are presumed present in processed foods at the same level authorized on raw commodities, unless a published section 409 tolerance exists. In this case, the level that the section 409 tolerance specifies is incorporated into the TAS. Thus, if the EPA has established a tolerance for pesticide *X* on apples but not in apple juice, the TAS presumes a residue level in apple juice equal to the published tolerance for raw apples. The TAS also contains conversion factors designed to adjust exposure to allow for residue concentration during processing. When a raw commodity tolerance is applied to a processed food in the TAS, the resulting exposure is multiplied by a conversion factor to incorporate the assumption that residues will concentrate during processing. These conversion factors generally are estimates, however, and are not based on scientific data. Therefore, the committee *did not use TAS conversion factors* in calculating any exposure or risk estimates in this report.

The TAS further elaborates on the published tolerances by disaggregating section 408 and section 409 tolerances by food type, particularly for processed foods. For the hypothesized pesticide *with no section 409 tolerances* used on apples, the TAS would assume residues equal to the published raw food tolerance for several forms of processed apples: applesauce, apple juice, and dried apples.

The TAS makes a similar assumption for pesticides *with* section 409 tolerances. Often, section 409 tolerances appear in the CFR as tolerances on, for example, processed apple products. The TAS expands this single section 409 tolerance by duplicating the section 409 tolerance level for each distinct processed apple product shown in the TAS. Therefore, a pesticide with one section 408 and one section 409 tolerance on apples in the CFR may have one section 408 and four section 409 tolerances in the TAS. This adjustment produces many more processed-food tolerances in the TAS than in the CFR. Nonetheless, these expanded or duplicated section 409 tolerances are easily distinguished from the processed-food residue estimates created in the TAS when no section 409 tolerance exists in the CFR (see Appendix B).

These methodological refinements yield some significant insights. For all 289 pesticides considered by the committee, the TAS contains tolerances or residue estimates for some 3,178 distinct processed-food forms. For the same 289 pesticides, section 409 tolerances cover only 239 food forms, which is about 1 approved tolerance for every 13 processed-food forms. Consequently, pesticide residues that may be consumed in 12 out of 13 processed foods are incorporated in TAS-based exposure and risk assessments only through the assumption that residues in processed foods will equal section 408 raw food tolerance levels. A list of all oncogenic pesticides with section 409 food or feed additive tolerances is presented in Table 3-7.

For oncogenic pesticides, the TAS contains 809 distinct estimates of residues in processed foods. Yet for the same pesticides, there are only 31 processed foods associated with published section 409 tolerances. Table 3-8 compares the number of TAS residue estimates for processed foods with the number of published section 409 tolerances for these same

TABLE 3-7 Presumed Oncogenic Pesticides with Section 409 Tolerances

Food-Additive Tolerances	Feed-Additive Tolerances
Benomyl	Acephate
Captan	Amitraz
Chlordimeform	Benomyl
Daminozide	Captan
Glyphosate	Chlordimeform
Azinphos-methyl	Cyromazine
Dicofol	Daminozide
Maleic hydrazide	Glyphosate
Mancozeb	Azinphos-methyl
Oryzalin	Linuron
Paraquat	Mancozeb
Toxaphene	Methanearsonic acid
Trifluralin	Paraquat
	Tetrachlorvinphos
	Thiodicarb
	Thiophanate-methyl

processed foods. The committee believes this discrepancy deserves attention.

Although the TAS residue estimates may overestimate exposure to some residues in processed foods and underestimate exposure to others, TAS is the best available tool for estimating pesticide residues in the diet. The consumption data the TAS incorporates, together with published and presumed residue levels, provide a reliable characterization of the relative magnitude and distribution of dietary exposure to pesticides. The range of error in TAS exposure estimates is well characterized compared to the uncertainties encountered at other steps in the risk assessment process.

ESTIMATION OF ONCOGENIC RISK

Like the EPA, the committee calculates oncogenic risk to humans by a seemingly simple formula: estimated exposure is multiplied by a pesticide's estimated oncogenic potency, which is a single number representing its tendency to induce tumors. This formula is expressed in the following equation:

dietary oncogenic risk =
exposure (food consumption × pesticide residues) × oncogenic potency

This potency factor, or Q*, is derived from mathematical models that

TABLE 3-8   Processed Foods in the Tolerance Assessment System (TAS) Compared with Section 409 Tolerances

Pesticide	TAS Processed Food Forms	Section 409 Tolerances[a]
Pesticides with food tolerances	3,178	239
All oncogens	809	31
All oncogenic herbicides, insecticides, and fungicides	755	24
All oncogens with Q*'s	502	25
All oncogenic herbicides, insecticides, and fungicides with Q*'s	490	19
All oncogens on—		
Corn	16	0
Grapes	37	3
Oranges	142	0
Soybeans	60	0
Tomatoes	100	8

[a]The numbers in this column represent tolerances published in the CFR plus additional processed food forms in the TAS to which these section 409 tolerances have been applied. For example, in the CFR the fungicide benomyl has one section 409 tolerance for processed tomato products. In the TAS this section 409 tolerance level is applied to five distinct processed tomato products resulting in four additional section 409 tolerances.

extrapolate from data derived from animal experiments to estimate human cancer risk (see the boxed article "The 'Q Star' "). Despite much effort to develop accurate models, there is a margin of error in the Q*'s, as well as a significant degree of uncertainty regarding their importance to human cancer risk estimates. For example, although the *models* used to develop Q*'s make the assumption that the potency of the carcinogen extends to the low dose, the *data* do not exclude the possibility that a threshold dose exists for certain compounds that exhibit oncogenicity in animal studies.

The Q* value is a probabilistic estimate of the upper bound on incidence of extra instances of tumor formation in humans that can be expected following dietary ingestion, or exposure by other routes, of a given level of a particular chemical over a 70-year human lifetime. The Q*'s used by the committee were calculated by EPA scientists and have not been formally peer reviewed. The methods for calculating risks that the EPA and the committee use estimate extra cases of tumor formation in humans above existing average expectations. While uncertain, these methods are used widely by essentially all governments and international organizations faced with assessing the health consequences of human exposure to animal oncogens.

It is important to understand what the risk estimates developed by these extrapolation models represent. First, the reported risk of cancer is typically expressed as a conservative upper-bound estimate of the number of additional cancer cases per 10,000 (10^{-4}), 100,000 (10^{-5}), or 1 million (10^{-6}) individuals. Risk refers to incidence or frequency of cancer cases, not cancer deaths. The risk is over and above the 1 in 3.85 to 1 in 4, or about 2.5×10^{-1}, lifetime risk of cancer now expected for members of the U.S. population.[9]

Oncogenic risks associated with pesticide residues in the diet have been calculated in many different ways for many crops and pesticides. The highest risks ever calculated for a pesticide are 1 additional cancer case in every 100 people (10^{-2}) following a lifetime's exposure. Such a risk estimate, if accurate, would mean that the odds that an average individual would contract cancer in a lifetime would rise from about 25 percent to 26 percent.[10] Further, potential cancer risk is estimated by identifying a conservative upper bound on potential human risk. The estimated risks reported in this chapter, which incorporate many conservative assumptions regarding crops consumed and pesticide residues, are no greater than 1×10^{-3}. This figure represents an increase in average individual human risk from 25 percent to 25.1 percent.

The risk estimates offered here incorporate many assumptions that *may* overstate actual risk. These include

• Conservative assumptions in the models used for extrapolating high-dose tumor incidence data in animal tests to expected low-dose incidence;

• Assumptions that all acres of all crops are treated with all pesticides for which they have tolerances;

• Assumptions that residues are always present at the tolerance when in fact they are usually at lower levels; and

• Assumptions that daily exposure to these residues occurs over the course of a 70-year lifetime.

On the other hand, several other factors *may* work to understate the dietary risks posed by these compounds. They include

• A lack of toxicological data for some active ingredients and most inerts, degradation products, and metabolites;

• The possibility that the models used for extrapolating the results of animal experiments may be insufficiently conservative in certain respects;

• The omission of certain routes of exposure; and

• Possible synergy of compounds and metabolites.

Further, the committee's rather mechanical calculation of risk, which multiplies total exposure by a pesticide's Q* value, leads to a purely quantitative estimate of the distribution and magnitude of these risks. A more sophisticated weight-of-the-evidence approach would be desirable and would improve confidence in quantitative estimates of risk. The risk estimates for linuron and permethrin are two good examples when a weight-of-the-evidence approach probably would alter determinations of human dietary risk. (For a more detailed discussion of the committee's risk assessment procedures, see Appendix B.) Such an approach generally yields somewhat different empirical results that provide a firmer sense of a compound's actual cancer risk to humans.

To indicate the relative hazard of animal oncogens to humans, the EPA has developed a classification system (see the boxed article "The EPA's Classification System for Carcinogens" for further discussion). This system, adapted from the approach of the International Agency for Research on Cancer (IARC), is designed to characterize the qualitative weight of the evidence for a carcinogenic compound. The system contains five basic categories: (A) human carcinogen, (B) probable human carcinogen, (C) possible human carcinogen, (D) not classifiable as to human carcinogenicity, and (E) evidence of noncarcinogenicity for humans.

The EPA's weight-of-the-evidence classification for the 28 pesticides is presented in certain tables to provide greater perspective of the relative human oncogenic hazard of these compounds. The committee did not use the carcinogen classification system to estimate risks or their distribution or to calculate the impacts of the scenarios described in Chapters 4 and 5.

An Analysis of Estimated Oncogenic Risk

Table 3-9 presents the estimates of dietary oncogenic risk for the 28 pesticides the committee was able to examine. The estimates are arranged in descending order of risk. As stated earlier, the committee examined these compounds by

• Raw versus processed food;
• Risk from categories of foodstuffs, including animal products;
• Pesticide type (herbicides, insecticides, and fungicides);
• Active ingredients; and
• The date tolerances were granted.

In addition, estimated risks were aggregated for combinations of these factors. For example, residues of old and new pesticides were analyzed by pesticide type in fresh and processed food. The data base compiled by

---

The EPA's Classification System for Carcinogens

The EPA classification system for carcinogens is adapted from a similar system developed by the International Agency for Research on Cancer. It is used by the EPA to classify all potential human carcinogens, not just pesticides. The purpose of the system is to characterize a compound's carcinogenic hazard to humans. Substances are classified based on the evaluation of such factors as the results of mutagenicity tests, consideration of any negative oncogenicity results, the types and diversity of tumors induced, the structural similarity of the compound to other carcinogens, and whether positive results have been replicated.

GROUP A—**Human carcinogen**
Sufficient evidence from epidemiologic studies to support a causal association between exposure to agents and cancer

GROUP B—**Probable human carcinogen**
B[1]—Sufficient evidence of carcinogenicity from animal studies with limited evidence of carcinogenicity from epidemiologic studies
B[2]—Sufficient evidence of carcinogenicity from animal studies, with inadequate or no epidemiologic data

GROUP C—**Possible human carcinogen**
Limited evidence of carcinogenicity in the absence of human data

GROUP D—**Not classifiable as to human carcinogenicity**
Inadequate or no human and animal data for carcinogenicity

GROUP E—**Evidence of noncarcinogenicity for humans**
No evidence of carcinogenicity in at least two adequate animal tests in different species in adequate epidemiologic and animal studies. This classification is based on available evidence and does not mean that the agent will not be a carcinogen under any circumstances.

---

the committee is designed to allow analyses of dietary pesticide residue risks according to any combination of these factors.

DISTRIBUTION OF RISK BY TOLERANCE TYPE: SECTION 408 VERSUS SECTION 409

The distribution of estimated oncogenic risk by tolerance type (raw versus processed food) is important because the Delaney Clause applies only when residues concentrate in processed foods above the levels allowed in raw foods. As noted in Chapter 2, the EPA has about 2,500 section 408 tolerances for oncogenic pesticides. It has approved only 31

TABLE 3-9   Estimated Oncogenic Risk from Dietary Exposure to 28 Pesticides

Active Ingredient	Food Crop Uses (number)	Type of Pesticide	Risk	Weight-of-the-Evidence Classification	Year of First Tolerance
Linuron (Lorox)	20	Herbicide	1.52×10^{-3}	C	1966
Zineb	83	Fungicide	7.17×10^{-4}	B_2[a]	1955
Captafol (Difolatan)	34	Fungicide	5.94×10^{-4}	B_2	1959
Captan	83	Fungicide	4.74×10^{-4}	B_2	1955
Maneb	56	Fungicide	4.42×10^{-4}	B_2[a]	1957
Permethrin (Ambush, Pounce)	43	Insecticide	4.21×10^{-4}	C	1978
Mancozeb (Dithane M-45)	44	Fungicide	3.38×10^{-4}	B_2[a]	1962
Folpet	41	Fungicide	3.24×10^{-4}	B_2	1955
Chlordimeform (Fundal, Galecron)	24	Insecticide	3.22×10^{-4}[b]	B_2	1968
Chlorothalonil (Bravo)	47	Fungicide	2.37×10^{-4}	NA	1961
Metiram	11	Fungicide	1.15×10^{-4}	B_2[a]	1967
Benomyl	101	Fungicide	1.13×10^{-4}	C	1972
O-Phenylphenol	22	Fungicide	9.99×10^{-5}	NA	1955
Acephate (Orthene)	34	Insecticide	3.73×10^{-5}	NA	1972
Alachlor (Lasso)	25	Herbicide	2.42×10^{-5}[c]	B_2	1969
Parathion	98	Insecticide	1.47×10^{-5}	C	1955
Metolachlor (Dual)	40	Herbicide	1.44×10^{-5}	C (pending)	1976
Oxadiazon (Ronstar)	26	Herbicide	1.21×10^{-5}	B_2	1977
Oryzalin (Surflan)	57	Herbicide	1.14×10^{-5}	C	1974
Pronamide (Kerb)	25	Herbicide	7.77×10^{-6}	C	1972
Cypermethrin (Ammo, Cymbush)	7	Insecticide	3.73×10^{-6}	C	1984
Ethalfluralin (Sonalan)	18	Herbicide	3.56×10^{-6}	NA	1982
Diclofop methyl (Holelon)	5	Herbicide	2.04×10^{-6}	NA	1980
Cyromazine (Larvadex)	4	Insecticide	3.58×10^{-7}	NA	1984
Terbutryn	4	Herbicide	2.86×10^{-7}	C	1959
Glyphosate (Roundup)	134	Herbicide	2.73×10^{-7}	C	1976
Fosetyl Al (Aliette)	1	Fungicide	3.29×10^{-8}	C	1983
Azinphos-methyl (Guthion)	78	Insecticide	1.68×10^{-9}	D	1956

NOTE: In this table and in those following, risk estimates are based on EPA data and methods using the TAS U.S. mean consumption estimates. They assume that residues are at the tolerance level, that 100 percent of all acres are treated, and that exposure occurs over a 70-year lifetime.

B_2 indicates a probable human carcinogen. C indicates a possible human carcinogen. D indicates not classifiable as to human carcinogenicity. NA indicates that the pesticide has not been classified by EPA.

[a]The classification is for the EBDC metabolite ethylene thiourea.

[b]This risk estimate assumes residues at the level of detection, or 0.05 ppm, for all meat, poultry, and dairy products with tolerances for chlordimeform.

[c]This risk estimate does not include the use of alachlor on potatoes because this use was withdrawn by the registrant when these risk estimates were calculated.

TABLE 3-10 Estimated Oncogenic Risk Distribution by Pesticide Type on Fresh and Processed Foods

Type of Pesticide	Fresh Food		Processed Food	
	Risk	Percentage[a]	Risk	Percentage[a]
Fungicides	2.53×10^{-3}	54.5	9.33×10^{-4}	77.8
Herbicides	1.44×10^{-3}	31.0	1.40×10^{-4}	11.6
Insecticides	6.73×10^{-4}	14.5	1.27×10^{-4}	10.6
Total		100.0		100.0
Estimated risk/percent total estimated risk	4.64×10^{-3}	79.4[b]	1.20×10^{-3}	20.6[b]

NOTE: These risk estimates are derived using EPA data and methods described on pages 50–66 and in Appendix B.
[a]These percentages represent fresh or processed food risk by pesticide type.
[b]These are percentages of total dietary risk.

section 409 tolerances for the same compounds. Many of these oncogenic pesticide residues probably will be found to concentrate. If they do, the EPA will have to establish many additional food and feed additive tolerances or consider revocation of the underlying raw commodity tolerances.

For the 28 oncogenic compounds included in the committee's assessment of current risks, the TAS identifies 490 processed foods. Only 19 section 409 tolerances have been approved for these foods. For the remaining 471 processed foods with no section 409 tolerances, the TAS assigns the section 408 tolerance as the assumed residue level. Based on the assumption that residues in processed foods without approved tolerances do not concentrate but are present at the same level allowed on the raw commodities, about 80 percent of estimated oncogenic risk is associated with raw foods. Processed foods account for about 20 percent (see Table 3-10).

This assumed contribution of risk from raw foods suggests that the Delaney Clause will not affect many pesticide uses or substantially reduce risk. The clause's potential impact could be larger, however, for the following reasons:

• In most cases, revoking processed-food tolerances would mean revoking section 408 raw-food tolerances for the crop from which the processed foods are derived. The EPA denies raw-commodity tolerances for new oncogenic active ingredients if it determines that their residues will concentrate in processed foods, which would ban them under the Delaney Clause. When the estimated oncogenic risk derived from residues in processed foods is added to the estimated risk from residues in or on their parent raw commodities, the total accounts for more than one-half of the estimated current oncogenic risk from all residues in all foods.

• Under current regulations all meat, milk, and poultry products have no processed food forms. Consequently, residues in them are not subject to the Delaney Clause. Yet, the clause could indirectly reduce the dietary risk associated with these foods if residues concentrate in processed feed such as soybeans and corn and tolerances for the feeds are revoked.

Because the food additives law applies only to concentrated residues in

TABLE 3-11 Crop Requirements for Processing Studies Under Current EPA Guidelines

Not Required		Required
Almonds	Lettuce	Apples
Apricots	Loganberries	Barley
Avocados	Mangoes	Beans
Beet greens	Milk	Corn, sweet
Beets	Mushrooms	Cottonseed
Blackberries	Muskmelons	Grapefruit
Blueberries	Mustard greens	Grapes
Boysenberries	Nectarines	Lemons
Broccoli	Nuts	Limes
Brussel sprouts	Onions, dry bulbs	Oats
Cabbage, sauerkraut	Onions, green	Oranges
Cantaloupes	Papayas	Peanuts
Carrots	Peaches	Pineapples
Cattle, meat, fat	Pears	Plums
Cauliflower	Peas	Potatoes
Celery	Peppers	Rice
Cherries	Pimientos	Rye
Collards	Poultry	Soybeans
Crab apples	Pumpkins, squash	Tomatoes
Cranberries	Quinces	Wheat
Cucumbers, pickles	Raspberries	
Dewberries	Rhubarb	
Eggplant	Rutabagas	
Eggs	Shallots	
Garlic	Strawberries	
Goats	Summer squash	
Hogs	Sweet potatoes	
Honeydew melons	Tangerines	
Horses	Taros	
Kale	Turnips	
Kohlrabi	Winter squash	
Leeks		

TABLE 3-12 Worst-Case Impact of the Delaney Clause

Type of Pesticide	Estimated Risk Reduction (number/%)[a]	Number of Crops Affected (number/%)[b]
Fungicides	$2.45 \times 10^{-3}/70.7$	27/19
Herbicides	$5.75 \times 10^{-4}/36.4$	34/20
Insecticides	$2.12 \times 10^{-4}/26.5$	25/16
Total	$3.23 \times 10^{-3}/55.4^c$	38/20[d]

NOTE: These risk estimates are derived using EPA data and methods described on pages 50–66 and in Appendix B. This scenario assumes that tolerances for all processed foods and the parent raw commodities are revoked.

[a]These percentages represent reduction in estimated dietary oncogenic risk by type of pesticide.

[b]These are percentages of all crop registrations for oncogenic herbicides, insecticides, or fungicides by pesticide type.

[c]This percentage represents the total estimated oncogenic risk eliminated.

[d]This is the percentage of all crop registrations for pesticides comprising total estimated risk.

processed foods, residues on crops with no processed-food forms escape the zero-risk standard of the Delaney Clause. Unprocessed fruits, vegetables, and animal products account for the majority of section 408 tolerances. From Table 3-11 it is apparent that the Delaney Clause will not revoke or deny tolerances for many fruit and vegetable crops, all currently defined as minor crops, unless the EPA changes its definition of a processed food.

The maximum impact of the Delaney Clause on the 28 pesticides can be estimated by assuming that residues concentrate in processed-food forms for all crops that have these forms. If section 408 and section 409 tolerances for oncogens were revoked or denied for all these crops pursuant to the Delaney Clause, 55.4 percent of current estimated risk would be eliminated (see Table 3-12). It is noteworthy that such a significant percentage of estimated oncogenic risk could be eliminated by tolerance revocations affecting only 20 percent of all crops. But it is also significant that residues accounting for nearly 45 percent of total estimated risk would remain in the diet.

ONCOGENIC RISK DERIVED FROM RESIDUES IN ANIMAL FEEDS

Although pesticide tolerances for most fruits and vegetables currently escape the Delaney Clause because these crops have no recognized

TABLE 3-13 Industry Recommendations of
Processed By-products Requiring Tolerances

Commodity	Estimated Waste Used for Livestock Feed[a]	
	Percentage	Tons, Wet
Apricots	47	4,897
Asparagus	44	15,272
Bananas[b]		
Beets, garden	20	19,733
Cabbages	9	8,024
Carrots	72	161,758
Cauliflower	80	25,326
Celery[b]		
Cherries	16	6,696
Cucumbers	25	7,447
Mung beans[b]		
Onions, bulb[b]		
Papayas[b]		
Passion fruit[b]		
Peaches	17	32,725
Pears	64	89,126
Peppers[b]		
Pimientos[b]		
Plums[b]		
Spinach	75	20,844
Sweet potatoes	90	52,052

[a]These figures were calculated in J. L. Cooper (1976, The Potential of Food Processing Solid Wastes as a Source of Cellulose for Enzymatic Conversion, pp. 251–271 in Biotechnology and Bioengineering Symposium No. 6) from data collected by A. M. Katsuyama (1973, Solid Waste Management in the Food Processing Industry, NTIS Report No. PB 219 019, Springfield, Va.: National Technical Information Service) by questionnaire and site visitation.
[b]Figures were not available for these commodities.

processed-food form, by-products from some of these crops are increasingly fed to animals. The EPA currently does not recognize many of these by-products as processed animal feeds. The National Food Processors Association has suggested requiring food-processing studies to verify the need for section 409 tolerances for processed by-products of 21 crops fed to animals (see Table 3-13). The EPA has not required such studies or yet considered the need for corresponding tolerances. If the suggested residue studies confirmed the presence of concentrated residues in by-products fed to animals, section 409 tolerances for these residues would be required. For oncogenic pesticides, the Delaney Clause would make these feed additive tolerances difficult for the EPA to grant or, in the case of old compounds, to continue. (The FDA's sensitivity-of-the-method approach might sustain some uses, however.) Section 408 tolerances for residues of these pesticides in animal food products could also be required.

The Delaney Clause would have still greater impact if feed-additive tolerances were required for residues that concentrate in hays and fodders that (1) do not leave the farm or (2) result from certain food-manufacturing processes. The EPA's current definition of processed feed does not include these feed sources. Only certain by-products that result from specific processes such as canning, milling, or hulling are now subject to the feed-additive tolerances when residues concentrate during these processes. Thus, pesticide residues in nonprocessed feeds such as fodders and hays do not require section 409 tolerances, *even when residues concentrate* during the drying of these feeds. Section 408 regulates residues in these feeds instead. Some fodders and hays not subject to feed-additive regulations are listed in Table 3-14.

Table 3-15 describes the oncogenic risk from meat, milk, dairy, and poultry products and major feed sources of residues. Were additional feed additive and food tolerances required, estimated oncogenic risk from animal products would probably increase. Because animal products have no processed-food forms under current EPA regulations, the Delaney Clause has smaller current and potential impacts on animal products than on other foods.

TABLE 3-14 Animal Feeds Not Subject to Feed-Additive Regulations

Alfalfa hay	Lespedeza hay	Rice straw
Almond hulls	Millet forage (dry)	Rye straw
Bean hay	Milo fodder	Safflower fodder
Clover	Mint hay	Sainfoin hay
Corn fodder	Oat hay, fodder, straw	Sorghum hay (fodder)
Cotton forage, by-products	Peanut hay	Soybean hay, straw
Cowpea fodder (dry vines)	Pea vine hay	Spearmint hay
Flax straw	Peppermint hay	Sugarcane fodder
Grass straw	Pigeon pea hay	Sunflower forage (dry)
Hops (dried)	Pineapple fodder (if dried)	Trefoil hay
Hop vines (dehydrated)	Rape straw	Vetch hay
Lentil hay	Rendered meat (cattle, poultry, swine, etc.)	Wheat straw

NOTE: Feed-additive tolerances are not required even in cases where residues concentrate during the drying of hays or forage.

TABLE 3-15   Estimated Oncogenic Risk from Meat, Milk, Dairy, and Poultry Products

Type of Pesticide	Estimated Risk		Major Sources of Residues
	Number/Percent[a]	Percentage Total Estimated Risk	
Herbicides	$7.73 \times 10^{-4}/69.9$	13	Corn, soybeans, various hays
Insecticides	$3.31 \times 10^{-4}/29.9^{*}$	6	Corn, cotton, soybeans
Fungicides	$1.59 \times 10^{-6}/00.1$	Negligible	
Total	$1.10 \times 10^{-3}/99.9$	19	

NOTE: These risk estimates are derived using EPA data and methods described on pages 50–66 and in Appendix B. There are no processed-food tolerances for meat and animal products. Processed meat (such as salami) and dairy products (such as cheese) are considered by the EPA as unique raw agricultural products.

[a]These figures represent risk and percent of risk from meat, milk, dairy, and poultry products.

DISTRIBUTION OF ESTIMATED RISK BY TYPE OF PESTICIDE

Table 3-16 and Figure 3-2 present the distribution of estimated oncogenic risk by fungicides, herbicides, and insecticides. Nearly 60 percent of all estimated risk is from fungicides, 27 percent is from herbicides, and 13 percent is from insecticides. Almost all estimated herbicide risk is from a single compound, linuron, which in large part reflects that compound's relatively high tolerances. Two active ingredients, chlordimeform and permethrin, account for nearly all estimated dietary oncogenic risk from insecticides. Estimated risk from fungicides is

TABLE 3-16   Distribution of Estimated Oncogenic Risk by Pesticide Type

Type of Pesticide	Risk (number/%)
Fungicides	$3.46 \times 10^{-3}/59.2$
Herbicides	$1.58 \times 10^{-3}/27.1$
Insecticides	$8.00 \times 10^{-4}/13.7$
Total	$5.84 \times 10^{-3a}/100$

NOTE: These risk estimates are derived using EPA data and methods described on pages 50–66 and in Appendix B.

[a]This number is the total of all upper-bound estimates of dietary oncogenic risk for the 28 compounds examined by the committee. It does not represent a total estimated dietary oncogenic risk to individuals in the population, but rather serves as a benchmark from which to measure distribution and reduction of risk.

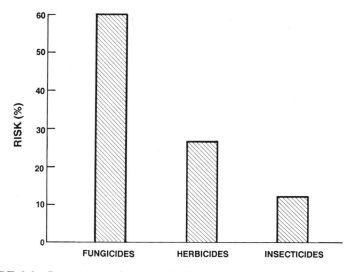

FIGURE 3-2 Percentage of estimated dietary oncogenic risk from fungicides, herbicides, and insecticides.

fairly evenly distributed among the nine compounds presenting the greatest estimated risks.

The committee found that roughly 20 percent of the current estimated total dietary oncogenic risk is associated with consumption of processed foods; fungicides account for three-fourths of this risk and nearly 60 percent of total oncogenic risk (see Table 3-10). This contribution is extraordinary. Most dietary risk from fungicides is attributable to crops that account for only 15 percent of all planted acres, and fungicides comprise only about 10 percent of all pesticides applied to food crops.

DISTRIBUTION OF ESTIMATED RISK BY ACTIVE INGREDIENT

When the risks attributable to individual active ingredients are analyzed, the markedly different distribution of risks within the categories of herbicides, insecticides, and fungicides is obvious. One herbicide, linuron, represents more than 98 percent of all estimated oncogenic risk from herbicides (see Table 3-17). Two insecticides, chlordimeform and permethrin, contribute more than 95 percent of all estimated dietary risk from insecticides (see Table 3-18). For the nine principal oncogenic fungicides, however, no single active ingredient accounts for more than 20 percent of all estimated fungicide risk (see Table 3-19).

Reducing dietary risk from insecticides and herbicides is primarily a matter of reducing or eliminating exposure to several presumably high-

TABLE 3-17 Estimated Oncogenic Risk from Dietary Exposure to Selected Herbicides

Active Ingredient	Number of Food Uses	TMRC[a] (mg pesticide)	Q*	Estimated Dietary Oncogenic Risk	Weight-of-the-Evidence Classification
Linuron (Lorox)	20	4.65×10^{-3}	3.28×10^{-1}	1.52×10^{-3}	C
Alachlor (Lasso)	25	4.08×10^{-4}	5.95×10^{-2}	2.42×10^{-5}	B_2
Metolachlor (Dual)	40	6.88×10^{-4}	2.10×10^{-3}	1.44×10^{-5}	C pending
Oxadiazon (Ronstar)	26	9.38×10^{-5}	1.3×10^{-1}	1.21×10^{-5}	B_2
Oryzalin (Surflan)	57	3.37×10^{-4}	3.4×10^{-2}	1.14×10^{-5}	C
Pronamide (Kerb)	25	4.86×10^{-4}	1.6×10^{-2}	7.77×10^{-6}	C
Ethalfluralin (Sonalan)	18	4.09×10^{-5}	8.7×10^{-2}	3.56×10^{-6}	NA
Diclofop methyl (Hoelon)	5	1.86×10^{-4}	1.1×10^{-2}	2.04×10^{-6}	NA
Terbutryn	4	1.53×10^{-4}	1.87×10^{-3}	2.86×10^{-7}	C
Glyphosate (Roundup)	134	4.63×10^{-3}	5.9×10^{-5}	2.73×10^{-7}	C

NOTE: These risk estimates are derived using EPA data and methods described on pages 50–66 and in Appendix B. B_2 indicates a probable human carcinogen. C indicates a possible human carcinogen. NA indicates that the pesticide has not been classified by the EPA.

[a]This column expresses the theoretical maximum residue contribution in the diet. See Appendix B for further discussion of TMRC.

risk compounds. Risks that might be posed by likely replacement chemicals must also be considered. If exposure to this one herbicide and these two insecticides were significantly reduced, the estimated dietary oncogenic risk would fall by about 30 percent. If this step were taken, the share of the remaining estimated risk contributed by fungicides would increase to nearly 99 percent. In this circumstance, the 10 agents presenting the greatest estimated oncogenic risk would all be fungicides. Unlike herbicides and insecticides, major reductions in estimated fungicide risk cannot be attained by reducing or eliminating use of any single agent.

DISTRIBUTION OF ESTIMATED RISK BY CROP

Examination of the risk from herbicides, insecticides, and fungicides on crops reveals a similar pattern. In each case the same herbicide (linuron) and the same insecticides (chlordimeform and permethrin) represent more than 99 percent of the total estimated herbicide and insecticide risk

TABLE 3-18 Estimated Oncogenic Risk from Dietary Exposure to Selected Insecticides

Active Ingredient	Number of Food Uses	TMRC[a] (mg pesticide)	Q*	Estimated Dietary Oncogenic Risk	Weight-of-the-Evidence Classification
Permethrin (Ambush, Pounce)	50	1.40×10^{-2}	3.0×10^{-2}	4.21×10^{-4}	C
Chlordimeform (Fundal, Galecron)	24	7.19×10^{-3}	9.4×10^{-1}	3.22×10^{-4}	B_2
Acephate (Orthene)	34	5.41×10^{-3}	6.9×10^{-3}	3.73×10^{-5}	C
Parathion	98	8.19×10^{-3}	1.8×10^{-3}	1.47×10^{-5}	C
Cypermethrin (Ammo, Cymbush)	7	1.97×10^{-4}	1.9×10^{-2}	3.73×10^{-6}	C
Cyromazine (Larvadex)	4	1.49×10^{-4}	2.4×10^{-3}	3.58×10^{-7}	NA
Azinphos-methyl (Guthion)	78	1.13×10^{-2}	1.5×10^{-7}	1.68×10^{-9}	D

NOTE: These risk estimates are derived using EPA data and methods described on pages 50–66 and in Appendix B. B_2 indicates a probable human carcinogen. C indicates a possible human carcinogen. D indicates not classifiable as to human carcinogenicity. NA indicates that the pesticide has not been classified by the EPA.

[a]This column expresses the theoretical maximum residue contribution in the diet.

TABLE 3-19 Estimated Oncogenic Risk from Dietary Exposure to Selected Fungicides

Active Ingredient	Number of Food Uses	TMRC[a] (mg pesticide)	Q*	Estimated Dietary Oncogenic Risk	Weight-of-the-Evidence Classification
Zineb	83	4.08×10^{-2}	1.76×10^{-2}	7.17×10^{-4}	$B_2{}^b$
Captafol	34	2.38×10^{-2}	2.5×10^{-2}	5.94×10^{-4}	B_2
Captan	77	2.06×10^{-1}	2.3×10^{-3}	4.74×10^{-4}	B_2
Maneb	56	2.52×10^{-2}	1.76×10^{-2}	4.42×10^{-4}	$B_2{}^b$
Mancozeb	44	1.92×10^{-2}	1.76×10^{-2}	3.38×10^{-4}	$B_2{}^b$
Folpet	41	9.26×10^{-2}	3.5×10^{-3}	3.24×10^{-4}	B_2
Chlorothalonil (Bravo)	47	9.91×10^{-3}	2.4×10^{-2}	2.37×10^{-4}	NA
Metiram	11	6.58×10^{-3}	1.76×10^{-2}	1.15×10^{-4}	$B_2{}^b$
Benomyl (Benlate)	101	5.49×10^{-2}	2.07×10^{-3}	1.13×10^{-4}	C
O-Phenylphenol	22	6.37×10^{-2}	1.57×10^{-3}	9.99×10^{-5}	NA
Fosetyl Al (Aliette)	1	7.67×10^{-6}	4.3×10^{-3}	3.29×10^{-8}	C

NOTE: These risk estimates are derived using EPA data and methods described on pages 50–66 and in Appendix B. B_2 indicates a probable human carcinogen. C indicates a possible human carcinogen. NA indicates that the pesticide has not been classified by the EPA.

[a]This column expresses the theoretical maximum residue contribution in the diet. See Appendix B for further discussion of TMRC.

[b]The classification is for the EBDC metabolite ethylene thiourea.

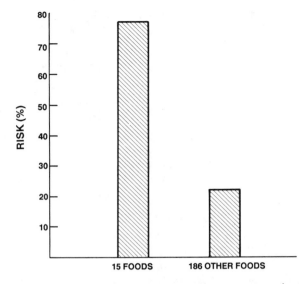

FIGURE 3-3   Concentration of total estimated dietary oncogenic risk in selected foods. (Also see Table 3-20.)

TABLE **3-20**   Fifteen Foods with the Greatest Estimated Oncogenic Risk

Food	Total Dietary Oncogenic Risk Estimates	
	Number	Percentage
Tomatoes	8.75×10^{-4}	14.9
Beef	6.49×10^{-4}	11.1
Potatoes	5.21×10^{-4}	8.9
Oranges .	3.76×10^{-4}	6.4
Lettuce	3.44×10^{-4}	5.8
Apples	3.23×10^{-4}	5.5
Peaches	3.23×10^{-4}	5.5
Pork	2.67×10^{-4}	4.5
Wheat	1.92×10^{-4}	3.3
Soybeans	1.28×10^{-4}	2.2
Beans	1.23×10^{-4}	2.1
Carrots	1.22×10^{-4}	2.1
Chicken	1.12×10^{-4}	1.9
Corn (bran, grain)	1.09×10^{-4}	1.9
Grapes	1.09×10^{-4}	1.9
Total		78.0

NOTE: These worst-case risk estimates are derived using EPA data and methods described on pages 50–66 and in Appendix B. They assume residues are at the tolerance level, although actual residues may be different. These numbers are the totals of the committee's upper-bound estimates of dietary oncogenic risk for oncogenic pesticides with tolerances on these crops. As more accurate data are received by the EPA, crops may move on or off the list.

TABLE 3-21   Estimated Oncogenic Risk from
Herbicides in Major Foods

Crop	Estimated Risk	
	Number	Percentage
Beef	5.38×10^{-4}	10.0
Potatoes	3.89×10^{-4}	6.7
Pork	2.17×10^{-4}	3.7
Soybeans	1.22×10^{-4}	2.1
Wheat	1.22×10^{-4}	2.1
Carrots	5.95×10^{-5}	1.0
Corn	4.98×10^{-5}	0.9
Asparagus	1.48×10^{-5}	0.3
Celery	1.04×10^{-5}	0.2
Milk	7.87×10^{-6}	0.1
Percentage of total risk from herbicides, insecticides, and fungicides		27.1

NOTE: These worst-case risk estimates are derived using EPA
data and methods described on pages 50–66 and in Appendix B.
They assume residues are at the tolerance level, although actual
residues may be different. These numbers are the totals of the
committee's upper-bound estimates of dietary oncogenic risk for
oncogenic herbicides with tolerances on these crops. As more
accurate data are received by the EPA, crops may move on or off
the list.

associated with most crops. With fungicides, estimated risk is again more
evenly distributed among active ingredients and among crops; no single
fungicide accounts for more than 43 percent of total fungicide risk from
any crop. Further, the ranking of estimated risk from fungicides varies
from crop to crop.

When estimated risks from individual foods are ranked, 15 crops and
animal products contribute nearly 80 percent of all estimated dietary
oncogenic risk from pesticide residues (see Figure 3-3 and Table 3-20).

Tables 3-21, 3-22, and 3-23 show estimated crop risk broken down
among fungicides, herbicides, and insecticides. Fungicide residues on just
10 crops represent 42 percent of total estimated dietary risk.

In general, relatively few pesticides account for high percentages of total
estimated risk in selected high-risk foods (see Tables 3-24, 3-25, 3-26, and
3-27). About 99 percent of herbicide risk from estimated residues in beef is
from one herbicide; 72 percent of estimated tomato risk is from five
fungicides (see the boxed article "Concentration of Residues in Processed
Foods"). Many of these fungicides are close substitutes in controlling a
range of diseases.

TABLE 3-22   Estimated Oncogenic Risk from Insecticides in Major Foods

Crop	Estimated Risk	
	Number	Percentage
Lettuce	1.59×10^{-4}	2.5
Chicken	1.11×10^{-4}	1.9
Beef	1.10×10^{-4}	1.9
Cottonseed	9.95×10^{-5}	1.7
Milk	5.19×10^{-5}	0.9
Tomatoes	5.17×10^{-5}	0.9
Pork	5.02×10^{-5}	0.9
Peaches	3.50×10^{-5}	0.6
Spinach	2.80×10^{-5}	0.5
Cabbage	1.82×10^{-5}	0.3
Percentage of total risk from herbicides, insecticides, and fungicides		12.1

NOTE: These worst-case risk estimates are derived using EPA data and methods described on pages 50–66 and in Appendix B. They assume residues are at the tolerance level, although actual residues may be different. These numbers are the totals of the committee's upper-bound estimates of dietary oncogenic risk for oncogenic insecticides with tolerances on these crops. As more accurate data are received by the EPA, crops may move on or off the list.

TABLE 3-23   Estimated Oncogenic Risk from Fungicides in Major Foods

Crop	Estimated Risk	
	Number	Percentage
Tomatoes	8.23×10^{-4}	14.1
Oranges	3.72×10^{-4}	6.3
Apples	3.18×10^{-4}	5.4
Peaches	2.86×10^{-4}	4.9
Lettuce	1.81×10^{-4}	0.1
Potatoes	1.29×10^{-4}	2.2
Beans	1.17×10^{-4}	2.0
Grapes	1.08×10^{-4}	1.8
Wheat	6.65×10^{-5}	1.1
Celery	6.04×10^{-5}	1.1
Percentage of total risk from herbicides, insecticides, and fungicides		42.0

NOTE: These worst-case risk estimates are derived using EPA data and methods described on pages 50–66 and in Appendix B. They assume residues are at the tolerance level, although actual residues may be different. These numbers are the totals of the committee's upper-bound estimates of dietary oncogenic risk for oncogenic fungicides with tolerances on these crops. As more accurate data are received by the EPA, crops may move on or off the list.

Concentration of Residues in Processed Foods

The data in the Tolerance Assessment System (TAS) indicate that under EPA's worst-case assumptions the estimated dietary oncogenic risk from tomato products may be 15 percent of the total dietary oncogenic risk from pesticide residues. The committee was greatly interested in the finding that one crop may constitute such a significant percentage of total dietary risk. Further, more than 90 percent of this estimated risk is attributable to fungicides and is derived assuming that residues *do not* concentrate in processed tomato products.

Most oncogenic fungicides have no section 409 tolerances for processed tomato products. The EPA has never considered the need for section 409 tolerances because it has not yet received the data required to set such tolerances. The committee expects concentration to occur for many crops whenever food processing involves drying, removing water, or extracting oils or other fractions of raw agricultural commodities.

To illustrate the potential impact that residue concentration could have on the distribution and character of dietary oncogenic risk, the committee undertook several analyses of fungicide use on tomatoes.

The method was simple. The committee made assumptions regarding the expected residue level on the raw crop as well as the expected level of concentration in processed products from this raw residue level. The committee then computed the ensuing worst-case risks. The results are presented below.

If one assumes that all acres are treated, that residues on raw tomatoes are at the current tolerance level, and that these residues in processed tomato products undergo a 10-fold concentration, then total estimated oncogenic risk from all fungicide residues in tomatoes would increase more than 300 percent above the committee's risk estimates, which assume no concentration of residues in processed foods. If residues on raw tomatoes are assumed to be one-tenth the published tolerance and to undergo a 10-fold concentration, then estimated oncogenic risk from fungicide residues would decline about 51 percent. Alternatively, if residues on raw tomatoes are present at one-half the tolerance level and concentrate by a factor of 10, estimated oncogenic risk from fungicides in tomato products would increase more than 118 percent.

As the residue chemistry data base and tolerance profile are modernized for all older products, the committee expects the following compared to current risk estimates:

• The actual residues likely to be found on the vast majority of fresh foods will decrease;

- The percentage of dietary oncogenic risk associated with processed-food forms will increase; and
- The share of dietary risk stemming from relatively few foods and pesticides will increase.

Assumed Levels

Raw Residue	Concentration in Processed Products (from raw residue)	New Risk[a]/% Change
CFR	None	6.19×10^{-4}
CFR tolerance	10×	2.67×10^{-3}/ + 331
1/2 CFR tolerance	10×	1.35×10^{-3}/ + 118
1/10 CFR tolerance	10×	3.02×10^{-4} / − 51
CFR tolerance	2×	8.47×10^{-4} / + 36
1/2 CFR tolerance	2×	4.43×10^{-4}/ − 28

[a]Risk assumes U.S. mean consumption estimates from the TAS, that residues are at the raw food tolerance, that all acres are treated, and that exposure occurs over a 70-year lifetime. The oncogenic fungicides metiram, folpet, O-phenylphenol, and zineb were not included in this analysis due to limited commercial use.

Herbicide residues on three foods account for more than 20 percent of estimated dietary risk. Nearly all of this risk is from residues at the tolerance level of one compound, linuron. Risks from insecticides, on the other hand, are evenly distributed among the top 10 crops.

Several conclusions emerge in considering the distribution of risks by crop and active ingredient. Where one chemical dominates risk, estimated dietary risk can be significantly reduced through action on tolerances for that chemical. For example, estimated dietary oncogenic risk from beef (about 11 percent of the total), could be reduced by 90 percent through actions lowering or revoking tolerances for linuron on beef products. Revoking all tolerances for linuron would reduce the committee's total estimate of dietary oncogenic risk by about 30 percent.

By contrast, estimated risk from tomatoes is primarily from fungicide residues. No single compound accounts for more than 38 percent of the total. Reducing residues from a single chemical will not significantly reduce estimated risk from tomatoes, because the oncogenic fungicides used in tomato production generally substitute for one another. The same generalization applies when one considers *all* fungicide active ingredients

TABLE 3-24   Estimated Oncogenic Risk from All Active Ingredients
Used on Selected Foods

Active Ingredient	Estimated Risk			Total Crop Risk (%)
	Raw Food	Processed Food	Total	
Tomatoes				
Captafol	1.90×10^{-4}	1.23×10^{-4}	3.14×10^{-4}	36
Chlorothalonil	6.09×10^{-5}	3.95×10^{-5}	1.00×10^{-4}	11
Folpet	4.44×10^{-5}	2.88×10^{-5}	7.32×10^{-5}	8
Metiram	3.58×10^{-5}	2.32×10^{-5}	5.89×10^{-5}	7
Beef				
Linuron	5.34×10^{-4}	0	5.34×10^{-4}	82
Chlordimeform	7.77×10^{-5}	0	7.77×10^{-5}	12
Permethrin	2.98×10^{-5}	0	2.98×10^{-5}	6
Oxadiazon	2.12×10^{-6}	0	2.12×10^{-6}	0.3
Alachlor	1.94×10^{-6}	0	1.94×10^{-6}	0.3
Potatoes				
Linuron	3.87×10^{-4}	5.64×10^{-7}	3.88×10^{-4}	74
Captan	6.79×10^{-5}	9.88×10^{-8}	6.80×10^{-5}	13
Mancozeb	2.08×10^{-5}	3.03×10^{-8}	2.08×10^{-5}	4
Captafol	1.48×10^{-5}	2.15×10^{-8}	1.48×10^{-5}	3
Metiram	1.04×10^{-5}	1.51×10^{-8}	1.04×10^{-5}	2

NOTE: These risk estimates are derived using EPA data and methods described on pages
50–66 and in Appendix B.

across *all* of their uses. Eliminating residues of a single fungicide
compound will not achieve dramatic reductions in estimated risks.

EPA'S INTERPRETATION OF THE DELANEY CLAUSE TO DATE

The EPA has applied the Delaney Clause unevenly to the 289 pesticides
examined here. It has never invoked the clause to repeal an existing
tolerance. (Many of these tolerances were established in the absence of
oncogenicity data or information indicating residue concentration.) Con-
versely, the agency has enforced the Delaney Clause strictly to refuse
section 408 and section 409 tolerances on all crops when section 409
tolerances are needed for new oncogenic active ingredients registered
since 1978. This has been the policy since the agency required more
complete data before granting initial tolerances. This policy helps explain
why most estimated dietary oncogenic risk is associated with tolerances

TABLE 3-25 Foods with the Greatest Estimated Oncogenic Risk from Herbicides

Active Ingredient	Estimated Risk			Risk from Herbicides on Crop (%)
	Raw Food	Processed Food	Total	
Beef				
Linuron	5.34×10^{-4}	0	5.34×10^{-4}	99
Oxadiazon	2.12×10^{-6}	0	2.12×10^{-6}	0.4
Alachlor	1.94×10^{-6}	0	1.94×10^{-6}	0.4
Terbutryn	5.92×10^{-7}	0	5.92×10^{-7}	Negligible
Glyphosate	7.23×10^{-10}	0	7.23×10^{-10}	Negligible
Potatoes				
Linuron	3.87×10^{-4}	5.64×10^{-7}	3.88×10^{-4}	99
Oryzalin	2.01×10^{-6}	2.72×10^{-9}	2.01×10^{-6}	0.5
Glyphosate	1.39×10^{-8}	2.0×10^{-11}	1.40×10^{-8}	Negligible
Pork				
Linuron	2.16×10^{-4}	0	2.16×10^{-4}	99
Oxadiazon	8.54×10^{-7}	0	8.54×10^{-7}	Negligible
Alachlor	7.82×10^{-7}	0	7.82×10^{-7}	Negligible
Terbutryn	2.27×10^{-7}	0	2.27×10^{-7}	Negligible
Glyphosate	1.68×10^{-10}	0	1.68×10^{-10}	Negligible

NOTE: These risk estimates are derived using EPA data and methods described on pages 50–66 and in Appendix B.

TABLE 3-26 Foods with the Greatest Estimated Oncogenic Risk from Insecticides

Active Ingredient	Estimated Risk			Risk from Insecticides on Crop (%)
	Raw Food	Processed Food	Risk	
Lettuce				
Permethrin	1.43×10^{-4}	0	1.43×10^{-4}	90
Acephate	1.54×10^{-5}	0	1.54×10^{-5}	10
Parathion	4.30×10^{-7}	0	4.30×10^{-7}	Negligible
Chicken				
Chlordimeform	1.11×10^{-4}	0	1.11×10^{-4}	99
Permethrin	7.06×10^{-7}	0	7.06×10^{-7}	0.1
Acephate	3.25×10^{-7}	0	3.25×10^{-7}	Negligible
Beef				
Chlordimeform	7.77×10^{-5}	0	7.77×10^{-5}	71
Permethrin	2.98×10^{-5}	0	2.98×10^{-5}	27
Cypermethrin	1.55×10^{-6}	0	1.55×10^{-6}	1.4
Acephate	1.12×10^{-6}	0	1.12×10^{-6}	1
Azinphos-methyl	2.04×10^{-11}	0	2.04×10^{-11}	Negligible

NOTE: These risk estimates are derived using EPA data and methods described on pages 50–66 and in Appendix B.

TABLE 3-27 Foods with the Greatest Estimated Oncogenic Risk from Fungicides

Active Ingredient	Estimated Risk			Risk from Fungicides on Crop (%)
	Raw Food	Processed Food	Total	
Tomatoes				
Captafol	1.90×10^{-4}	1.23×10^{-4}	3.14×10^{-4}	38
Chlorothalonil	6.09×10^{-5}	3.95×10^{-5}	1.00×10^{-4}	12
Folpet	4.44×10^{-5}	2.88×10^{-5}	7.32×10^{-5}	9
Metiram	3.58×10^{-5}	2.32×10^{-5}	5.89×10^{-5}	7
Captan	2.92×10^{-5}	1.89×10^{-5}	4.81×10^{-5}	6
Oranges				
Zineb	2.07×10^{-5}	1.42×10^{-4}	1.62×10^{-4}	43
Captan	9.68×10^{-6}	6.62×10^{-5}	7.58×10^{-5}	20
Folpet	8.84×10^{-6}	6.04×10^{-5}	6.92×10^{-5}	9
Benomyl	3.48×10^{-6}	2.38×10^{-5}	2.72×10^{-5}	7
O-Phenylphenol	2.64×10^{-6}	1.81×10^{-5}	2.07×10^{-5}	6
Apples				
Mancozeb	5.97×10^{-5}	3.08×10^{-5}	9.05×10^{-5}	28
Folpet	4.24×10^{-5}	2.19×10^{-5}	6.43×10^{-5}	20
Captan	2.79×10^{-5}	1.44×10^{-5}	4.22×10^{-5}	13
O-Phenylphenol	1.90×10^{-5}	9.81×10^{-6}	2.88×10^{-5}	9
Metiram	1.71×10^{-5}	8.79×10^{-6}	2.59×10^{-5}	8

NOTE: These risk estimates are derived using EPA data and methods described on pages 50–66 and in Appendix B.

for older pesticides. In this report, new chemicals are those registered since 1978, and old chemicals are those registered earlier. In 1978, FIFRA amendments imposed new data demands, as well as other regulatory requirements, on registrants.

The distribution of estimated oncogenic risk associated with tolerances granted over time indicates that most risk comes from old chemicals, particularly old fungicides (Table 3-28). For herbicides, one active ingredient registered in 1965 contributes most of the risk. For fungicides, old pesticides account for 97.7 percent of the estimated risk. Tolerances for one insecticide, permethrin, granted after 1978 account for slightly more than half of all insecticide risk and less than 5 percent of total estimated dietary oncogenic risk. As shown in Figure 3-4, more than 90 percent of all estimated dietary oncogenic risk is associated with tolerances granted before 1978. When all pesticides are considered (see Table 3-28), the trend is clear: the estimated dietary oncogenic risk associated with tolerances granted after 1978 is very small when compared with the risk associated

TABLE 3-28   Estimated Oncogenic Risk from Tolerances over Time

Type of Pesticide	Tolerance Type					
	Raw Food		Processed Food		Total	
	Number	Percent[a]	Number	Percent[a]	Number	Percent[a]
Fungicides						
Pre-1970	1.20×10^{-3}	76.1	1.14×10^{-4}	7.26	1.31×10^{-3}	83.4
1970–1977	2.04×10^{-4}	12.9	2.20×10^{-5}	1.39	2.26×10^{-4}	14.3
1978–1985	1.54×10^{-5}	0.97	2.66×10^{-6}	0.16	1.81×10^{-5}	1.14
Total					1.55×10^{-3}	98.84[b]
Insecticides						
Pre-1970	2.82×10^{-6}	0.3	1.17×10^{-8}	0.001	2.83×10^{-6}	0.35
1970–1977	2.57×10^{-4}	32.1	1.01×10^{-4}	12.6	3.58×10^{-4}	44.8
1978–1985	4.04×10^{-4}	50.6	2.11×10^{-5}	2.6	4.26×10^{-4}	53.2
Total					7.86×10^{-4}	98.35[b]
Herbicides						
Pre-1970	4.50×10^{-4}	13.0	4.94×10^{-5}	1.42	5.00×10^{-4}	14.46
1970–1977	1.69×10^{-3}	49.0	6.57×10^{-4}	18.9	2.35×10^{-3}	68.0
1978–1985	1.25×10^{-5}	0.36	3.89×10^{-5}	1.1	5.15×10^{-5}	1.4
Total					2.90×10^{-3}	83.86[b]

NOTE: These risk estimates are derived using EPA data and methods described on pages 50–66 and in Appendix B.

[a]These columns express the percent of total risk by pesticide type.
[b]Numbers do not equal 100 percent because petition numbers indicating the year of a tolerance petition were not available for all tolerances.

with tolerances granted before 1978. The reasons for this are (1) the fact that the few oncogenic pesticides registered since 1978 generally present less dietary oncogenic risk than those registered before 1978 and (2) the EPA's application of the Delaney Clause.

The distribution of estimated risk between raw- and processed-food tolerances by time also is presented in Table 3-28. About one-fifth of all estimated dietary oncogenic risk is associated with residues of pesticides in processed food; nearly 80 percent of this risk is derived from tolerances granted before 1978.

EPA Application of the Delaney Clause to New Active Ingredients

From 1975 through 1981 the EPA issued a series of standards and requirements for data to support pesticide registrations. In 1982 the EPA published a proposed rule consolidating all testing requirements. The EPA's final rule, which did not differ significantly from the 1982 proposal, became effective in April 1985. Although the EPA had required oncogenicity testing for many pesticides before the development of these formal data requirements, it was clear for the first time which studies would be routinely required, which criteria would govern exemptions from data requirements, and which testing protocols registrants would have to follow.[11]

In the late 1970s, pesticide oncogenicity and residue concentration data became available for newly registered pesticides. The EPA began exploring the regulatory ramifications of the Delaney Clause in the granting of tolerances for new active ingredients. Simultaneously, the agency began confronting questions about the applicability of the Delaney Clause in the review and reregistration of old pesticides.

To explore the history of the EPA's use of the Delaney Clause, the committee wrote to the agency, seeking confirmation of a list of decisions in which the clause had been discussed or relied on. In response, the EPA identified six regulatory actions on petitions for new tolerances in which the Delaney Clause was specifically cited. These cases are presented in Table 3-29. (Detailed case studies of these pesticides are contained in Appendix C.) The EPA also noted 10 additional pesticides that the Delaney Clause may affect in the review of existing registrations. These cases are presented in Table 3-30.

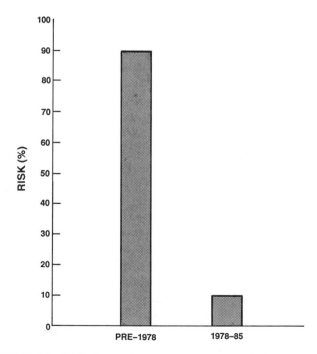

FIGURE 3-4   Risk from tolerances granted before and after 1978.

TABLE 3-29   Tolerance Actions for Which the Delaney Clause Was Cited

Chemical Name/ Regulatory Action	Concern Related to Delaney Clause	Risk Associated with Tolerance Application	Agency Decision
Fosetyl Al			
Application for section 408 tolerance in hops	Need for section 409 tolerance and oncogenicity of fosetyl Al	1×10^{-8}	Denied: Delaney Clause cited
Amitraz			
Application for section 408 tolerance in apples, pears	Need for section 409 tolerance in apples and oncogenicity of amitraz	1×10^{-6}	Denied: apples, Delaney Clause cited Allowed: pears, no processed food form
Dicamba			
Application for section 408 tolerance in sugarcane	Need for section 409 tolerance and oncogenicity of nitrosamine contaminant	1×10^{-10}	Allowed: FDA constituents policy cited
Larvadex			
Application for section 408 tolerance in eggs/poultry	Need for section 409 tolerance and oncogenicity of metabolite acetamide	1×10^{-8}	Allowed: SOM[a]/FDC Act cited
Permethrin			
Application for section 408 tolerance in tomatoes	Need for section 409 tolerance and oncogenicity of permethrin	1×10^{-4}	Denied: Delaney Clause cited[b]
Thiodicarb			
Application for section 408 and 409 tolerances in cotton	Need for section 409 tolerance and oncogenicity of metabolite acetamide	1×10^{-8}	Allowed: SOM/FDC Act cited

NOTE: These risk estimates are derived using EPA data and methods described on pages 50–66 and in Appendix B.

[a]SOM is the sensitivity-of-the-method procedure. This has been used in cases where the residue of an oncogenic chemical in an animal product is deemed to present an additional oncogenic risk of less than 1 in 1 million (1×10^{-6}) and can be reliably detected using modern residue chemistry techniques. In these cases the Delaney Clause has been bypassed. (For further discussion, see Chapter 2 and the case studies in Appendix C.)

[b]Section 408 tolerances for tomatoes grown in Florida and destined only for fresh market were granted.

TABLE 3-30 Pesticide Active Ingredients Under Review for Which the Delaney Clause Has Been a Concern

Pesticide	Major Uses and Pesticide Type	Estimated Oncogenic Risk	Volume of Use[a] (pounds AI/year)
Special Review			
Alachlor (Lasso)	Corn, soybean herbicide	2.42×10^{-5}	85,100,000
Dicofol (Kelthane)	Citrus, cotton acaricide/insecticide	No risk assessment performed	1,200,000
Captan	Fruit, vegetable fungicide	4.74×10^{-4}	10,000,000
Daminozide (Alar)	Select fruit, vegetable growth regulator	8.30×10^{-3}	825,000
Registration Standards			
Benomyl (Benlate)	Multiple-use systemic fungicide	1.13×10^{-4}	2,000,000
EBDCs (mancozeb, maneb, metiram, zineb)	Group of four widely used fruit and vegetable fungicides	1.11×10^{-3}	28,000,000
Chlorobenzilate	Citrus acaracide	No risk assessment performed	1,600,000
Metolachlor (Dual)	Corn, soybean herbicide	1.44×10^{-6}	38,000,000
Oryzalin (Surflan)	Citrus, field crop herbicide	1.14×10^{-5}	1,600,000
Thiophanate-methyl (Topsin M)	Fruit, vegetable fungicide	No risk assessment performed	28,000

NOTE: These risk estimates are derived using EPA data and methods described on pages 50–66 and in Appendix B.

[a]The pounds active ingredient/year are averaged from selected years and are derived from Webb, S.E.H., 1981, "Preliminary Data: Pesticide Use on Selected Deciduous Fruits in the United States, 1978," Economic Research Service Staff Report No. AGES810626, Washington, D.C.: U.S. Department of Agriculture; Ferguson, W. L., 1984, "1979 Pesticide Use on Vegetables in Five Regions," Springfield, Va.: National Technical Information Service; Parks, J. R., 1983, "Pesticide Use on Fall Potatoes in the United States, 1979," Economic Research Service Staff Report No. AGES830113, Washington, D.C.: U.S. Department of Agriculture; Gianessi, L. P., 1986, "A National Pesticide Usage Data Base," Washington, D.C.: Resources for the Future, photocopy; and unpublished data from the EPA for the years 1981 through 1985.

The agency's policy in recent years of not approving tolerances for oncogenic *active ingredients* that concentrate in processed foods is amply demonstrated in Table 3-30. The EPA has denied all applications for section 409 tolerances since 1978 that involve oncogenic active ingredients, including at least one active ingredient with very small estimated risk (10^{-8}).

Another important conclusion can be drawn from Table 3-29. In at least three cases involving old and new ingredients, the EPA granted new tolerances when it determined that oncogenic potential came from an impurity, metabolite, or contaminant of the parent active ingredient (dicamba, cyromazine, and thiodicarb). In these cases, the EPA relied on the FDA's interpretations of the Delaney Clause. From these cases, it is clear that the EPA will consider applying, in appropriate cases, the FDA's constituents policy and sensitivity-of-the-method procedures in granting food- and feed-additive tolerances for oncogenic pesticides. (For a more detailed discussion, see Chapter 2.)

The estimated additional risk sanctioned by these EPA tolerances for dicamba, cyromazine, and thiodicarb is far less than the estimated risk associated with tolerances that have been denied. These include permethrin tolerances on tomatoes and amitraz tolerances on apples. Risks allowed are on the order of 1×10^{-8} or less. Tolerances denied had risks between 1×10^{-4} and 1×10^{-8}.

The agency also gave the committee a list of 10 active ingredients for which it suspects that manufacturer or registrant concern about the impact of the Delaney Clause significantly influenced the content of tolerance applications (see Table 3-31). In each case, the agency is aware of section 408 and section 409 tolerance petitions that a registrant withdrew or declined to file because of concerns about the Delaney Clause. The committee believes that the Delaney Clause has been more influential than this table reveals.

Once a pesticide is determined to be oncogenic, most registrants withdraw or do not submit petitions for section 409 tolerances. One reason is that tolerance petitions must be accompanied by a fee that must be paid regardless of the agency's decision. Companies will often attempt to obtain registrations, however, when they regard evidence of oncogenicity as equivocal or believe that the oncogenic risks are very low

TABLE 3-31   Pesticides with Retracted or Unpursued Tolerance Applications

Amitraz (Bamm)	Fosetyl Al (Aliette)
Benomyl (Benlate)	Metolachlor (Dual)
Captan	Permethrin (Pounce, Ambush)
Cypermethrin (Ammo, Cymbush)	Vinclozolin (Ronilan)
EBDCs (mancozeb, maneb, metiram, zineb)	

NOTE: In these cases, the EPA believes the petitioners either retracted or failed to pursue applications for tolerances under section 408 or 409 because of potential problems from the Delaney Clause.

and the use proposed may fall within an exception to the Delaney Clause. Another strategy is to change a pesticide's use pattern in a way that keeps residues below the level detectable on raw agricultural commodities (see Appendix E).

CASE STUDIES OF POTENTIAL POLICY PRECEDENTS

Tolerances for New Active Ingredients

Recent reports have criticized the EPA for not articulating a clear policy for application of the Delaney Clause in the tolerance-setting and reassessment process.[12] In fact, the need for such a policy was the reason the EPA initated this project. Even in cases when the EPA has applied the constituents policy or the sensitivity-of-the-method procedure, it has stressed that such action does not represent a formal change in policy. The agency has defended its authority to use these options on a case-by-case basis until a more definitive policy is adopted.

In this section, recent agency actions are analyzed to determine what patterns emerge from the EPA's application of the Delaney Clause in the tolerance process. First, the application of the Delaney Clause to new pesticides and pesticide uses seems clear-cut. New section 409 tolerances are not approved for clearly oncogenic pesticides. New section 408 tolerances are not approved for crops routinely processed into food forms in which oncogenic residues are expected to concentrate. The agency is willing to approve new tolerances for very low risk oncogens if there is a reasonable basis for doing so within FDA precedents, however.

The greatest area of uncertainty is how the EPA will proceed in cases involving currently registered pesticides that have been found to be oncogens and have several existing section 409 tolerances *or* are shown to need these tolerances as residue chemistry data requirements are satisfied. The committee finds no convincing legal or scientific basis for the EPA, as it completes the special review and reregistration processes, to avoid applying the standards of section 409, including the Delaney Clause, to currently registered compounds.

Prior-Sanctioned Pesticides

The prior-sanction exception to the Food Additives Amendment of the FDC Act would arguably render the Delaney Clause inapplicable to any pesticide residue in processed foods approved before 1958. (The FDC Act's definition of a food additive excludes substances regulated as food additives before 1958 from the food additive amendments of 1958, including the Delaney Clause.) Because of this, some pesticide residues could technically escape the current requirements for food additives (including the Delaney Clause) if it could be shown that the FDA or the USDA sanctioned these residues before 1958.

The committee briefly attempted to determine the number of pre-1958 tolerances to which the prior-sanction exception might apply. The committee could find no tolerances issued between 1954 and 1958 that could be described as food-additive tolerances by current standards. Nevertheless, such tolerances may have been issued and there may have been earlier approvals of residue-producing uses of agents still in use. The committee believes, however, that the number of prior-sanctioned residues that might technically escape the strict standards of the food-additive regulation is quite small. Even when the prior-sanction exception might be invoked to preserve a tolerance, the committee can discern no health or scientific basis for treating residues sanctioned before 1958 differently from those sanctioned after 1958.

The following review of seven case studies sheds some light on how the agency may resolve the issues surrounding Delaney Clause applications.

Tolerance Actions and New Active Ingredients

FOSETYL AL

Fosetyl Al is a systemic organophosphorous fungicide used to control downy mildew and other diseases. It is currently widely used in Europe. In this country, the only registered use of fosetyl Al is on pineapples.

The registrant, Rhone-Poulenc, in 1983 applied for tolerances for fosetyl Al on hops. Fosetyl Al residues were determined to concentrate during the drying of hops, and it has demonstrated weak but positive oncogenic effects in animals. Therefore, the EPA cited the Delaney Clause in denying section 408 and section 409 tolerances for residues in or on hops.

Significantly, the risk presented by fosetyl Al residues in hops would have been far less than the risk from fungicides currently used on hops. According to the EPA, the additional risk presented by fosetyl Al residues on hops would have been 1×10^{-8}, or 1 in 100 million or less. This risk is several orders of magnitude less than the estimated risk from ethylenebisdithiocarbamate (EBDC) fungicide residues widely used on hops, which is between 1×10^{-4} and 1×10^{-5}.

PERMETHRIN

Permethrin is a widely used synthetic pyrethroid insecticide. In setting tolerances for permethrin, the EPA granted a section 408 tolerance for the fresh-market portion of tomato crops, but denied section 409 tolerances for the processed portion. This was the first time the EPA had set a tolerance for an oncogenic pesticide only on the raw portion of a crop with the knowledge that this pesticide's residues concentrate during processing. The EPA's general policy is to deny a raw agricultural tolerance for an oncogen when a section 409 tolerance is also needed. The agency departed from this policy in approving the use of permethrin on fresh tomatoes grown in Florida, because 98 percent of the Florida tomato crop is produced for the fresh market. In this case the agency was prepared to consider fresh tomatoes from Florida a distinct crop from processed tomatoes grown elsewhere. No tolerances for the use of permethrin on tomatoes grown outside Florida have been granted. Under the terms of the EPA's approval, surplus Florida tomatoes may not be processed.

The agency has not drawn similar distinctions for other pesticides or tolerance applications. This may be because providing proof that a crop would be sold exclusively through the fresh market would be very difficult.

Section 408 tolerances granted for the use of permethrin on corn and soybeans provide other insights. In these cases, the agency initially denied petitions for section 408 and section 409 tolerances because of residue concentrations in processed soybean and corn products. After further testing, the agency granted section 408 tolerances based on proposed changes in the label directions designed to reduce residues in the raw form of the crop below a level detectable by widely accepted analytical methods. The key change was extension of the time between application and harvest, allowing residues to degrade below detection levels by harvest. With residues theoretically eliminated from the raw commodity, the issue of concentration in the processed foods was moot.

THIODICARB

Thiodicarb is a newly registered carbamate insecticide, effective on a range of insect pests. Thiodicarb itself is not oncogenic. A metabolite of thiodicarb, acetamide, is oncogenic when administered to test animals at relatively high doses (12,500 to 80,000 ppm). Animals fed treated crops metabolize thiodicarb residues into acetamide. Residues of acetamide are then present in minute amounts in animal products. For example, 1.8 parts per billion (ppb) are present in beef liver, assuming that thiodicarb residues are at the tolerance level and that all feed is treated.

In issuing section 409 feed-additive tolerances for thiodicarb, the EPA adopted the FDA's sensitivity-of-the-method procedure. This interpretation requires the applicant for a feed-additive tolerance for an oncogenic substance to prove that the risk to humans from eating animals fed treated feed is less than 1 in 1 million or 1×10^{-6}. (See Chapter 2 and the thiodicarb case study in Appendix C for further examination of these issues.)

On the basis of EPA calculations, meat and poulty could contain up to 90 ppb of acetamide and the risk would be below 10^{-6}; milk and eggs could contain up to 30 and 90 ppb, respectively. Expected residues in meat and poultry, milk, and eggs were 1.8, 0.3, and 0.07 ppb, respectively, resulting in risk far less than 10^{-6}. In every case, even at the highest allowable levels, the risk from acetamide in food as a result of thiodicarb use is well below the 10^{-6} standard.

For purposes of the committee's work, it is noteworthy that the risks involved here were insufficient to trigger a special review of thiodicarb. As stated by the EPA in the final rule:

There are no regulatory actions pending against the registration of thiodicarb. On the basis of the available studies on acetamide and the chronic oncogenicity studies for thiodicarb, the agency has concluded that the human risks posed by the use of thiodicarb on cotton and soybeans does [sic] not raise prudent concerns of unreasonable adverse effects and that a special review under 40 CFR 162.11 is not warranted. (*Federal Register* 50(No. 128):27464)

In the agency's opinion, the regulatory actions surrounding thiodicarb arise entirely from the Delaney Clause and concern the issuance of tolerances, not the granting of product registration. In the absence of the Delaney Clause, therefore, the risk associated with thiodicarb tolerances would not have warranted agency review.

DICAMBA

Dicamba is a broadleaf herbicide widely used in the production of soybeans, corn, and other row and field crops. Studies submitted to the EPA do not show dicamba as oncogenic. However, studies have shown a contaminant of dicamba, dimethylnitrosamine (DMNA), to be an animal oncogen. The EPA relied on the FDA's constituents policy in granting section 409 tolerances for dicamba residues in or on sugarcane molasses. The FDA articulated its constituents policy in the April 2, 1982 *Federal Register* (bracketed phrases are added to describe how the EPA applied the constituents policy to dicamba): "The constituents policy states that the safety of any undesired [in this case oncogenic] nonfunctional constituents [in non-oncogenic substances] should be judged under the general safety clause of the FDC Act [not the Delaney Clause], using risk assessment as one of the decision-making tools."

The FDA has interpreted the general safety clause of the FDC Act as allowing an additional risk no greater than 1×10^{-6}. The EPA assessed the additional risk from exposure to DMNA in sugarcane molasses as no greater than 2.9×10^{-8}. Accordingly, the agency approved section 409 tolerances. The EPA explained its policy as follows:

EPA does not regard deliberately added active or inert ingredients, or metabolites thereof, as potential candidates for clearance under the constitutents policy rationale. Rather, EPA will only consider applying this rationale to impurities arising from the manufacture of the pesticide (residual reactants, intermediates, and products of side reactions and chemical degradates). Furthermore the Agency will consider using this rationale in issuing a food additive regulation only where the potential risk from the impurity is extremely low.[13]

(The *Federal Register* notice did not define low potential risk. The FDA criteria, however, is 1×10^{-6}.)

Tolerance Actions and Old Active Ingredients

DICOFOL AND CHLOROBENZILATE

Dicofol and chlorobenzilate are insecticides, acaricides, and miticides registered before the creation of the EPA in 1970. They are widely used in citrus production. Dicofol is also extensively used on cotton. Both compounds have demonstrated oncogenic effects in animal experiments. The agency has scrutinized each for several years. Residues of both pesticides at concentrated levels have been found in food products, primarily citrus oil. The EPA has not altered the citrus tolerance for either chemical, however, because it believes that the oncogenic potential of the pesticides is so weak, and citrus oil is consumed in such small quantities, that a quantitative assessment of the oncogenic risk from consumption of citrus oil cannot be supported by the available data. In essence, the agency has chosen to defer action on these tolerances indefinitely. These cases suggest that there is a de minimis risk standard below which the agency will not calculate risks.

BENOMYL

Benomyl is the most widely used *systemic* fungicide in the world. It is important because its existing section 409 tolerances will probably be the first to force an EPA decision on retroactive application of the Delaney Clause. Benomyl is one of the most extensively studied pesticides in use. It has been through the EPA's special review process and then through its registration standards procedure. The data supporting its current registrations are generally of high quality. The registrant and the EPA agree that benomyl causes an oncogenic response in animal experiments, and that it concentrates in certain processed foods. It appears that existing

TABLE 3-32   Number of Cancer Studies Due for
Pesticide Active Ingredients, 1986–1990

Year	Oncogenicity	Chronic Feeding	Total
1986	10	5	15
1987	27	16	43
1988	21	17	38
1989	24	28	52
1990	3	3	6
Total	85	69	154

SOURCE: U.S. Environmental Protection Agency. 1986. Data
Generation Schedule Status Report. Washington, D.C.

section 409 tolerances for benomyl violate the Delaney Clause. The
agency has deferred action on these tolerances pending public comment
on the benomyl registration standard, recently invited by notice in the
Federal Register.

The resolution of the benomyl issue could provide a basis for agency
actions in the future. The impact of tolerance revocations for benomyl
and other oncogenic active ingredients included in the committee's risk
estimates is projected in the next section and discussed in further detail in
Chapter 5.

PROJECTING PAST ACTIONS INTO THE FUTURE

Over the next five years, the EPA will receive new data on the
oncogenicity of many agriculturally important chemicals through the data
call-in, special review, and registration standards programs. The approaches the EPA devises for reassessing tolerances in light of the
Delaney Clause will have a tremendous impact on how these new data are
evaluated and incorporated into the pesticide reregistration process.[14]

Table 3-32 shows an approximate schedule for the submission of new
chronic feeding and oncogenicity bioassay results for major food-crop
pesticides in response to data call-in letters issued from 1982 to 1986.
From 1987 through 1989, the EPA should receive about 40 to 50 new tests
each year.

In completing the call-in, the EPA gave priority to data on chronic
health effects. It has requested relatively few new residue concentration
studies. The agency has recently begun to seriously evaluate the complexity and cost of modernizing residue chemistry data. It is already clear

that the costs can be sizable. They may exceed the cost of a complete new chronic toxicology data base for active ingredients used on many foods.

THE SHORT-TERM POTENTIAL IMPACT OF THE DELANEY CLAUSE

Tables 3-33 and 3-34 show the approximate dates the EPA is expected to have enough information to compel decisions on certain pesticide tolerances. The committee's criteria for including specific compounds on these lists are that the pesticides are oncogenic compounds used on foods for which a special review *and* a registration standard will be complete by the date listed.[15]

The committee's analysis supports several important conclusions. First, the EPA will soon be faced with several significant decisions regarding section 409 tolerances for oncogenic pesticides. These decisions involve commercially important chemicals, which present sizable estimated risks. Second, the estimated dietary risk associated with these pesticides represents approximately 85 percent of all estimated dietary oncogenic pesticide risks. Third, agency actions could have the greatest impact on fungicide use and on associated dietary risk. Over the next three years the EPA is scheduled to make decisions on active ingredients that account for about 85 percent of fungicide use. Fourth, most fungi-

TABLE 3-33 Potential Short-Term Impact of the Delaney Clause on Selected Fungicides

Active Ingredient	Possible Date for Tolerance Revocation	Action	Estimated Risk on Commodities			Fungicide Market Share (% acre treatments)
			Raw	Processed	Total	
Benomyl	1986	RS[a]	3.42×10^{-5}	7.91×10^{-5}	1.13×10^{-4}	15
EBDCs						35
Mancozeb	1987	RS	2.43×10^{-4}	9.44×10^{-5}	3.38×10^{-4}	
Maneb	1987	RS	3.90×10^{-4}	5.22×10^{-5}	4.42×10^{-4}	
Metiram	1987	RS	7.65×10^{-5}	3.91×10^{-5}	1.15×10^{-4}	
Zineb	1987	RS	4.71×10^{-4}	2.45×10^{-4}	7.17×10^{-4}	
Captafol	1987	SR[b]	4.34×10^{-4}	1.59×10^{-4}	5.94×10^{-4}	5
Folpet	1987	RS	1.81×10^{-4}	1.43×10^{-4}	3.24×10^{-4}	5
Captan	1988	SR	2.80×10^{-4}	1.93×10^{-4}	4.74×10^{-4}	15
Chlorothalonil	1988	SR	1.89×10^{-4}	4.82×10^{-5}	2.37×10^{-4}	10

NOTE: These risk estimates are derived using EPA data and methods described on pages 50–66 and in Appendix B.

[a]RS is registration standard.
[b]SR is special review.

TABLE 3-34   Potential Short-Term Impact of the Delaney Clause on Selected Herbicides

Active Ingredient	Possible Date for Tolerance Revocation	Action	Estimated Risk on Commodities			Herbicide Market Share (% pounds applied)
			Raw	Processed	Total	
Pronamide (Kerb)	1986	RS[a]	7.14×10^{-6}	6.28×10^{-7}	7.77×10^{-6}	<1
Terbutryn	1986	RS	2.86×10^{-7}		2.86×10^{-7}	<1
Trifluralin (Treflan)	1986	RS	No risk assessment conducted			8
Paraquat	1986	RS	No risk assessment conducted			<1
Alachlor (Lasso)	1986	SR[b]	1.36×10^{-5}	1.06×10^{-5}	2.42×10^{-5}	18
Linuron (Lorox)	1987	SR	1.12×10^{-3}	3.96×10^{-4}	1.52×10^{-3}	1

NOTE: These risk estimates are derived using EPA data and methods described on pages 50–66 and in Appendix B.

[a]RS is registration standard.
[b]SR is special review.

cides have few section 409 tolerances; some will have to be granted if certain uses on food crops are to continue.

The EPA faces an especially difficult challenge with the fungicides. To guarantee that its regulatory actions actually reduce real risks, the agency must carefully assess all fungicides registered for each crop and base its actions on reducing risk after predictable substitutions have been made. One principle should guide the EPA's actions to reduce dietary oncogenic risks. It should focus its efforts on *all* oncogenic pesticides used on the most widely consumed crops that in turn present the greatest dietary risk.

NOTES

1. National Agricultural Chemical Association. 1986. Industry Profile Survey: 1985. Washington, D.C.
2. Gianessi, L. P. 1986. A National Pesticide Usage Data Base. Washington, D.C.: Resources for the Future.
3. Ballard, G., W. Cummings, M. Luther, and N. Pelletier. 1980. Fungicides: An Overview of Their Significance to Agriculture and Their Pesticide Regulatory Implications. Washington, D.C.: U.S. Environmental Protection Agency.
4. U.S. Department of Agriculture. 1985. Economic Indicators of the Farm Sector: Farm Sector Review, 1984. ECIFS 4-2. Washington, D.C.: U.S. Government Printing Office.
5. U.S. Environmental Protection Agency. 1986. Guidelines for Carcinogenic Risk Assessment. *Federal Register* 51(185): 33992–34003.
6. Paynter, O. E. 1984. Standard Evaluation Procedures for Oncogenicity Potential:

Guidance for Analysis and Evaluation of Long-term Rodent Studies. Washington, D.C.: U.S. Environmental Protection Agency.

7. U.S. Environmental Protection Agency. 1985. Captan Special Review Position Document 2/3. Washington, D.C.

8. U.S. General Accounting Office. October 1986. Pesticides: Need to Enhance FDA's Ability to Protect the Public From Illegal Residues. GAO/RCED-87-7. Washington, D.C.

9. National Research Council. 1984. Cancer Today: Origins, Prevention, and Treatment. Washington, D.C.: National Academy Press.

10. U.S. Environmental Protection Agency. 1983. Ethylene Dibromide Special Review Position Document 4. Washington, D.C.

11. 40 CFR Part 158 (1986).

12. U.S. General Accounting Office. 1986. Pesticides: EPA's Formidable Task to Assess and Regulate Their Risks. GAO/RCED-86-125. Washington, D.C.

13. U.S. Environmental Protection Agency. 1984. Tolerances for Pesticides in Food Administered by the Environmental Protection Agency; Animal Drugs, Feeds, and Related Products; Tolerances for Pesticides in Animal Feeds; Dicamba; Denial of Stay. *Federal Register* 49(235): 47481–47483.

14. U.S. Environmental Protection Agency. 1986. Data Generation Schedule Status Report. Washington, D.C.

15. U.S. Environmental Protection Agency. 1986. Report on the Status of the Chemicals in the Special Review Program, Registration Standards Program, and Data Call-In Program. Washington, D.C.

4

The Scenarios and the Results

INTRODUCTION

This chapter describes the results of four scenarios, or policy constructs, that represent plausible strategies for the EPA to follow when reregistering oncogenic pesticides that are known or suspected to leave residues in raw or processed foods. The consequences of applying each of these scenarios to all existing tolerances are expressed as changes in estimated dietary risk and pesticide use from the committee's baseline (see Chapter 3). It should be kept in mind that this baseline consists of the estimated dietary oncogenic risk derived from only 28 of the 53 compounds identified by the EPA as oncogenic. The scenarios were developed to estimate the relative impacts on human health and on pesticide use of alternative approaches to controlling dietary oncogenic risk. Each scenario falls within an interpretation of section 409 of the Food, Drug and Cosmetic (FDC) Act. The committee emphasizes, however, that it does not endorse any of the scenarios, nor was it asked to offer any opinion on the compatibility of any of these scenarios with current law or interpretation.

These scenarios are theoretical policy constructs. As such, they differ in important ways from the policy options the EPA might follow. First, all the estimated changes in risk and pesticide use assume that all pesticides and tolerances are brought immediately into compliance with the risk levels and criteria articulated in each scenario and that no other criteria influence EPA decision making. In practice, the EPA regulates one pesticide at a time and with current resources carries out between 10 and 20 reviews of major active ingredients each year.[1]

At its current level of activity, the EPA would need perhaps a decade to bring the 150 most widely used pesticides applied to foods into compliance with any single policy. As reported in Chapter 3, however, virtually all pesticides that pose sizable oncogenic risks are scheduled for regulatory review in the next few years. Any new policy the EPA chooses can have a major impact—by either reducing or maintaining existing risk—in the next two to five years.

The projected effects of the scenarios are based on the committee's estimates of *dietary* risks and pesticide use. Although the committee used EPA data and methods, it had limited resources to analyze pesticide risks and benefits. In carrying out actual regulatory reviews, the EPA assesses a much larger body of scientific data with a much more complicated set of tools and criteria. In particular, the EPA generally uses a weight-of-the-evidence approach in estimating *all* risks posed by pesticides, not just dietary or oncogenic risks. At each step in the risk assessment process, the EPA considers whether other data and knowledge about a pesticide should alter either a quantitative estimate or the confidence placed in a given calculation. For some chemicals, the agency's concern about the risks is lessened after review of further data. For other chemicals, the EPA's concern is reinforced or heightened.

In spite of these limitations, the committee believes the results in this chapter show what could happen after the EPA chooses a policy for complying with the Delaney Clause in the tolerance-setting and regulatory review processes. The results indicate the impact of the Delaney Clause on currently registered pesticides. Future impacts are not projected.

Within each scenario, impacts are analyzed at several levels and from alternate points of reference. First, impacts on risk reduction and changes in use patterns are estimated for the 53 pesticides identified by the EPA as oncogens, and then for the herbicides, insecticides, and fungicides included in these 53 compounds. Results approximate the distribution of existing dietary risk and pesticide uses that might be eliminated under policies corresponding to the various scenarios.

A second level of analysis focuses on individual pesticides. This chapter examines the impacts of each scenario on the dietary risks and crop uses associated with all the registered uses of a given pesticide. Analyses of individual pesticides are useful because the EPA routinely focuses on the risks of individual active ingredients when deciding how to respond to tolerance petitions and registrations. This perspective is also important to manufacturers and users who are concerned about the continued commercial viability of a pesticide.

Last, changes in dietary risks and pesticide use patterns on a crop-by-crop basis are explored. The crops analyzed in-depth were chosen with the help of EPA officials. Each of these crops is commonly processed into other foods in which the EPA has found or suspects concentrated residues. Consequently, existing and future tolerances for oncogenic pesticides in these crops may need to be brought into compliance with the Delaney Clause.

Selection of Pesticide-Crop Combinations

Because of the time required to gather data on pesticide use and expenditures, only a limited number of crop-level analyses were undertaken. The committee purposely selected crop-pesticide combinations that might present the EPA with difficult decisions regarding application of the Delaney Clause. Crops were chosen based on dietary consumption, economic importance, the volume and value of pesticides currently used on the crop, the availability of alternative pesticide and pest control methods, and the likelihood of concentrated residues in processed foods. On the basis of these criteria, eight crop-pesticide combinations were selected for detailed analysis:

- Corn and soybean herbicides;
- Cotton insecticides; and
- Apple, grape, peanut, potato, and tomato fungicides.

These eight combinations account for about 35 percent of total estimated dietary oncogenic risk.

ANALYTICAL METHODS

Dietary Risk

Crop-level analyses in this chapter use a different method for assessing dietary risk than the one used in Chapter 3. In Chapter 3, estimates of dietary risk were based on the assumption that 100 percent of all acres of every crop were treated with each pesticide having tolerances for that crop. The crop-level analyses presented here, however, take account of the actual percentage of planted acres that were treated with each oncogenic pesticide. Estimated risk at the crop level is derived by multiplying the total estimated crop risk by the average percentage of crop acres that were actually treated with each oncogenic pesticide during three of the past five years (not including 1983 for commodity support crops due to acreage reduction under the Payment-in-Kind program). The committee recognizes that adjusting risk estimates by the percentage of acres treated may incorrectly reduce estimated risk to individuals in regions where a higher percentage of a given crop contains residues of a certain pesticide. On the other hand, this method generally gives a more accurate estimate of risk faced by a population than the method discussed in Chapter 3.

The committee adjusted crop-level risk by the percentage of acres treated to calculate the impact of the scenarios on current patterns of pesticide use and to estimate changes in risk based on subsequent pesticide use patterns. It is important to understand that all calculations of dietary risk *reduction* at the crop level are from risk estimates that take into account the percentage of acres treated. (This adjustment in risk estimates is not used in Chapter 3 or in any but the crop-level analyses in Chapter 4. Information was not available on the percentage of acres treated for all crops with pesticide tolerances.)

Pesticide Use

In the context of the crop-level analyses, determining the effect of tolerance revocation on the total acre treatments and expenditures associated with oncogenic active ingredients is also possible. Data on acre treatments and expenditures are used as proxy indicators of the benefits of pesticide use. The committee selected these proxies on the assumption that the amount farmers spend on and use a pesticide reflects the gross benefits they receive from the use of that pesticide. The committee is aware that in most situations these proxies do not account for the substitution of pest control methods. Nonetheless, with the available data and time, the committee could identify no more realistic way for approximating changes in benefits.

DESCRIPTION OF THE SCENARIOS AND RESULTS

Four policy scenarios are analyzed. Each contains a distinct set of criteria governing the establishment and evaluation of tolerances for residues of pesticides considered to pose an oncogenic hazard. The scenarios fall along a policy continuum. At one extreme, scenario 1 is strict and aggressive in eliminating all dietary residues of known or suspected oncogenic pesticides. At the other extreme, under scenario 4, most existing tolerances for oncogenic pesticides would fall within an "acceptable" range of risk. The impact of these scenarios on active ingredients not yet registered or on new tolerances sought for active ingredients currently registered is not estimated. The focus here is on oncogenic pesticides currently registered for use on food crops. A description of these scenarios is presented in Table 4-1.

TABLE 4-1   Key Features of the Four Scenarios Examined by the Committee

Tolerances	Scenario			
	1	2	3	4
	Risk Standard			
Section 408	Zero risk	Risk/ benefit	10^{-6} risk trigger for each crop, processed and raw form combined; no consideration of benefits	Risk/benefit for raw foods with no processed form
Section 409	Zero risk	Zero risk for processed foods (tied to parent raw commodities)	See above	10^{-6} risk trigger for processed foods (tied to parent raw commodities); no consideration of benefits
	Consistent Treatment of Section 408 and Section 409 Tolerances			
	Yes	No	Yes	No

Scenario 1

Scenario 1 applies a zero-risk standard to oncogenic residues in or on all raw and processed foods. The impact is simple—whenever the agency determines that a pesticide poses an oncogenic risk, all existing food tolerances for the pesticide are revoked.

Under this scenario, no distinction is made between residues in or on raw or processed foods. Hence, neither the agency nor the pesticide registrants would have to determine whether a pesticide concentrated in processed foods. Moreover, because any finding of oncogenicity would trigger tolerance revocation, there would be no need to quantify oncogenic risk. In essence, this scenario applies the historic understanding of the Delaney Clause to residues in processed foods and extends it to residues in or on raw commodities.

RESULTS

Scenario 1 would eliminate all dietary exposure to pesticides that have caused an oncogenic response in test animals. The magnitude of dietary risk reduction accomplished would depend on how risks were estimated. For any method of estimating risk, 100 percent of it would be eliminated. (See Table 4-2 for risk reduction based on the committee's baseline risk estimates developed in Chapter 3.)

TABLE 4-2   Scenario 1—Reduction in Estimated Risk

Type of Pesticide	Risk		Total Expenditures (%)^b
	Reduction	Percentage^a	
Fungicides	3.46×10^{-3}	100	90
Herbicides	1.58×10^{-3}	100	38
Insecticides	8.00×10^{-4}	100	40
All oncogenic fungicides, herbicides, and insecticides	5.84×10^{-3}	100^c	45^d

NOTE: Risk estimates are derived from the 28 herbicides, insecticides, and fungicides constituting the committee's total dietary risk estimate. They are derived using EPA data and methods described on pages 50–66 and in Appendix B.

^{a}These figures express the percentage of risk reduction for herbicides, insecticides, *or* fungicides.

^{b}These figures express the percentage of total expenditures for all herbicides, insecticides, *or* fungicides.

^{c}This figure expresses the percentage of risk reduction for herbicides, insecticides, *and* fungicides.

^{d}This figure expresses the percentage of total expenditures for all herbicides, insecticides, *and* fungicides.

Food-use tolerances would be revoked for all 53 pesticide active ingredients that EPA has determined, conclusively or preliminarily, to be oncogens. The number and distribution of tolerances revoked and crops affected are reported in Table 4-3. A total of 3,769 raw and processed food forms with approved tolerances or assumed residues in the Tolerance Assessment System (TAS) would be affected, which is about 25 percent of the total number. Almost 200 crops would lose tolerances, which equals about 95 percent of all crops with pesticide tolerances. The fungicides would be particularly affected; 44 percent of all existing fungicide tolerances would be revoked. As shown in Table 4-3, herbicides and insecticides are less severely affected.

Crop-Level Analysis   As shown in Table 4-4, the impact of scenario 1 on individual crops varies greatly. Tolerances associated with 18 percent of all grape fungicide acre treatments and 91 percent of all potato fungicide acre treatments would be revoked. Measured by the percentage of total expenditures associated with lost tolerances, the range is from 8 percent for grape fungicides to 83 percent for peanut fungicides.

Another significant difference for the eight crops examined is the number of registered pesticides remaining as viable substitutes. The key indicator is the percentage of acre treatments eliminated when oncogenic pesticides are barred from use on food crops. The greater the percentage of acre treatments affected, the greater the presumed impact on the "benefits" of pesticide use.

A more accurate estimate of scenario 1's impact on these crops can be gained by judging the ease of switching from oncogenic to non-oncogenic pesticides. A crude indication of substitution is the number of registered alternatives available to replace oncogenic pesticides. It is generally more difficult to find substitutes for fungicides than for herbicides and insecticides. Under scenario 1, from one-third to one-half of all fungicides with tolerances for the crops discussed would be lost. For insecticides and herbicides, the tolerances lost are always less, ranging from 8 to 20 percent. Actual substitutability, however, must be considered on a case-by-case basis; some herbicides and insecticides may be effective on only a small percentage of weed and insect species.

This analysis suggests clearly that crops heavily dependent on fungicides would suffer the most severe consequences under scenario 1. (This observation will be documented further in Chapter 5.) Administratively, scenario 1 would be simple to implement. The only issue of possible contention—an issue common to all scenarios—is whether a given pesticide is or is not an oncogen. Once that judgment is made, the implications of scenario 1 are clear: all food tolerances are revoked. Traditional risk/benefit assessments following the approaches in Chapter 2 would be undertaken for non-oncogenic pesticides. It is possible, of course, that other public health or environmental risks of such pesticides

TABLE 4-3   Scenario 1—Effect on Active Ingredients, Tolerances, and Crops

	Effect on —		
Type of Pesticide	Active Ingredients (number)	Tolerances and Residue Estimates (number/%)[a]	Crops Losing Tolerances
Herbicides	17	1,295/26	172
Insecticides	19	1,222/17	152
Fungicides	14	1,111/44	137
Other	3	141	NA
All oncogens	53	3,769/25[b]	186

NOTE: The effect on tolerances and crops are for the 53 active ingredients the EPA identified as oncogenic. The tolerances and crops associated with the 28 active ingredients where risk estimates were available to the committee are used as a basis for comparison in tables describing the results of scenarios 3 and 4.

[a]These figures express the percentage of all herbicide, insecticide, *or* fungicide tolerances and residue estimates in the TAS.

[b]This figure expresses the percentage of all tolerances and residue estimates in the TAS.

TABLE **4-4** Impacts of Scenario 1 on Major Crop Uses for Registered Pesticides

Crop	Number of Active Ingredients—		Estimated Reduction in Crop Risk (number/%)	Percent Acre Treatments Lost	Percent Expenditures Affected
	With Tolerances	Losing Tolerances			
Fungicides					
Apples	21	10	4.28×10^{-5}/100	59	53
Grapes	15	7	5.56×10^{-6}/100	18	8
Peanuts	14	9	3.83×10^{-7}/100	86	83
Potatoes	15	10	6.47×10^{-5}/100	91	80
Tomatoes	20	11	8.28×10^{-5}/100	50	51
Herbicides					
Corn	39	8	1.31×10^{-6}/100	39	40
Soybeans	40	11	1.59×10^{-5}/100	67	58
Insecticides					
Cotton	45	9	1.29×10^{-5}/100	80	60

NOTE: These risk estimates are derived using EPA data and methods described on pages 50–66 and in Appendix B. Risk estimates in this table are adjusted (multiplied) by the percentage of acres treated.

might outweigh the benefits, leading to some regulatory action. That outcome is equally likely under existing law, however.

Scenario 2

This scenario applies a zero-risk standard to all oncogenic pesticide residues in processed foods. No detectable residue of an oncogenic pesticide in a processed food would be allowed. Because the mere presence of a residue in a processed food would trigger tolerance revocation under this scenario, the percentage of tolerances and crops affected is expressed as a percentage of tolerances and crop uses for all 53 oncogenic compounds. Reductions in risk, as with all scenarios, are derived from the 28 pesticides for which risk estimates were available to the committee. Because concentration of residues is not required to trigger tolerance revocation under this scenario, it is stricter or more risk averse than current law. In applying the zero-risk standard to residues in processed foods under scenario 2, there is no consideration of benefits.

For the purpose of calculating risk reduction, this scenario assumes there is no practical way to separate the portions of a crop grown only for fresh markets from those destined for processing. Thus, scenario 2 requires revocation of section 408 and section 409 tolerances to enforce the zero-risk standard in processed foods. The EPA has taken a similar approach in the past, routinely linking approval of section 408 raw food and section 409 processed-food tolerances. The only exceptions to this practice occur when there is a practical way to ensure that a crop is marketed exclusively in its fresh or raw form. This rarely occurs, however. (See the permethrin case study in Chapter 3 and Appendix C.)

Scenario 2 differs from scenario 1 in its application to crops such as lettuce, other vegetables, some fruits, and all meat, poultry, and dairy products that have no processed form under current EPA guidelines. These foods require only section 408 tolerances. In contrast, under scenario 1, residues of all oncogenic pesticides on all foods are disallowed. Oncogenic residues are disallowed in scenarios 1 and 2 for all crops with recognized processed forms.

RESULTS

Scenario 2 would reduce total estimated dietary oncogenic risk by about 55 percent. Risk is reduced unevenly among insecticides, herbicides, and fungicides, however. More than 70 percent of all risk from fungicides would be eliminated, compared with only about 26 percent of all insecticide risk and about 36 percent of herbicide risk (see Table 4-5). In contrast, Table 4-6 shows that the percentage of all oncogenic pesticide tolerances and residue estimates affected is quite uniform, ranging from 56 percent for fungicides to 50 percent for insecticides.

Section 408 tolerances associated with 45 percent of all oncogenic risk would remain unaffected under scenario 2. This share of the total estimated risk is from foods with no currently recognized processed forms, including vegetables, fruits, eggs, and all meat and dairy products.

TABLE 4-5   Scenario 2—Reduction in Estimated Risk

| | Risk | |
Type of Pesticide	Reduction	Estimated (%)[a]
Fungicides	2.45×10^{-3}	70.7
Herbicides	5.75×10^{-4}	36.4
Insecticides	2.12×10^{-4}	26.5
All oncogenic fungicides, herbicides, and insecticides	3.23×10^{-3}	55.4[b]

NOTE: Risk reduction is measured from the 28 herbicides, insecticides, and fungicides constituting the committee's total dietary risk estimate. These risk estimates are derived using EPA data and methods described on pages 50–66 and in Appendix B.

[a]These figures express the percentage of risk reduction for herbicides, insecticides, *or* fungicides.

[b]This figure expresses the percentage of risk reduction for herbicides, insecticides, *and* fungicides.

TABLE 4-6 Scenario 2—Effect on Active Ingredients, Tolerances, and Crops

| | Effect on — | | |
Type of Pesticide	Active Ingredients (number)	Tolerances and Residue Estimates (number/%)[a]	Crops (number/%)[b]
Fungicides	11	627/56	27/20
Insecticides	6	648/53	25/16
Herbicides	9	659/50	34/20
All oncogenic fungicides, herbicides, and insecticides	26	1,934/51[c]	38/20[d]

[a]These figures express the percentage of all *oncogenic* herbicide, insecticide, *or* fungicide tolerances and TAS residue estimates.

[b]These figures express the percentage of all crops treated with *oncogenic* herbicides, insecticides, *or* fungicides.

[c]This figure expresses the percentage of all *oncogenic* herbicide, insecticide, *and* fungicide tolerances and TAS residue estimates.

[d]This figure expresses the percentage of all crops treated with *oncogenic* herbicides, insecticides, *and* fungicides.

Under scenario 2, these uses would be reviewed in the traditional fashion, which could lead to some risk reduction beyond the assured 55 percent risk reduction under this scenario. The committee is unable to project the outcome of these individual risk/benefit decisions in this and all other scenarios. The reader can gain some perspective on the crops and foods that lack processed forms and hence are not under any circumstances affected by the Delaney Clause from Table 3-11 in the previous chapter.

From the standpoint of agricultural producers, scenario 2 has a relatively narrow effect. Not more than one in five crops would lose tolerances, although 51 percent of all tolerances for oncogenic herbicides, insecticides, and fungicides would be lost. Some crops that would lose tolerances are major commodities.

Effects on Individual Active Ingredients Dietary risk reduction under this scenario is efficient in that a 55 percent reduction in risk is achieved through tolerance revocations affecting only about 20 percent of all crops for which these oncogenic compounds are registered (see Table 4-6). For example, with the widely used fungicide benomyl, a 93 percent reduction in dietary risk would be achieved through tolerance revocations affecting only 17 crops with processed forms, or 17 percent of the 101 foods (including meats) for which benomyl has tolerances. For another major fungicide, captan, revocations on 19 crops with processed forms, or 25 percent of all captan registrations, account for a 71 percent reduction in dietary oncogenic risk from this pesticide. For a major herbicide, alachlor, a 50 percent reduction in risk is attained by revoking tolerances for only four crops, or 16 percent of all alachlor tolerances.

The degree of risk reduction under this scenario, however, depends greatly on the crop on which a pesticide is used. The impact on the crop then stems from whether and to what extent it is processed. Under this scenario, residues in raw agricultural products are approved under a different standard than residues in processed foods. These different standards account for the fact that some crops and types of pesticides are preferentially targeted. For example, dietary risk from benomyl is reduced by 93 percent with a corresponding loss of benefits. Dietary risk from linuron and maneb, however, is reduced by only 36 and 43 percent, respectively.

This inconsistency reveals the significance of judgments on which crops are considered not processed. Currently, many crops, such as raspberries and other small fruits, are in this category even though jams, jellies, candies, and other foodstuffs made from such fruits are clearly processed-food forms. The need to redefine the processed and not processed categories could put considerable administrative and resource strains on the agency. Residues in animal feeds and food products pose particular problems. Any policy with significantly different definitions of processed and not processed food could lead to markedly different regulatory outcomes.

Crop–Level Impacts   Impacts on seven of the eight crops examined under scenario 2 are identical to scenario 1. All risk is eliminated and all tolerances are revoked (see Table 4-7) except for peanut fungicides. This result occurs for all the crops studied except peanuts because TAS assumes no processed peanut food forms *for the 53 oncogens examined*. This anomaly is a result of the TAS tolerance expansion process and does not imply that residues will not be present or that peanuts have no processed forms. Peanut butter and peanut oil are clearly processed-food forms. The TAS contains peanut oil tolerances for other pesticides. This example highlights the critical relationship between the definition of a processed food and the application of the Delaney Clause to food tolerances. As pointed out above, when a zero-risk standard precludes establishment of a processed-food tolerance, this generally means that tolerances for the parent raw commodity must also be revoked.

Scenario 3

Scenario 3 applies a 1 in 1 million (1×10^{-6}) risk standard to section 408 and section 409 tolerances, that is, to all processed and raw foods. Dietary risk estimates are calculated using the sum of TAS residue estimates for

TABLE 4-7   Impacts of Scenario 2 on Major Crop Uses for Registered Pesticides

Crop	Number of Active Ingredients— With Tolerances	Losing Tolerances	Estimated Reduction in Crop Risk (number/%)	Percent Acre Treatments Lost	Percent Expenditures Affected
			Fungicides		
Apples	21	10	4.28×10^{-5}/100	59	53
Grapes	15	7	5.56×10^{-6}/100	18	8
Peanuts	14	No impact	No impact	No impact	No impact
Potatoes	15	10	6.47×10^{-5}/100	91	80
Tomatoes	20	11	8.28×10^{-5}/100	50	51
			Herbicides		
Corn	39	8	1.31×10^{-6}/100	39	40
Soybeans	40	11	1.59×10^{-5}/100	67	58
			Insecticides		
Cotton	45	9	1.29×10^{-5}/100	80	60

NOTE: These risk estimates are derived using EPA data and methods described on pages 50–66 and in Appendix B. Risk estimates in this table are adjusted (multiplied) by the percentage of acres treated.

each use of a pesticide on raw and processed forms of a given crop. When the total dietary risk from the residues of any pesticide found on the raw and processed forms of a crop exceeds 10^{-6}, all tolerances for that pesticide on that crop would be revoked or denied. There would be no consideration of benefits once risk went above this level. The use would be automatically disapproved. Because this scenario is based on quantitative levels of risk, it could only be applied to the 28 compounds that comprise the committee's estimate of dietary oncogenic risk.

An important feature of this scenario is that dietary risk is calculated at the crop level, as opposed to current EPA practice in which dietary risk is calculated for an active ingredient across all of its uses. In this scenario, for example, exposure to an oncogenic pesticide on fresh tomatoes is added to the exposure to these residues in all processed tomato products in determining whether the 10^{-6} risk trigger is met for that crop use. When the trigger is exceeded *for tomatoes,* there would be no consideration of benefits from that pesticide's use *on tomatoes.* Tolerances for these uses would be revoked. Dietary risks less than 10^{-6} from a pesticide's use on a crop would be evaluated using standard procedures.

This scenario applies the same standard to tolerances for both raw and processed commodities. In contrast to current EPA practice, this scenario implies a stricter regulatory stance on section 408 raw agricultural commodity tolerances, particularly those with no associated section 409 tolerances, because benefits are not considered when risks exceed 10^{-6}.

It is less strict, however, than the current zero-risk standard for section 409 processed-food tolerances and their associated section 408 tolerances; tolerances for processed foods are not prohibited unless risks from the whole crop exceed the 10^{-6} standard.

RESULTS

This scenario and scenario 4, below, demonstrate the impact of simple assumptions in the calculation of exposure and how these assumptions affect dietary risk estimates across different food products and crop uses.

The most striking result of scenario 3 is that although 98 percent of total estimated dietary risk would be eliminated, only 32 percent of all tolerances for oncogens and 38 percent of all crops would be affected. Scenario 3 would achieve only 2 percent less risk reduction than scenario 1, while revoking 1,500 fewer tolerances for the 28 compounds that constitute the committee's risk estimate (see Tables 4-8 and 4-9).

Scenario 3 is efficient in that it targets crop uses posing dietary risks greater than 10^{-6} and revokes the associated tolerances, but still leaves untouched nearly 70 percent of all tolerances and nearly two-thirds of all crops (see Table 4-8). For example, 99 percent of all herbicide risk would be eliminated, but only 16 percent of all herbicide tolerances would be revoked. Just 12 percent of all crops treated with oncogenic herbicides would be affected. For fungicides, the percentage and numbers of tolerances and crops affected are higher. Yet, more than 98 percent of dietary risk is eliminated through revocation of 53 percent of fungicide tolerances affecting 42 percent of the 137 crops on which fungicides are used.

TABLE 4-8   Scenario 3—Reduction in Estimated Risk

Type of Pesticide	Risk	
	Reduction	Percentage[a]
Fungicides	3.41×10^{-3}	98.5
Herbicides	1.56×10^{-3}	98.9
Insecticides	7.79×10^{-4}	97.4
All oncogenic fungicides, herbicides, and insecticides	5.75×10^{-3}	98.5[b]

NOTE: Risk reduction is measured from the 28 herbicides, insecticides, and fungicides constituting the committee's total dietary risk estimate. These risk estimates are derived using EPA data and methods described on pages 50–66 and in Appendix B.

[a]These figures express the percentage of risk reduction for herbicides, insecticides, *or* fungicides.

[b]This figure expresses the percentage of risk reduction for herbicides, insecticides, *and* fungicides.

TABLE 4-9   Scenario 3—Effect on Active Ingredients, Tolerances, and Crops

| | Effect on— | | |
Type of Pesticide	Active Ingredients (number)	Tolerances and Residue Estimates (number/%)[a]	Crops (number/%)[b]
Fungicides	10	502/53	58/42
Insecticides	5	132/21	27/20
Herbicides	7	122/16	20/12
All oncogenic fungicides, herbicides, and insecticides	22	756/32[c]	68/38[d]

[a]These figures express the percentage of herbicide, insecticide, *or* fungicide tolerances and TAS residue estimates for the 28 compounds constituting the committee's total dietary risk estimate.

[b]These figures express the percentage of crops treated with the herbicides, insecticides, *or* fungicides for the 28 compounds constituting the committee's total dietary risk estimate.

[c]This figure expresses the percentage of all herbicide, insecticide, *and* fungicide tolerances and TAS residue estimates for the 28 compounds constituting the committee's total dietary risk estimate.

[d]This figure expresses the percentage of all crops treated with the 28 compounds constituting the committee's total dietary risk estimate.

Impacts on Individual Active Ingredients   A notable feature of scenario 3 is that it has no impact on certain widely used oncogenic pesticides when the oncogenic risk from any individual crop does not exceed 10^{-6}. For instance, the widely used but weakly oncogenic herbicides glyphosate and metolachlor would not experience any tolerance revocations. Under scenario 2, the same herbicides would suffer many tolerance revocations because of the presence of residues in processed foods. Further, for certain compounds, scenario 3 achieves a greater or equal reduction of risk by revoking fewer tolerances than do other scenarios. In the case of the fungicide benomyl, scenario 3 achieves the same percentage reduction in risk as the next best scenario (2), while affecting 5 percent fewer crops.

Crop-Level Impacts   The difference between scenario 2 and 3 is particularly striking at the crop level (see Tables 4-7 and 4-10). Whereas scenarios 1 and 2 eliminate all tolerances associated with processed crops, scenario 3 would affect only those crop uses where the combined dietary risk from fresh and processed food residues is greater than 10^{-6}. Scenario 3 is more discriminating.

TABLE 4-10   Impacts of Scenario 3 on Major Crop Uses for Registered Pesticides

Crop	Number of Active Ingredients—		Estimated Reduction in Crop Risk (number/%)	Percent Acre Treatments Lost	Percent Expenditures Affected
	With Tolerances	Losing Tolerances			
			Fungicides		
Apples	21	4	4.21×10^{-5}/98	54	46
Grapes	15	1	3.38×10^{-6}/70	10	4
Peanuts	14	No impact	No impact	No impact	No impact
Potatoes	15	1	4.36×10^{-6}/68	31	29
Tomatoes	20	5	8.22×10^{-5}/99	49	51
			Herbicides		
Corn	39	2	1.31×10^{-6}/99.9	30	27
Soybeans	40	2	1.59×10^{-5}/99.9	27	20
			Insecticides		
Cotton	45	1	1.28×10^{-5}/99	9	7

NOTE: These risk estimates are derived using EPA data and methods described on pages 50–66 and in Appendix B. Risk estimates in this table are adjusted (multiplied) by the percentage of acres treated.

For some crops, scenario 3 eliminates a high percentage of risk with a modest loss of benefits. For example, dietary risk from cotton insecticides is reduced by 99 percent and grape fungicides by 70 percent, even though in each case tolerances for only one compound are revoked. Each pesticide affected accounts for less than 10 percent of acre treatments and expenditures.

These cases suggest that scenario 3 offers a considerable opportunity for sizable risk reductions with relatively modest loss of benefits, at least for some crops. This feature of scenario 3 is not shared by scenario 2. Under scenario 2, six more oncogenic corn herbicides would lose tolerances, resulting in an additional reduction in dietary oncogenic risk from corn of less than one-tenth of 1 percent.

Scenario 4

Under scenario 4, tolerances for a crop would be revoked when the risk from all the various processed forms of a particular crop exceeds 10^{-6}. Scenario 4 is conceptually similiar to scenario 2 in one respect; a specified level of risk associated with the processed-food forms of a crop triggers tolerance revocations. The risk level of 10^{-6} for scenario 4 differs from the zero-risk standard for scenario 2. As in scenario 2, when the specified risk level (10^{-6}) is exceeded by residues in or on the processed portion of the crop, section 408 and section 409 tolerances are revoked.

RESULTS

Scenario 4 reduces the estimated dietary risk derived from 28 herbicides, insecticides, and fungicides by about 36 percent. The relatively modest degree of risk reduction in this scenario is partially explained by the fact that all crops with no processed form are exempt. In other words, for raw foods this scenario reflects the current interpretation of section 408. As evident in Table 4-11, the effects of scenario 4 are highly variable. Herbicide risk is reduced by about 11 percent, while nearly 51 percent of fungicide risk is eliminated. There is a high degree of variability from pesticide to pesticide as well. Ten pesticides suffer no tolerance revocations at all. For the rest, the risk reduction ranges from 6 percent for acephate to 80 percent for benomyl.

Scenario 4 affects few crops and a small percentage of all tolerances (Table 4-12). Only 12 percent of all tolerances and 10 percent of all crops treated with oncogenic herbicides, insecticides, and fungicides are affected under this scenario. Apples and tomatoes, which are often consumed in processed forms, are much more vulnerable under this scenario than other crops.

Crop-Level Impacts   The results of scenario 4 at the crop level are shown in Table 4-13. Scenarios 3 and 4 have identical effects on cotton and tomato tolerances, yet for all other crops the results are quite different. In scenario 4, current risk from processed corn and potato

TABLE 4-11   Scenario 4—Reduction in Estimated Risk

	Risk	
Type of Pesticide	Reduction	Percentage[a]
Fungicides	1.75×10^{-3}	50.7
Herbicides	1.76×10^{-4}	11.1
Insecticides	1.54×10^{-4}	19.2
All oncogenic fungicides, herbicides, and insecticides	2.08×10^{-3}	35.7[b]

NOTE: Risk reduction is measured from the 28 herbicides, insecticides, and fungicides constituting the committee's total dietary risk estimate. These risk estimates are derived using EPA data and methods described on pages 50–66 and in Appendix B.

[a]These figures express the percentage of risk reduction for herbicides, insecticides, *or* fungicides.

[b]These figures express the percentage of risk reduction for herbicides, insecticides, *and* fungicides.

TABLE 4-12 Scenario 4—Effect on Active Ingredients, Tolerances, and Crops

Type of Pesticide	Effect on—		
	Active Ingredients (number)	Tolerances Lost (number/%)[a]	Crops (number/%)[b]
Fungicides	10	207/21	12/9
Herbicides	4	44/6	4/2
Insecticides	4	20/3	4/3
All oncogenic fungicides, herbicides, and insecticides	18	271/12[c]	14/10[d]

[a]These figures express the percentage of herbicide, insecticide, *or* fungicide tolerances and TAS residue estimates for the 28 compounds constituting the committee's total dietary risk estimate.

[b]These figures express the percentage of crops treated with the herbicides, insecticides, *or* fungicides for the 28 compounds constituting the committee's total dietary risk estimate.

[c]This figure expresses the percentage of all herbicide, insecticide, *and* fungicide tolerances and TAS residue estimates for the 28 compounds constituting the committee's total dietary risk estimate.

[d]This figure expresses the percentage of all crops treated with the 28 compounds constituting the committee's total dietary risk estimate.

TABLE 4-13 Impacts of Scenario 4 on Major Crop Uses for Registered Pesticides

Crop	Number of Active Ingredients—		Estimated Reduction in Crop Risk (number/%)	Percent Acre Treatments Lost	Percent Expenditures Affected
	With Tolerances	Tolerances Lost			
Fungicides					
Apples	21	3	4.00×10^{-5}/93	49	42
Grapes	15	2	2.40×10^{-5}/93	10	4
Peanuts	14	No impact	No impact	No impact	No impact
Potatoes	15	No impact	No impact	No impact	No impact
Tomatoes	20	5	8.22×10^{-5}/99	49	51
Herbicides					
Corn	39	No impact	No impact	No impact	No impact
Soybeans	40	1	1.49×10^{-5}/94	9	7
Insecticides					
Cotton	45	4	1.28×10^{-5}/99	9	7

NOTE: These risk estimates are derived using EPA data and methods described on pages 50–66 and in Appendix B. Risk estimates in this table are adjusted (multiplied) by the percentage of acres treated.

products is less than 10^{-6}; therefore no tolerances are revoked. Peanuts are protected because TAS assumes no processed peanut food forms for the 53 oncogens examined. Soybean producers, on the other hand, would lose the use of one compound that accounts for more than 94 percent of the risk from soybean herbicides, but for less than 10 percent of all acre treatments and expenditures.

Summary

The performance of these scenarios will be discussed in detail in the next chapter. However, several key observations are relevant to all of them.

• Uniform treatment of raw and processed food tolerances appears to result in more consistent risk reduction for all pesticides and foods.

• A nonzero-risk standard, consistently applied to raw and processed foods, can reduce risk significantly by selecting out high-risk pesticide and food combinations. Any risk standard (including zero risk) applied differently to raw and processed foods cannot achieve such selective risk reduction.

• For insecticides and herbicides, risk can be greatly reduced by revoking tolerances for only one or two compounds—often those that present high risks and relatively low benefits. For fungicides, however, this is not the case. There are few compounds that present high risk and low benefits. Therefore, actions against one or two compounds often will not result in substantial risk reduction.

NOTE

1. Special reviews set for fiscal year 1987 listed. 1986. *Pesticide and Toxic Chemical News* 14(October):9–10.

5

Comparing the Impact
of the Scenarios

This chapter compares the four scenarios by their effects on herbicides, insecticides, and fungicides; individual pesticide active ingredients; and selected crop-pesticide combinations.

The previous chapter describes the scenarios and their impacts. This chapter highlights the important convergent and divergent effects of these scenarios on oncogenic pesticides as measured by changes in estimated dietary oncogenic risk, acre treatments, and expenditures.

THE IMPACTS OF THE SCENARIOS ON HERBICIDES, INSECTICIDES, AND FUNGICIDES

The four scenarios have markedly different impacts on the major classes of pesticides. In each scenario, fungicides suffer the greatest percentage of canceled crop uses and tolerance revocations; the revocations account for the greatest percentage of total risk reduction. In each case, more than 50 percent of all fungicide risk is eliminated, and half or more of existing fungicide uses are affected.

These scenarios have more diverse effects on insecticides and herbicides. The risk reduction for insecticides ranges from 19 percent in scenario 4 to 99 percent in scenario 3. For herbicides the range is from 11 percent in scenario 4 to 99 percent in scenario 3. Table 5-1 arrays the percentage of estimated risk reduction across the scenarios for each type of pesticide.

A chief reason for the disparity among the scenarios' risk reduction is

118

TABLE 5-1 Estimated Risk Reduction for Each Type of Pesticide by Scenario (in percent)

Risk Standard	Scenario			
	1	2	3	4
Tolerances				
Section 408	Zero risk	Risk/benefit	10^{-6} risk trigger for each crop, processed and raw form combined; no consideration of benefits	Risk/benefit for raw foods with no processed form
Section 409	Zero risk	Zero risk for processed foods tied to parent raw commodities	See above	10^{-6} risk trigger for processed foods (tied to parent raw commodities); no consideration of benefits
Pesticides				
Fungicides	100	71	98	51
Herbicides	100	36	99	11
Insecticides	100	26	99	19
All pesticides	100	55	98	36

that much of the dietary risk from herbicides and insecticides examined in this study stems from residues in food derived from animals. The EPA does not currently recognize these foods as having processed forms. Any scenario that revokes or denies tolerances on the basis of oncogenic risk in processed foods will not touch tolerances for residues in beef, milk, poultry, or pork products. Thus, even though dietary risk from exposure to residues in animal products may exceed that associated with the human food forms of the major feed crops, tolerances for animal products will not be revoked under scenarios 2 or 4. For example, in a case where meat from animals fed pesticide-treated corn presents a greater risk than corn oil derived from the same treated corn, tolerances for meat would not be revoked.

Of the compounds the committee examined, about 50 percent of all herbicide risk and 40 percent of all insecticide risk are derived from tolerances for animal products. This partially explains the difference in the treatment of herbicides and insecticides in scenarios 2 and 4 compared with scenario 3. On the other hand, less than 1 percent of all risk from fungicide residues is from tolerances for animal products. This helps explain the comparatively consistent treatment of fungicides across all scenarios.

Although the EPA's criteria currently attribute very little oncogenic risk to fungicide residues in animal products, the committee is suspicious of this low estimate. Indeed, much evidence suggests that many fungicide-treated crops whose by-products are fed to animals lack legally mandated feed-additive tolerances. Modern residue chemistry data are likely to demonstrate the need for such tolerances. If these tolerances are set, overall estimated risk would rise, as would the percentage of risk derived from meat, poultry, and dairy products, currently all defined as raw foods. The percentage reduction in fungicide risk under scenarios 2 and 4, on the other hand, would decline. This change in depiction of the baseline would not greatly change the overall performance of the scenarios, however.

Further, the committee is aware that confirmation of residues in processed food or feed could result in the loss of tolerances for the major animal feed crops. This in turn could reduce the residue level in all food products derived from animals fed these crops, leading to a de facto reduction in risk without the loss of food tolerances for these crops. It is important to note, however, that total elimination of this risk is not certain in these cases. Crops with animal feed uses could retain both food and feed tolerances through the sensitivity-of-the-method procedure if it were demonstrated that residues of these oncogenic pesticides in human food posed very low risks. (See Appendix C for the thiodicarb case study.) Scenarios 2 and 4, which do not directly affect tolerances for animal products, ensure less risk reduction than does scenario 3, which is not limited to finding residues in a processed food.

THE IMPACTS OF THE SCENARIOS ON INDIVIDUAL ACTIVE INGREDIENT RISK

Among individual pesticides, fungicides are the most heavily affected under all scenarios. This does not mean, however, that all scenarios have equal effects. In fact, the same scenario can have quite disparate impacts on different fungicides, herbicides, and insecticides.

A single scenario can have very different impacts on two similar types of pesticides. For example, under scenario 3, tolerances accounting for more than 93 percent of all risk from benomyl and 98 percent from maneb are revoked. Scenario 4 treats the two fungicides quite differently: 80 percent of benomyl risk and 25 percent of maneb risk are eliminated.

When one examines the effect of the different scenarios on all tolerances for the same active ingredient, scenario 3 stands out sharply. It consistently revokes tolerances for pesticides presenting relatively high risks, but does not affect relatively low-risk compounds. Scenario 3 achieves only 2 percent less risk reduction than scenario 1 while revoking 1,500 fewer food tolerances for the 28 compounds that constitute the

TABLE 5-2   Impact of Scenarios on Different Pesticide Active
Ingredients

Pesticide	Reduction in Risk from Total Estimated Risk in Three Scenarios (%)		
	2	3	4
Herbicides			
Alachlor (Lasso)	50	77	50
Linuron (Lorox)	36	99	11
Metolachlor (Dual)	30	0	0
Insecticides			
Chlordimeform (Galecon)	31	99	31
Cypermethrin (Cymbush, Ammo)	5	77	0
Permethrin (Pounce, Ambush)	24	98	12
Fungicides			
Benomyl (Benlate)	93	93	80
Captan	71	98	48
Maneb	43	98	25

committee's risk estimate. Scenario 3 achieves greater risk reduction than
either scenario 2 or 4. Scenario 1, of course, eliminates all dietary
oncogenic risk.

Sizable differences in risk reduction between scenarios 3 and 4 are
apparent for many compounds, as shown in Table 5-2. For the insecticide
permethrin, scenario 3 reduces dietary risk by 98 percent, whereas
scenario 4 reduces risk by only 12 percent. For the herbicide linuron,
scenario 3 reduces risk by 99 percent; scenario 4 reduces risk by 11
percent. The selectivity of scenario 3 is also highlighted at this level of
analysis, particularly when contrasted with scenario 2.

Scenario 2 (which allows no risk in processed foods) does not discriminate between active ingredients that pose more significant and relatively
insignificant risks. Even though scenario 2 achieves a higher degree of
risk reduction than scenario 4, it fails to do so efficiently—particularly
when compared with scenario 3. This is because the rigorous zero-risk
standard in scenario 2 applies only to the processed portion of the food
supply. As a result, tolerances for pesticides accounting for sizable
estimated oncogenic risks, such as linuron and maneb, are relatively
unaffected under scenario 2 because many foods on which they are found
lack processed forms. At the same time, several pesticides presenting
relatively low estimated dietary risks, such as glyphosate and
metolachlor, lose tolerances under scenario 2 because they are presumed
to be present in certain processed foods. This failure to discriminate

TABLE 5-3 Risk, Acre Treatment, and Expenditure Reductions for Selected Crop-Pesticide Combinations (in percent)

| | Scenarios | | | | | | | | | | | |
| | 1 | | | 2 | | | 3 | | | 4 | | |
Type of Pesticide	Risk Reduction	Acre Treatment Reduction	Expenditure Reduction	Risk Reduction	Acre Treatment Reduction	Expenditure Reduction	Risk Reduction	Acre Treatment Reduction	Expenditure Reduction	Risk Reduction	Acre Treatment Reduction	Expenditure Reduction
Fungicides for—												
Apples	100	59	53	100	59	53	98	54	46	93	50	42
Grapes	100	18	8	100	18	8	70	10	4	70	10	4
Peanuts	100	86	83	0	0	0	0	0	0	0	0	0
Potatoes	100	91	81	100	91	81	68	31	29	0	0	0
Tomatoes	100	50	52	100	50	52	99	49	51	99	49	51
Herbicides for—												
Corn	100	39	40	100	39	40	99	30	27	0	0	0
Soybeans	100	67	58	100	67	58	99	27	20	94	9	7
Insecticides for—												
Cotton	100	80	61	100	80	61	99	9	7	99	9	7

between high- and low-risk exposures to residues is the principal flaw in this scenario.

Scenario 4 displays greater consistency than scenario 2 because it revokes relatively few tolerances for either high- or low-risk residues in food. Consequently scenario 4 results in less risk reduction than any other scenario.

In sum, an analysis by individual active ingredients reveals that scenario 3 reduces more risk from herbicides, fungicides, and insecticides than do scenarios 2 and 4, while allowing continued use of several relatively low-risk compounds. Scenario 2 revokes more tolerances for these low-risk active ingredients by eliminating all tolerances for all crops with processed forms. Scenario 2 also revokes fewer tolerances for certain high-risk compounds applied to foods with no processed form, resulting in less overall risk reduction. Scenario 4 allows most tolerances for high- and low-risk compounds to continue. Scenario 1, of course, eliminates all tolerances for all oncogenic active ingredients.

A CROP-LEVEL ANALYSIS: THE IMPACTS OF THE SCENARIOS ON BENEFITS AND RISKS

This section examines the immediate impact of the four scenarios on risks and benefits associated with eight crop-pesticide combinations. Longer-term impacts on crop production and the effect of the Delaney Clause on new product development are discussed in the next chapter.

All calculations of risk in the following crop-level analyses reflect estimated total risk for a crop adjusted (multiplied) by the percentage of planted acres actually treated with the pesticides in question. Risk reduction estimates are based on this adjusted risk estimate. Only the crop-level analyses in this chapter and Chapter 4 incorporate the percentage of planted acres treated.

Benefits are measured by several rough indicators of pesticide use and expenditures. The impact of the scenarios is measured by the acre treatments and expenditures associated with pesticides that lose tolerances as a percentage of all herbicide, insecticide, or fungicide use on that crop. The committee believes that a better measure of a pesticide benefit is the difference between the total benefits received from its use, minus the total benefits of using the next best pest control method. It lacked the time and resources to perform such estimates, however.

The committee decided to study crops having processed-food forms. Because of this choice, scenarios 1 and 2 produce nearly identical results. Scenarios 3 and 4, on the other hand, differ markedly. Table 5-3 displays the effects of the scenarios on these eight crops in terms of risk reduction and acre treatments lost.

Corn and Soybean Herbicides

Because of their zero-risk standards, scenarios 1 and 2 would revoke tolerances for eight active ingredients, which account for 39 percent of all corn herbicide acre treatments and 40 percent of expenditures.

Under scenario 3, however, corn tolerances for only one of the four active ingredients for which risk estimates were possible would be revoked. Eliminating use of this single pesticide would reduce dietary risk from corn herbicides by 99 percent while affecting 30 percent of all corn herbicide acre treatments and 27 percent of expenditures. Scenario 4 leaves all corn herbicide tolerances untouched because oncogenic risk from herbicide residues in processed corn products in no case exceeds 10^{-6}.

Soybean producers would be harder hit than corn producers under scenarios 1 and 2. Both scenarios would revoke tolerances for 11 herbicides, which currently account for 67 percent of all acre treatments and 58 percent of all expenditures. Scenario 3 would eliminate two herbicides, resulting in 99 percent risk reduction. Scenario 4 would eliminate tolerances for only one herbicide, linuron, but this would eliminate 94 percent of the estimated dietary risk from soybean herbicides. This substantial risk reduction is striking considering linuron's share of total acre treatments (9 percent) and expenditures (7 percent).

Because of the availability of a range of new, effective, non-oncogenic herbicides, the impact of tolerance revocations on corn and soybean producers would probably be modest even under scenarios 1 and 2, which would repeal tolerances for all oncogenic compounds. It is also true, however, that this result would eliminate less than 1 percent of total estimated dietary risk.

Cotton Insecticides

Scenarios 1 and 2 would end the use of eight insecticides accounting for about 80 percent of all cotton insecticide acre treatments and 61 percent of all expenditures. The loss of cypermethrin, which accounts for about 45 percent of all acre treatments, would produce most of this impact. The repeal of all cotton tolerances for oncogenic insecticides would reduce total estimated dietary risk by only about 0.2 percent.

The loss of eight active ingredients accounting for nearly 80 percent of all acre treatments would require a sizable adjustment in insect control for cotton. Although state agricultural experiment stations and extension entomologists recommend many of the 35 remaining registered compounds for control of the Heliothis complex and other cotton insect pests, a number of these compounds are not as economical as the agents that would lose tolerances—particularly the synthetic pyrethroid cypermethrin.

It is also important to note that virtually all estimated dietary risk from insecticides used on cotton is from chlordimeform, which accounts for only 9 percent of all cotton acre treatments and 7 percent of cotton insecticide expenditures. Eliminating the most widely used oncogenic cotton insecticides, cypermethrin and parathion, under scenarios 1 and 2 would reduce estimated dietary risk from cotton insecticides by less than 1 percent and total risk by only 0.0002 percent.

Scenarios 3 and 4, which apply to the six cotton insecticides for which risk estimates were possible, would revoke tolerances for only one insecticide, chlordimeform. As in the case of the herbicide linuron on soybeans, actions against one pesticide could dramatically reduce estimated dietary risk from cotton, while affecting a relatively small share of total expenditures on, and acre treatments with, cotton insecticides.

Apple Fungicides

Ten oncogenic active ingredients currently account for more than 50 percent of all expenditures on apple fungicides. Scenarios 1 and 2 would eliminate all the benefits associated with this use. Chemicals accounting for 59 percent of all acre treatments and 53 percent of all expenditures on apple fungicides would lose tolerances. Total baseline risk would be reduced by more than 5 percent. Applied to these same 10 fungicides, scenarios 3 and 4 would affect fewer active ingredients and achieve slightly less risk reduction by revoking tolerances representing 54 and 50 percent of acre treatments, respectively (see Table 5-3). In each scenario, a significant percentage of all apple fungicides would be lost, creating the possible need for replacement compounds or other control methods.

A substantial number of presumably non-oncogenic apple fungicides are in development, currently registered, or both. Copper, sulfur, and the fungicide triadimefon are the primary currently registered non-oncogenic alternatives. The committee's survey of compounds in development identified a relatively high rate of product discovery for new apple fungicides. At least nine compounds are now being field tested for control of the major apple fungal diseases. Nearly all appear to be better than the best commercially available standard for *eradicating* apple scab and powdery mildew. However, more than half of these are poor in *protecting against* apple scab. None of the new compounds was found to be as good as the commercial standard for treating the seven summer diseases: bitter rot, black rot, white rot, sooty blotch, fly speck, brooks spot, and black pox.

The revocation of tolerances for all oncogenic apple fungicides in scenarios 1 and 2 would be felt hardest in the Southeast, where adequate replacement fungicides currently do not exist for all diseases. In the northeastern and north central growing regions, apple production also currently relies on oncogenic fungicides; however, non-oncogenic replacements for the dominant fungal diseases, powdery mildew and apple scab, are more readily available.

The 10^{-6} risk standard of scenarios 3 and 4 would initially preserve tolerances for certain oncogenic fungicides on apples. It is likely, however, that over time, few oncogenic apple fungicides would retain tolerances. This would occur when the use of agents that do not now trigger the 10^{-6} risk criterion increases after tolerances for other fungicides are revoked.

Even under scenario 4, which would initially revoke tolerances for only two active ingredients, a substitution pattern could emerge in which risk from residues of each remaining oncogenic apple fungicide would eventually exceed 10^{-6} and trigger tolerance revocation. In fact, revocation of tolerances for the apple fungicides that currently present the greatest risk could increase the total dietary risk if little-used, more potent fungicides come into broader use. Several scenarios that could increase estimated risk are presented below in the section on tolerance reduction. This finding highlights the importance of ensuring that regulatory actions at the crop level actually reduce risk, taking into account the probable actions of growers to find and apply substitute chemicals.

Potato Fungicides

Nine oncogenic fungicides currently account for around 81 percent of all expenditures and nearly 91 percent of all acre treatments for potato diseases. Scenarios 1 and 2 would terminate uses of these agents, eliminating all potato fungicide risk and reducing overall estimated risk by 2 percent.

The complete loss of all oncogenic fungicides currently used in potato production would again have different regional impacts. Northeastern potato growers currently apply around 55 percent of all oncogenic fungicides on potatoes; midwestern growers apply around 33 percent. Western potato growers apply less than 15 percent of the total, although they plant more than 50 percent of all potato acres. Partly because blight and other fungal diseases are not generally a problem in the West, potato production has been moving there over the past 20 years.[1]

Most of the oncogenic fungicides used in potato production are applied as preventatives on a routine basis. There is little field monitoring and forecasting to make more accurate determinations of when fungicide applications are necessary. It is increasingly possible, however, to use information about weather and crop conditions to prescribe the use of fungicides when most needed. This practice can reduce the use of fungicides up to 30 percent in some areas in some years. It has not become common practice, though, perhaps because growers lack confidence in these forecasts.

Currently registered non-oncogenic potato fungicides are little used. Generally these agents (triphenyltin hydroxide, metalaxyl, and sulfur) are far less effective than currently used fungicides. Further, some alternatives (triphenyltin hydroxide) pose other toxicological problems. Ridomil (metalaxyl) shows some control of potato blight but is far more expensive than the current fungicides of choice (EBDCs, chlorothalonil), is not widely used, and is known to have led to pathogen resistance in other crops.

Scenarios 3 and 4, which would apply to seven potato fungicides for which risk estimates were possible, would have much different results than scenarios 1 and 2. Scenario 3 would initially revoke tolerances for only one fungicide, mancozeb, which accounts for about 68 percent of potato fungicide risk and about 31 percent of acre treatments and expenditures. Over time, however, scenario 3 would probably have the same effect as scenarios 1 and 2. Because of the shortage of non-oncogenic substitutes, the elimination of one oncogenic fungicide would very likely increase the percentage of all acres that are treated with other registered oncogenic compounds. The risks posed by these alternatives would eventually exceed 10^{-6}, leading to the loss of all tolerances for all oncogenic potato fungicides.

Scenario 4, which revokes tolerances for a pesticide on a crop when the risk derived from the processed form of the crop is greater than 10^{-6}, would revoke no tolerances for fungicides used on potatoes. The EPA's Tolerance Assessment System (TAS) currently assumes that most potatoes are consumed in the nonprocessed form. They are usually cooked fresh and consumed as baked, boiled, or fried potatoes. In the average U.S. diet, the TAS calculates that less than 1 percent of all potatoes are consumed in processed forms, such as chips or dried instant potatoes. Accordingly, the risk from consumption of processed potatoes calculated on the percentage of acres treated is less than 10^{-6} for all fungicides. Even though the risk from at least one fungicide on whole potatoes exceeds 10^{-6}, scenario 4 would revoke no tolerances for potato fungicides.

Tomato Fungicides

Scenarios 1 and 2 would revoke tolerances for 11 oncogenic active ingredients accounting for approximately 50 percent of all acre treatments and 51 percent of all tomato fungicide expenditures. All dietary oncogenic risk from tomatoes would be eliminated, and 11 of the 20 fungicides registered for use on tomatoes would lose tolerances. Scenarios 3 and 4, which would apply to 10 of these 11 oncogenic fungicides for which risk estimates were possible, would revoke tolerances for only five active ingredients but the impact would be nearly the same. The estimated dietary oncogenic risk from fungicides on tomatoes would be reduced by 99 percent, and tolerances would be lost for active ingredients accounting for 49 percent of all acre treatments and 51 percent of expenditures. As with all the fungicide-crop combinations examined, the impact of scenarios 3 and 4 would most likely continue past these initial tolerance revocations. Tolerance revocations for the five compounds would result in the increased use of other oncogenic tomato fungicides. As this occurred, the risk from these replacement compounds would probably exceed 10^{-6} and trigger tolerance revocations for them as well.

The midwestern and southeastern growing regions would feel the loss of these oncogenic tomato fungicides the most. Growers in the Midwest, East, and Southeast apply 85 percent of all oncogenic fungicides to tomatoes, even though less than one-third of all tomatoes are grown in these regions.[2] Approximately 80 percent of these applications are made in southeastern states. Nearly two-thirds of all tomatoes consumed in the United States are grown in California, yet less than 10 percent of the total pounds of oncogenic fungicides used on tomatoes are applied there.[3]

The committee's survey of non-oncogenic tomato fungicides in development or in field testing indicates a moderate degree of activity in this area. Nonetheless, the committee is unable to judge the relative efficacy of these compounds. It appears that as many as eight new compounds are currently being tested for control of the eight major tomato diseases, however. This finding suggests that additional non-oncogenic alternative fungicides for control of tomato diseases may be available within several years.

Peanut Fungicides

Because TAS assumes no processed peanut food forms for the 53 oncogenic pesticides examined, the results of the scenarios on peanuts differ from the committee's other crop-level analyses. Neither scenario 2 nor 4 would result in any lost tolerances. Because no single fungicide risk exceeds 10^{-6}, no tolerances would be revoked under scenario 3. Only scenario 1 would revoke peanut fungicide tolerances.

Oncogenic compounds account for about 86 percent of all acre treatments and 83 percent of all expenditures for fungicides on peanuts. Under scenario 1, all benefits associated with these fungicides would be lost. Because peanuts are grown entirely in the Southeast, and federal marketing orders bar expansion or movement of peanut cultivation to other regions, the impact of scenario 1 would be concentrated in these southeastern states.

The committee's survey of plant pathologists and examination of the most recent test results in *Fungicide and Nematicide Tests* indicate that there are three or four new fungicides that control major peanut diseases as well as the currently used oncogenic fungicides.[4] Although none of these have tolerances for use on peanuts yet, it appears that non-oncogenic fungicides could become available in the near future.

ALTERNATIVES TO THE SCENARIOS

On the basis of an analysis of the eight crops discussed, the potential agricultural impact of all scenarios seems severe when measured by the percentage of acre treatments and expenditures associated with revoked tolerances. Efforts to eliminate oncogenic residues in fungicide-treated crops could yield the greatest public health benefits, but could also force significant adjustments in agricultural practices. In light of this finding, the committee decided to explore the impact of cropwide tolerance reduction as a way to reduce risk from fungicide residues in food.

Fungicides: A Special Case

Fungicide sales in 1985 totaled $269 million, or slightly more than 7 percent of all agricultural pesticides sales.[5] In contrast to their small market share, fungicides account for 60 percent of all estimated oncogenic risk. They also provide significant benefits per acre for producers of high-value fruit and vegetable crops. Many growers rely heavily on fungicides, particularly in humid regions.

Implementation of any of the scenarios could present problems because relatively few new fungicides have gained registration or been granted tolerances in recent years. Although 14 percent of all R&D expeditures by major U.S. pesticide manufacturers were spent on new fungicide research and development—a commitment roughly twice the percentage of fungicide sales—the fungicide market remains an elusive target for most major agrichemical firms.[6] Only four products registered since 1972 have gained market shares greater than 5 percent for any food crop.[7] In contrast, several herbicides and insecticides introduced during the same time have gained significant market shares, especially the pyrethroid insecticides for use on cotton and vegetables and several new corn and soybean herbicides.

Almost all newer fungicides are systemic in action; that is, the material translocates to another part of the plant from where it was applied and residues are generally found inside the plant rather than on its surface. Because of this, systemic fungicides often encourage pathogen resistance. On the other hand, fewer of the new fungicides are oncogenic, and those that are oncogenic tend to be less potent. Older oncogenic fungicides tend to be nonsystemic in action, and most have yet to develop any serious resistance problems.

The problems of resistance and the lack of product diversity and depth are complicated by the following circumstances peculiar to fungicides as a class:

• Approximately 90 percent of all fungicides used in agriculture are animal oncogens. Many of these compounds are substitutes for each other. Regulatory action taken to reduce oncogenic risks from use of one fungicide will often result in wider use of another oncogen. Indeed, unless the sequence and timing of regulatory actions are carefully planned, total dietary cancer risk from fungicide residues could rise.

• In general, raw commodity tolerances for most oncogenic fungicides (except benomyl and some EBDCs on certain crops) were established in the absence of modern residue chemistry data. These tolerances are generally well above actual residue levels and tend to overstate risks from residues of these fungicides on crops.

• The dietary risk from residues of these compounds in certain processed foods is probably understated, however, because of the scarcity of processing studies and consequent lack of processed-food tolerances. Complete data on residue concentration in processed foods exist only for benomyl. Except for tolerances for captan on raisins and mancozeb on raisins, rye, oats, and wheat, no oncogenic fungicide other than benomyl has any section 409 tolerances. Yet it is certain that fungicide residues concentrate in processed foods made from several crops. Fungicide tolerances for residues in animal products are also incomplete.

• The use of fungicides in agriculture is concentrated in humid regions of the country, principally the East and particularly the Southeast. Important regional implications need to be considered in evaluating alternative regulatory policies.

The combination of these factors makes regulation of oncogenic risk from fungicides a complex and delicate problem. The committee believes that the Delaney Clause, as traditionally interpreted, is not responsive to these considerations. Literal implementation could complicate EPA attempts to reduce dietary cancer risk from fungicides.

The following analyses are the results of the committee's effort to better understand the challenge confronting the EPA. The committee emphasizes the need for an approach to reduce fungicide risk that takes all the above factors into account. The approach considered here—cropwide tolerance reduction—differs significantly from the automatic tolerance revocations by the scenarios analyzed above and from current EPA practice.

Cropwide Tolerance Reduction

The most compelling argument for addressing the risk posed by all oncogenic pesticides of a given class, such as fungicides, on a given crop is the difficulty of ensuring that regulatory actions against a single compound will reduce dietary risks. Addressing the risk posed by all oncogenic agents in a single class used on a crop requires consideration of different risk reduction measures than those typically used for one compound. Strategies of tolerance reduction or even establishment of zero tolerances have particular appeal here for several reasons:

• Zero and level-of-detection tolerances, which are tolerances set when the only residue allowed is that undetectable at the limit of detection, as well as tolerance reductions, have been applied in regulating some of the oncogenic fungicides on tobacco and certain vegetable crops exported to Canada and elsewhere.

• The EPA has used level-of-detection tolerances to bypass the Delaney Clause (see the permethrin case study in Appendix C) and to allow the use of an economically valuable oncogenic compound.

• Tolerance revocations for individual fungicides, implemented one compound at a time, could actually cause estimated dietary risk to rise.

A cropwide tolerance reduction strategy is useful for fungicides because the market is dominated by oncogenic compounds that are ready substitutes for each other; few viable non-oncogenic alternative fungicides are in development; and tolerances for many of the widely used older compounds are well above the levels that properly treated crops at the time of harvest should have. In contrast, cropwide tolerance reduction is probably not the optimal strategy for reducing dietary oncogenic risk from corn and soybean herbicides and cotton insecticides because there are numerous non-oncogenic substitutes; risk is attributable to one or two compounds; and tolerances, because they are generally newer, more accurately reflect actual residue levels in food.

Table 5-4 presents the order in which the EPA will face regulatory decisions on oncogenic fungicides. As described in Chapter 3, these dates represent the time by which the EPA expects to have completed a special review *and* registration standard for each of these oncogenic fungicides. At the conclusion of these processes, the EPA will probably know with relative certainty whether a pesticide is an animal oncogen and whether

TABLE 5-4   Potential Short-Term Impact of the Delaney Clause on Selected Fungicides

Active Ingredient	Date of Possible Tolerance Action	Action	Estimated Risk			Fungicide Market Share (% pounds applied)
			Raw	Processed	Total	
Benomyl	1986	RS[a]	3.42×10^{-5}	7.91×10^{-5}	1.13×10^{-4}	10
Captafol	1987	SR[b]	4.34×10^{-4}	1.59×10^{-4}	5.94×10^{-4}	5
EBDCs						35
Mancozeb	1987	RS	2.43×10^{-4}	9.44×10^{-5}	3.38×10^{-4}	
Maneb	1987	RS	3.90×10^{-4}	5.22×10^{-5}	4.42×10^{-4}	
Metiram	1987	RS	7.65×10^{-5}	3.91×10^{-5}	1.15×10^{-4}	
Zineb	1987	RS	4.71×10^{-4}	2.45×10^{-4}	7.17×10^{-4}	
Folpet	1987	RS	1.81×10^{-4}	1.43×10^{-4}	3.24×10^{-4}	5
Captan	1988	SR	2.80×10^{-4}	1.93×10^{-4}	4.74×10^{-4}	15
Chlorothalonil	1988	SR	1.89×10^{-4}	4.82×10^{-5}	2.37×10^{-4}	10

NOTE: These risk estimates are derived using EPA data and methods described on pages 50–66 and in Appendix B.

[a]RS is registration standard.
[b]SR is special review.

residues of that pesticide concentrate in processed foods. With such information available, the EPA will have to decide whether or not to revoke or modify tolerances under the Delaney Clause.

To determine whether tolerance revocations might increase the risk presented by oncogenic fungicide residues in major fruit and vegetable crops, the committee performed a simple analysis for benomyl and the EBDCs. For selected crops, the percentage of acres treated with a fungicide is assumed to be zero to simulate the effect of tolerance revocation. Then, the shares of total acres treated with the likely replacements are raised to compensate for the loss of the compound eliminated. A new estimate of dietary risk is then computed.

All risk estimates analyzed below assume residues at the tolerance level, incorporate TAS residue estimates for processed foods for which no section 409 tolerances have been established, and are adjusted to reflect the percentage of planted acres assumed to be treated with each fungicide.

BENOMYL

The fungicide benomyl is the first fungicide active ingredient registered before 1978 for which complete residue and oncogenicity data are available. Benomyl residues concentrate in several processed foods, and

TABLE **5-5** Estimated Change in Dietary Oncogenic Risk in Some
Crops from Revoking Benomyl Tolerances

Benomyl Acres Treated with Replacement Fungicide (%)	Dietary Oncogenic Risk (%) in —			
	Apples	Peanuts	Potatoes	Tomatoes
No replacement	−4.8	−1.1	NA	−1.5
Captan (50) Mancozeb (50)	+26.4	NA	NA	+3.2
Chlorothalonil (100)	NA	+14.8	NA	+1.5

NOTE: NA means the pesticide is not used or is not considered a likely substitute pesticide on that crop.

benomyl is a confirmed animal oncogen. If benomyl tolerances were revoked pursuant to the Delaney Clause (residues are assumed to concentrate in all crops examined), little or no reduction in risk would be achieved (see Table 5-5). This is because, on the basis of current data, benomyl generally poses a lower dietary risk than the most likely substitute fungicides.

For each of the crops analyzed, substitution of other compounds for the revoked benomyl tolerances raised the estimated dietary oncogenic risk. Significant increases are evident in apples where benomyl-treated acres were evenly divided between captan and the EBDC fungicide mancozeb. Following this substitution, risk from apple fungicides rose more than 26 percent. In peanuts, dietary oncogenic risk would rise nearly 15 percent if all acres now treated with benomyl were subsequently treated with chlorothalonil.

EBDCs

Revocation of tolerances for the EBDC fungicides would yield mixed results. For some crops the dietary risk from fungicides would rise, for others it would stay about the same, and for some it would be reduced significantly.

Captafol and chlorothalonil are considered the most likely replacements for EBDC use on tomatoes. If the acres previously treated with EBDCs were evenly divided between captafol and chlorothalonil, the risk from fungicide residues in or on tomato products would rise almost 50 percent (see Table 5-6).

There are more replacement fungicides for use on apples than other crops; thus, many more substitution scenarios could unfold. In all cases examined by the committee, the risk from fungicide residues in apples

TABLE 5-6   Estimated Change in Dietary Oncogenic Risk in Some Crops from Revoking EBDC Tolerances

EBDC Acres Treated with Replacement Fungicide (%)	Dietary Oncogenic Risk (%) in —		
	Apples	Potatoes	Tomatoes
Chlorothalonil (50) Captafol (50)	NA	NA	+46
Captan (100)	−18	NA	NA
Captan (40) Folpet (60)	−6.7	NA	NA
Captan (60) Benomyl (40)	−33	NA	NA
Chlorothalonil (100)	NA	−62.1	NA

NOTE: NA means the pesticide is not used or is not considered a likely substitute pesticide on that crop.

was reduced. This reduction was not always significant, however. When captan was applied to 40 percent of EBDC acres and folpet to 60 percent, the result was a 6.7 percent risk reduction. The greatest risk reduction, 33 percent, would occur if 60 percent of the former EBDC acres were treated with captan and 40 percent with benomyl.

Revocation of EBDC tolerances achieved the greatest reduction in dietary oncogenic risk for potatoes. The committee assumed that all acres treated with EBDCs would be treated with chlorothalonil. This assumption reduced estimated risk by 62 percent.

The point of these projections is that any regulatory strategy, whether based on the Delaney Clause or any other standard, that attempts to reduce dietary oncogenic risk from fungicides by addressing compounds one at a time will not produce significantly lower risks. The one-pesticide-at-a-time approach may actually increase risk for many widely consumed crops that currently present significant dietary oncogenic risks. The Delaney Clause could worsen this phenomenon if the EPA revoked tolerances for oncogenic fungicides in the order in which data are available to make such decisions. The committee concludes that reducing tolerance levels for all oncogenic fungicides crop by crop will yield greater risk reductions than sequential actions to control individual fungicides across all of their uses. Furthermore, tolerance reductions and even zero tolerances are viable options that could be applied to many pesticides on many crops.

NOTES

1. U.S. Department of Agriculture. 1985. Agricultural Statistics 1985. Washington, D.C.: U.S. Government Printing Office.
2. U.S. Department of Agriculture. 1984. Vegetables. Washington, D.C.: U.S. Government Printing Office.
3. U.S. Environmental Protection Agency. 1986. Unpublished data. Washington, D.C.
4. Ritchie, D., ed. 1985. Fungicide and Nematicide Tests. Vol. 40. St. Paul, Minn.: American Phytopathological Society.
5. National Agricultural Chemicals Association. 1985. P. 3 in Impact of Current Law on Agricultural Pesticide Research Productivity. Washington, D.C. Photocopy.
6. *Ibid.*, p. 13.
7. U.S. Environmental Protection Agency. 1986. Unpublished data. Washington, D.C.

6

Pesticide Innovation and the Economic Effects of Implementing the Delaney Clause

The economic effects in the agricultural sector of regulatory actions taken pursuant to the Delaney Clause will depend on a number of factors. These include the availability of effective currently registered alternative chemicals and the extent and success of chemical and nonchemical new product innovation in pest control. This chapter examines the innovation process and seeks to determine whether the Delaney Clause has had or will have an impact on it. This chapter also assesses the status of pest control innovation in major areas such as plant breeding, genetic engineering, and biological, cultural, and chemical pest control.

As seen in Chapter 3, the committee's estimated current level of oncogenic risk is largely associated with old pesticides. Nearly all estimated herbicide and fungicide risk and more than half of the estimated insecticide risk are from pre-1978 products. If the Delaney Clause were applied to existing tolerances for currently registered, potentially oncogenic active ingredients, food tolerances for many economically valuable pesticides would be lost. The resulting void would create significant market opportunities for new non-oncogenic pesticides and other pest control technologies. The predictable losses in company income, however, might discourage overall investment in pesticide innovation research.

Chapters 4 and 5 discuss four scenarios and tolerance reduction approaches that the EPA might follow in regulating oncogenic pesticides. Each scenario would require the revocation of many tolerances for fungicides. Herbicides and insecticides would be affected to a lesser extent. The two chapters focus on the short-term effects of the scenarios; this chapter examines the scenarios' long-term effects on pest control innovation.

It is difficult to determine whether pest control R&D efforts are designed to eliminate oncogenic pesticide residues from the food supply. It is even harder to determine whether the Delaney Clause is causing the development of less-oncogenic or non-oncogenic pesticides. Experience from past changes in EPA policies provides some insight, but there have been few changes in federal regulation of cancer-causing agents. This lack of data prevents studies that attempt to correlate pesticide R&D invest-ments with different regulations on exposure to oncogens.

Another important issue is the possible effects of rapid pesticide cancellations on R&D. In the past, single compounds have been canceled. There are no data on the effects of the few pesticide cancellations on total R&D activity. To gain information, the committee questioned industry research directors, reviewed available studies on the impacts of EPA pesticide regulations and FDA drug regulations, compiled information from various sources on past levels and rates of pesticide innovation, and analyzed other innovation indicators such as the number of new pesti-cides for certain crops field tested recently.

THE INNOVATION PROCESS AND THE PESTICIDE INDUSTRY

The pesticide innovation process involves finding and developing new compounds that are effective and safe, improving formulations of older compounds, expanding uses of older compounds to more crops and pests, and satisfying regulatory data requirements. The pesticide innovation cycle goes beyond industry's discovery of new compounds. It includes the government's approval or acceptance of product registrations, grower awareness and adoption of new products, and long-term product viability. The last two phases depend on a new pesticide's profitability, successful integration with other farming practices, availability for minor crop use, and susceptibility to pest resistance.

The development of a new pesticide is a long and expensive process. The sequence of activities is shown in Figure 6-1. Usually 9 to 10 years will elapse from discovery to first registration. After registration, the market life for different pesticides varies greatly. Many pesticides widely used today, such as 2,4-D, parathion, and the ethylenebisdithiocarbamate (EBDC) fungicides, have been on the market for 35 years or more. But products may lose their market share and be removed from the market for many reasons. These include regulatory restrictions triggered by safety concerns; competition with more active, lower-cost pesticides or nonchemical pest controls; crop acreage adjustments; or pest resistance.

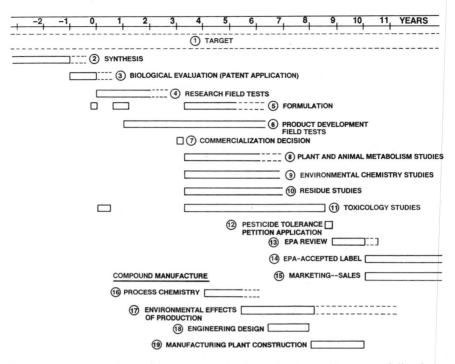

FIGURE 6-1 Pesticide development from production to commercialization. Source: Sharp, D. 1986. Metabolism of Pesticides—An Industry View. Paper presented at the Sixth International Congress of Pesticide Chemists, Ottawa, Canada, August 10-15, 1986.

Many of the organochlorine insecticides have been replaced for one or more of these reasons.

Besides the variability of a product's market life, economic returns from a pesticide company's R&D investments can be greatly affected by the uncertainty in the process of actually finding new pesticides. For certain pesticides, particularly insecticides, it is increasingly difficult to find new, effective products through conventional screening of available chemicals. About 23,000 new compounds are now screened for each new pesticide discovered; 10 years ago the figure was 10,000.[1]

It is not surprising that the pesticide industry devotes large sums of money to research. Multinational agrichemical companies spend from 9 to 15 percent of sales revenue on R&D.[2] Most R&D in pesticide and pharmaceutical companies is internally financed and conducted. Otherwise, the company's proprietary information may be leaked. The drawback with internal financing is that if products are unexpectedly canceled, funds available for R&D may shrink.

REVIEW OF INDUSTRY R&D AND STUDIES TO DATE

Although there have been no studies of how regulatory attempts to control carcinogens may affect pesticide innovation, there have been studies on how other EPA pesticide restrictions affect the total level and nature of R&D efforts.

The committee examined four major studies in this area: (1) a 1981 study by the Council on Agricultural Science and Technology (CAST); (2) a 1981 report by the Office of Technology Assessment (OTA); (3) a 1982 Ph.D. thesis by U. Hatch; and (4) a 1984 study by H. G. Grawbowski and W. K. Viscusi.

The four studies indicate how regulatory delay and uncertainty affect R&D activities. The CAST study found that from 1968 to 1978, direct costs of bringing a new pesticide to market increased; delays from discovery to first registration grew; and R&D expenditures shifted from synthesis, screening, and field testing to registration, environmental testing, and residue analysis.[3]

The OTA report emphasized that total pesticide R&D expenditures continued to rise following the 1972 amendments to the Federal Insecticide, Fungicide and Rodenticide Act (FIFRA). The increase in real R&D investments did not cause more new pesticide registrations, however.[4]

Hatch attempted to quantify the relationships among the following factors: delay from discovery to registration, FIFRA changes, and the number of new active ingredients registered per million dollars of R&D expenditures from 1967 to 1982. Total R&D expenditures and R&D expenditures allocated to new chemical discoveries were used for estimates. The estimated impact from a 10 percent longer delay in registration was a 7 to 9 percent decrease in products registered. The creation of the EPA in 1970 and the 1978 amendments to FIFRA seemed to have no effects on R&D productivity.[5]

Grawbowski and Viscusi showed that from 1971 to 1975, R&D allotments declined when compared to sales. These figures might have reflected rapidly rising pesticide sales rather than a reduction in investments in response to the EPA's early activities. Grawbowski and Viscusi also showed that the effective patent life for commercial pesticides fell from 15 years during 1971 to 1976 to 12 years during 1977 to 1982. They suggested that the delay in commercialization might reflect the longer time needed to develop new products or meet regulatory requirements for new technology compared with the regulation of variants of established products.[6] A related study on the pharmaceutical industry by Graw-bowski and Vernon found that stricter regulations induced innovation only in techniques for complying with regulatory requirements, such as improved equipment for detecting drug residues.[7] This indicates that the implementation of the Delaney Clause might not lead to development of non-oncogenic pest control methods.

The committee also addressed the extent to which unexpected product cancellations might reduce R&D investments. The regulatory scenarios examined in Chapter 4 contemplate tolerance revocation for existing product uses. Increased uncertainty of pesticide profits would reduce pesticide investments. Cancellations of existing uses of some pesticides could increase R&D investments only if they provided new sales opportunities for other pesticides and did not severely limit funds for internally financed reinvestment. Profit opportunities from cancellation of a competitor's products are affected by the availability of alternative pest controls and adjustments in crop patterns.

Survey of R&D Directors

The committee questioned the research directors of 20 pesticide companies. These directors are involved in planning investment responses to changes in regulations by the EPA and other federal agencies. They want a regulatory environment that will give farmers and consumers confidence that pesticide products and food are safe. They also want to sell their products. Thus, their responses may reflect a wish to reduce regulatory impacts. A few summaries of results from the survey are described here. The complete survey and results are presented in Appendix E.

Asked how many pesticides would be vulnerable to Delaney Clause restrictions during reregistration (assuming the EPA's current policies continue), the research directors responded that 24 percent of currently registered pesticides representing about 9 percent of total sales are in jeopardy. About half of the fungicides and 10 to 20 percent of the insecticides were cited as vulnerable. In addition to the loss of products, the research directors thought there would be a slight increase in testing costs (5 to 15 percent). More than half said that the EPA's implementation of the Delaney Clause had caused a one- to two-year delay in new product registrations. Companies often respond to a potential denial of registrations by attempting to change use patterns to reduce residues. They may not discontinue research or registration efforts for a potential new pesticide if initial testing indicates one with weak oncogenicity. The research directors viewed the Delaney Clause as an important regulation. They identified other problems such as groundwater contamination as more serious, however.

Historical Perspective of R&D

A pesticide firm needs a dynamic R&D program if it is to remain competitive. As shown in Table 6-1, total deflated expenditures on R&D have risen steadily during the last 20 years. In 1985, about 64 percent of all expenditures on pesticide R&D in the United States were for discovering and developing new products, 23 percent for expanding uses of existing products, and 13 percent for defending older products.[8] Industry experienced an increase of 14.4 percent for R&D expenditures in 1985 compared with 6 percent in 1983 (Table 6-1). This was in the face of a 9 percent drop in domestic pesticide sales between 1984 and 1985.

Most pesticide R&D in the United States takes place at about 20 multinational corporations that manufacture active ingredients for pesticides. Hundreds of middle-sized and small companies develop, produce,

TABLE 6-1   Pesticide Industry Total R&D Expenditures

Year	Undeflated (millions of dollars)	Deflated[a] (millions of dollars)	Annual Increase Deflated (%)
1967	$ 52.4	$ 65.9	
1968	58.2	70.6	7.1
1969	64.1	73.8	4.5
1970	69.9	76.4	3.5
1971	87.7	91.4	19.6
1972	98.5	98.5	7.8
1973	110.7	104.7	6.3
1974	134.8	117.1	11.8
1975	160.5	127.6	9.0
1976	195.2	147.5	15.6
1977	250.1	178.5	21.0
1978	289.6	192.5	7.8
1979	332.3	203.3	5.6
1980	395.1	221.2	8.8
1981	449.9	230.1	4.0
1982	526.9	254.3	10.5
1983	580.2	269.5	6.0
1984	730.6	327.0	21.3
1985	868.9	374.2	14.4
		Average	10.2

[a]This column expresses deflation by the GNP deflator (1972 = 100).

SOURCE: Hatch U., 1983, The Impact of Regulatory Delay on R&D Productivity and Costs in the Pesticide Industry, Ph.D. dissertation, University of Minnesota, St. Paul; National Agricultural Chemical Association, 1986, Industry Profile Survey: 1985, Washington, D.C. Photocopy.

and blend thousands of pesticide mixtures and retail products, but they conduct little research to develop new active ingredients. Smaller firms conduct more R&D in biological and genetically engineered pest control, however.[9]

Long- and short-term innovation prospects are important in assessing Delaney Clause implications. As discussed previously, the EPA schedule of pesticide reregistrations will require decisions in the next three to five years on many products that currently have large sales. This places an emphasis on pesticide development and marketing pesticides that have already entered field testing. Compounds being developed have the potential to lessen short-term effects of pesticide use cancellations. The next 9 to 10 years will probably be the shortest feasible time to bring new pesticide chemistry or biotechnology products to market. It will be even longer before the products are widely adopted by farmers.

One indication of innovation's rate and trend is the number of pesticides registered for the first time each year. This information for the past 20 years is shown in Table 6-2. (Only about two-thirds of these pesticides have agricultural uses.) Overall, the introduction of products for agricultural use decreased, even though firms submitted 25 new pesticide compounds for registration in 1985, which was 10 more than in 1984. Some promising new herbicides were also registered for use in 1986. However, new products must compete with the performance of and farmers' loyalties to existing products. As a result there are considerable differences in the adoption and sales of new products compared with older ones.

INSECTICIDES

In the last 40 years, the major three classes of pesticides—insecticides, herbicides, and fungicides—have evolved at different rates. The chemistry of insecticide products has developed through four generations: (1) organochlorines, such as DDT, chlordane, aldrin, and dieldrin; (2) organophosphates, such as parathion; (3) carbamates, such as carbaryl and carbofuran; and (4) pyrethroids, including permethrin and cypermethrin. Changes in use patterns were influenced by acute and chronic toxicity, environmental effects, and insect resistance to widely used compounds.

Regulatory actions based on chronic health and environmental effects have largely eliminated all uses of organochlorine insecticides on foods. Organophosphate and carbamate insecticides remain widely used; synthetic pyrethroids continue to gain market share. Pest resistance, however, has become a limiting factor in the success of chemical insecticides. Synthetic pyrethroids were widely considered a breakthrough when

TABLE 6-2 Number of Chemicals Registered for the First Time as Pesticides Under FIFRA (1967–1984)

Year	Pesticide Bactericide, Slimicide	Fungicide	Herbicide	Insecticide	Nematocide	Rodenticide	Other	Total	Agricultural or Forestry Uses
1967	5	2	2	4	0	2	1	16	NA
1968	4	5	2	6	0	0	1	18	NA
1969	2	0	4	7	0	0	1	14	NA
1970	3	2	2	1	0	0	2	10	NA
1971	1	1	0	0	0	1	1	4	NA
1972	5	6	5	4	0	0	1	21	11
1973	2	4	3	5	1	0	0	15	10
1974	0	6	8	6	1	1	0	22	14
1975	11	5	11	8	0	0	1	36	18
1976	4	2	3	2	0	0	1	12	7
1977	1	0	1	1	0	0	0	3	2
1978	0	1	2	2	0	0	1	6	5
1979	0	4	2	8	0	1	2	17	14
1980	0	1	3	4	0	2	1	11	6
1981	3	2	4	6	0	0	3	18	10
1982	5	2	7	5	0	2	1	22	15
1983	1	3	4	6	0	0	2	16	9
1984	2	1	1	6	0	1	2	13	7

SOURCE: U.S. Environmental Protection Agency. 1985. Chemicals Registered for the First Time as Pesticidal Active Ingredients Under FIFRA. Washington, D.C. Photocopy.

introduced in the 1970s. But the emergence of resistance of some pests to pyrethroids in some areas is worrisome. In particular, pockets of resistance to pyrethroids by the tobacco budworm have been shown in cotton-producing areas of Texas. Since the pyrethroids, no new major chemical class of insecticide has been commercialized. Several new classes of insecticide show promise for a wide range of agricultural and public health uses, but there are no new classes of proven materials for control of the budworm and the bollworm.

HERBICIDES

The invention of new herbicides has flourished during the past 40 years with the development and wide acceptance of many different chemical classes. These include phenoxy herbicides, such as 2,4-D; triazines, such as atrazine and cyanazine; benzoic acids, such as dicamba; acetanilides, such as alachlor and metolachlor; ureas, such as linuron; and the nonselective, broad-spectrum glyphosate. In the past few years, the number of newly registered herbicides introduced into the market substantially surpassed the number of new agents in all other major categories of pesticides combined.

Several new herbicides were registered in 1986. These compounds represent the first marketable results of new herbicide chemistry. The two most important classes of new herbicides are the imidazolinones and the sulfonylureas. Tests show that these herbicides are non-oncogenic. They are generally applied at rates lower than the herbicides in wide use today.

The principal factor behind the success in chemical herbicide innovation is the size of the herbicide market. Agricultural herbicide sales in the United States are about $2.7 billion. This is about two and one-half times the size of the domestic insecticide market and about 10 times greater than the fungicide market.

As discussed previously, some of the widely used herbicides are suspected or confirmed animal oncogens. Oncogenic herbicides account for about 60 percent of current expenditures for chemical weed control (see Chapter 3). Possible regulatory actions restricting the use of these herbicides could create opportunities for new herbicides or other weed control methods.

FUNGICIDES

The unique case of fungicides has been discussed at length in Chapters 3–5. Fungicides registered in the 1940s and 1950s currently dominate the market because they are relatively inexpensive, effective against a broad range of pathogens, less prone to pest resistance problems, and exhibit low acute toxicity. In addition, they are often important in integrated disease management programs. These factors give existing products a formidable competitive edge over new fungicidal compounds. Yet, it is in dealing with fungicides that a strict application of the Delaney Clause may most significantly affect current product use.

Ninety percent of all fungicide acre treatments are with potential animal oncogens. Furthermore, chronic toxicity to humans is likely to remain a problem because it is difficult to develop fungicides that are not toxic to genetic material. As a result, the fungicides, and growers who rely heavily on them, are particularly vulnerable to actions to restrict dietary exposure to potential oncogenic compounds. To aggravate this problem, the science involved in producing new fungicides is extremely complex, and developments in recent years have been minor.[10] For example, in the past 15 years, only four new fungicides have been introduced that account for more than 5 percent of sales in any food crop. This is not because fungicide research and development expenditures have lagged. These investments are nearly twice as high relative to sales as are investments for herbicides and insecticides. Because total fungicide sales are relatively small, however, total fungicide research is modest. Also, because individual fungicide markets are small, there is less economic incentive for innovation and product expansion. Further, the development of products for minor crops is not often profitable for pesticide companies. (The influence of market size on pesticide registration is discussed at greater length later in this chapter.) Some new product work in Europe has been directed toward combinations of old and new fungicides.

FUTURE PROSPECTS IN CHEMICAL PEST CONTROL

It is difficult to obtain an accurate count of the pesticides for which new registrations are being sought that will become available for commercial use. Using the number of tolerance petitions for this purpose can be misleading because the percentage of petitions for new active ingredient tolerances not granted is unknown.

Because of these uncertainties, the committee obtained information from specialists in crop protection and published reports of field tests to learn which unregistered pesticides are now being field tested. The inquiry concentrated on the production of selected crops that might be affected by the cancellation of currently marketed pesticides. Some of the pesticides being reviewed are already registered for use on other crops; others have no current registration. The results help clarify which compounds are being developed and provide some indication of chemical substitution possibilities in the next five years.

TABLE 6-3 Evaluation of Experimental and Unregistered Citrus Insecticides

Target Pest	Number of Compounds	Comparison to Best Commercially Available Standard		
		Better	Similar	Poorer
Thrips				
Compounds near registration	4	0	1	3
Compounds under evaluation	6	0	0	6
Red mite	10		3[a]	
California red scale	4	0	0	4

NOTE: A total of 19 insecticides were tested by insecticide and acaricide tests.

[a]Evaluations for only 3 of the 10 materials were adequate to provide a comparison to commercial standards. The remaining 7 need additional testing.

SOURCE: York, Alan C., ed. 1985. *Insecticide and Acaracide Tests*. Vol. 10. College Park, Md.: Entomological Society of America.

Citrus and Cotton Insecticides

The committee's findings for the citrus insecticides are presented in Table 6-3. Except for three products to control red mites and one to control thrips, the compounds being tested were judged less effective than currently available insecticides and acaricides.

Thirteen unregistered cotton insecticides were evaluated and reported in *Insecticide and Acaricide Tests*.[11] Some were tested on more than one pest. Eight new materials were tested on bollworms, eight on boll weevils, two on cotton fleahoppers, one on cotton aphids, and six on spider mites. Variability in results precluded a valid comparison with the best commercially available insecticides.

Cotton pest control research is inspired more by potential pest resistance than by the Delaney Clause. Currently available non-oncogenic cotton insecticides and integrated pest management programs appear adequate to sustain the U.S. cotton industry.

Corn and Soybean Herbicides

Several products representing new chemistry (most notably the imidazolinone and sulfonylurea compounds) have been commercially introduced in the past several years. Manufacturers now are more sophisticated in designing new molecules with herbicidal activity. Because one or more functional groups of chemicals are known to affect

TABLE 6-4   Number of Herbicides in Field Tests

Weeds/Stage	Corn	Soybeans
Broadleaf weeds		
Preplant	1	1
Preemergence	0	0
Pre- and postemergence	0	2
Postemergence	0	0
Grass weeds		
Preplant	1	3
Preemergence	0	0
Pre- and postemergence	0	3
Postemergence	1	1

SOURCE: Dexter, Alan G., ed. 1984. *North Central Weed Control Conference Research Report.* Vol. 41.

specific plant enzyme systems, the search for new herbicides is more logical today than 10 years ago.

The committee identified three new herbicides recently tested on corn (see Table 6-4). Their effectiveness in controlling weeds in the major groups of grasses and broadleaf weeds varied widely, as did the effectiveness of the commercially available herbicides with which they were compared. Because of the varied data, the new materials could not be ranked as superior, similar to, or poorer than the best herbicides now available. At present, more than 40 herbicides are registered for use on corn; about 10 are used on at least 1 million acres in the United States.

Ten herbicides were tested for weed control in soybeans: three for broadleaf weeds and seven for grasses (see Table 6-4). Here again, variability precluded a valid assessment of their effectiveness compared with that of the best commercially available standard. About 40 herbicides are now registered for use on soybeans, about 10 of which are used on at least 1 million acres in the United States.

Apple, Peanut, Potato, and Tomato Fungicides

New fungicides in the late stages of development were evaluated and compared with the best commercially available fungicides. The results are shown in Table 6-5. The data show that prospects are good for eradicants of apple scab and powdery mildew of apples and promising for two major diseases of peanuts. Prospects of new fungicides for summer diseases of apples, sclerotinia in peanuts, and nearly all potato diseases are poor, however. Several compounds are being evaluated and tested for control of tomato diseases, but performance results are not yet available.

TABLE 6-5 Evaluation of Experimental and Unregistered Fungicides

Target Pest Under Testing	Compounds (number)	Comparison to Best Commercially Available Standard		
		Better	Similar	Poorer
Apple Fungicides[a]				
Apple scab				
Eradicant	9	8	0	1
Protectant	8	0	3	5
Powdery mildew	9	7	1	1
Summer diseases[b]	9	0	0	9
Peanut Fungicides				
Leaf spot	9	2	4	3
Sclerotinia	2	0	1	1
Southern blight (white mold)	5	3	2	0
Potato Fungicides				
Early and late blight	3	0	3	0
Early blight	1	0	0	1
Late blight	2	0	0	2
Tomato Fungicides[c]				
Anthracnose	4			
Bacterial speck	6			
Bacterial spot	2			
Black rot	2			
Buckeye rot	4			
Early blight	2			
Rhizoctonia	1			
Root knot nematode	1			
Verticillium wilt	1			

[a]Nine fungicides were evaluated, some against more than one pest.

[b]Summer diseases include bitter rot, black rot, white rot, sooty blotch, fly speck, brooks spot, and black pox.

[c]Because only eight fungicides were tested, valid comparisons could not be made.

CHEMICAL PESTICIDE PROSPECTS RELATIVE TO DIETARY RISKS

Data on the effectiveness of pesticides now in the process of registration are limited. The EPA generally does not use such data to evaluate the pesticides. More testing must be done before the effectiveness of new materials can be compared with that of the best now commercially available. Some products have been tested for six to eight years without obtaining registration.

Non-oncogenic products now being developed are only one part of total innovation. Non-oncogenic products that are registered and might serve as substitutes for canceled products should also be included. When both are considered, the prospects for an adequate supply of pesticides for effective chemical pest control is good for herbicides, fair for insecticides, and poor for fungicides (Table 6-6). If past trends continue, prospects for future product development will depend primarily on anticipated market size and profitability. Firms are investing in fungicide R&D at a rate disproportionate to market share, however. This relatively high investment rate may reflect scale diseconomies and the likelihood of future cancellations.

Sales of all types of pesticides declined in 1985, but their market shares remained stable. Of total pesticide sales, herbicides, insecticides, and fungicides accounted for 66, 23, and 7 percent of the market, respectively. Herbicides, insecticides, and fungicides accounted for 48, 22, and 14 percent of R&D expenditures, respectively. Considering market share and R&D expenditures on these different classes of pesticides, it is not surprising that there are many alternative herbicides, a modest number of alternative insecticides, and few alternative fungicides.

Unfortunately, the rate of successful product innovation is almost inversely proportional to dietary oncogenic risk. Fungicides account for more than 60 percent of estimated risk, herbicides for about 27 percent, and insecticides for about 13 percent (Table 6-6 and Figure 6-2). Because market share and profitability strongly affect R&D, it is doubtful that resource allocations will change significantly in the future despite the need for new fungicides.

The committee believes that the EPA's implementation of the Delaney Clause *could* affect future profits and R&D investment by—

TABLE 6-6   Current Status of Pesticides and Available Alternatives

Type of Pesticide	Pesticide Sales (%)[a]	Industry R&D Expenditures (%)	Estimated Oncogenic Risk (%)[b]	Alternatives for Major Classes of Pest	
				Chemicals Available	Research[c]
Herbicide	66	48	27	Excellent	Good
Insecticide	23	22	13	Fair/good	Fair
Fungicide	7	14	60	Poor	Poor

[a]The percentages do not add to 100 percent because of other pesticide types (National Agricultural Chemicals Association. 1986. Industry Profile Survey: 1985. Washington, D.C. Photocopy).

[b]Percentages are from Chapter 3.

[c]This category represents the general level of research activity for the three major classes of pests: weeds, insects, and plant diseases. It is not intended to reflect long-term research for all classes of pests.

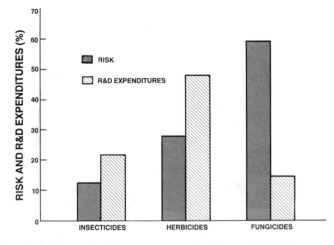

FIGURE 6-2 Estimated dietary oncogenic risk and R&D expenditures by pesticide type.

• Increasing costs for required test data to support tolerances for registration or reregistration;
• Shortening the commercial lives of pesticides through tolerance revocations or product cancellations;
• Increasing the borrowing costs when tests and other procedures prolong the time from discovery to marketing; and
• Increasing net return variability and thereby discouraging investment because of uncertainty about EPA implementation strategies.

INNOVATION PROSPECTS IN PEST CONTROL

Plant Breeding

Although plant breeding for resistance to pests began in the late nineteenth century, the development of crop varieties resistant to insect pests was not pursued energetically until recently. This lack of interest was primarily because resistance was difficult to achieve, and other low-cost, effective controls were often available. Nevertheless, plant breeders have developed more than 150 cultivars with insect resistance. The rewards of successful insect resistance research can be great. For example, federal, state, and private agencies spent about $9.3 million on developing resistance in wheat to the Hessian fly and wheat stem sawfly;

in alfalfa to the spotted alfalfa aphid; and in corn to the European corn borer. Savings to farmers from resistant varieties are estimated at several hundred million dollars annually, not including savings from eliminating pest control chemicals. Additional examples of insect-resistant crop cultivars include the resistance of rice to the brown planthopper, alfalfa to the pea aphid, and sorghum to the green bug.

Breeding for resistance to plant diseases has been pursued vigorously and to much greater advantage than for resistance to insects. This is in spite of the fact that some cultivars can resist only a few diseases, which enhances the possibility of an epidemic, such as the southern corn leaf blight in 1970. Resistant cultivars of cereal crops have been the mainstay of disease protection for many years. Success in crop breeding includes disease resistance of corn to southern corn leaf blight and other blights, wheat to stem rust, cucurbits to powdery mildew, cotton to *Fusarium* wilt, alfalfa to bacterial wilt, pears to fire blight, tobacco to bacterial wilt, and sugarcane to mosaic disease. Resistant cultivars have also been the major means of controlling parasitic nematodes, especially some species of root-knot, cyst-causing, and stem nematodes.

Some plants naturally produce chemicals that protect them against weeds and other pests. Cultivars are being developed that have traits for producing metabolites that are toxic to specific weeds, fungi, insects, or even grazing animals. For example, chemicals from the wild Bolivian potato have been correlated with its resistance to insect pests that attack potatoes cultivated in the United States. Scientists are working to breed these traits into U.S. potato varieties.

But, resistant cultivars do not necessarily stay resistant. Depending on crop management and biological factors, mutant organisms frequently develop. Therefore, different types of resistance must be incorporated into cultivars. Breeding for resistance requires no more time than the development of a new pesticide, and the expenditures of time and resources have been well worth it in many cases.

Genetic Engineering

Specific genetic characteristics can be manipulated in microbes and plants to achieve crop protection. (For an in-depth discussion, see *Agricultural Biotechnology: Strategies for National Competitiveness.*[12]) Genetic engineering could increase the potential for effective insect control via modification of bacteria, viruses, and fungi. For example, bacteria and viruses infecting insects could be genetically engineered to produce toxins that only kill specific insects. A possible candidate is the baculovirus, which infects only specific pests and is harmless to beneficial insects, vertebrates, and plants. However, development problems exist with baculoviruses, including the need to expand the range of particular viruses to encompass more than one pest species, the need to improve their environmental stability, and the facilitation of their large-scale commercial production.

Fungi also might be engineered as safe, effective insect and weed control agents. Many fungi produce specific toxins that act against insects or plants. Their "toxin" genes could be enhanced and transferred to new fungal hosts to create biological control agents that would attack only specific insects or weeds.

Plants themselves can be targets of genetic engineering. A crop can be genetically altered to express a specific, limited portion of a plant virus's genetic information, which would give the crop resistance to infection by that virus. Scientists have already achieved plant resistance to the tobacco mosaic virus, which causes large commercial losses of tomatoes and bell peppers as well as tobacco.

In a related strategy, the gene responsible for a plant's natural resistance to certain pathogens can often be transferred to a susceptible cultivar which might differ only by that single "resistance" gene.

Alternatively, the pathogen or its toxin can be used in the laboratory to select resistant cultivars from cell cultures. Intensive investigation on this front has led to isolation of some disease-resistant plants.

Research on herbicide-resistant crops is in progress. Resistant cultivars can be selected from cell cultures, a strategy that has been used to select imidazolinone-resistant corn. "Resistance" genes from other plants or even bacteria can be genetically engineered; glyphosate-resistant plants have been created by this technique. And, the two techniques are being combined to create crops resistant to sulfonylurea herbicides.

Fruit and vegetable seed markets, because they are small, will not stimulate rapid development of biotechnology products. Developments in pest control for minor crops from genetic engineering and conventional plant breeding are not likely to come soon enough to replace the many potential pesticide use cancellations in the next three to five years. Private genetic engineering firms will probably produce animal drugs and herbicide-resistant cultivars of major crops rather than alternative pest controls for those canceled by the Delaney Clause. Legal and regulatory issues have significantly curtailed development and testing of genetically engineered biological control agents. Until these issues are resolved, the benefits that these agents could provide will not be available to farmers in this country.

Biological Control

Biological control is the regulation of pest populations by natural enemies. In this report, biological pest control involves the intentional release or introduction of any biological organism, such as viruses, predators, pathogens, and parasites.

In the United States, biological control currently plays a limited but significant role in agriculture. In certain crops in some regions, biological control strategies are critical to continued production of important cash commodities. In many cases biological control methods have been integrated with selective use of chemical pesticides. For example, the release and establishment of predatory mites biologically controls spider mites on almonds in some areas of California. The predatory mites were selected in the laboratory for resistance to insecticides commonly used in almond production. This program has reduced the need to apply acaricide sprays and is less costly than total reliance on chemical pest control.

Compared with synthetic chemical pesticides, however, biological controls are applied against relatively few economically important agricultural pests. The potential for biological pest control has been significant for *specific* pests, as evidenced by valuable programs for certain crops. The development of biological control agents and systems is limited by the following factors:

• *The implementation and maintenance of effective management practices.* Biological control is complex compared with chemical spray treatments, schedules, and practices.

• *The specificity of biological control organisms.* Although some organisms may control a few pest species, usually a unique biological control is needed for each pest.

• *The mobility of certain control organisms.* This factor may lead to free benefits for some farmers from pest control paid for by other growers.[13]

Biological systems to manage insect pests have been established in several crops, most notably citrus, nuts, and apples. In addition, biological insect control agents are used as components of integrated pest control in cotton, citrus, rice, nuts, soybeans, fruits, vegetables, and deciduous fruit crops.

Several biological compounds are now registered or being considered for registration to control various insect pests. The use of *Bacillus thuringiensis* to control lepidopteran larvae is widespread. A few bacterial compounds are near final registration; among them are *Trichoderma* for the control of *Armillaria* root rot and *Agrobacterium radiobacter* for the control of crown gall.

Control can also be achieved by using insect pheromones, hormones, or their analogs to attract and trap pests, induce fruitless mating, or arrest development of insect larvae. Juvenile hormones are currently registered and sold to control flies, mosquitoes, fleas, and cockroaches. When applied as a spray, they arrest insect development at an immature stage, preventing reproduction as well as destructive adult-stage activities.

Although the genetically engineered *Pseudomonas syringae* protects crops from frost, not disease, it is a potentially significant biological control. Once field tests are permitted, tests with other genetically engineered organisms are expected to follow.

Nuclear polyhedrios viruses (NPVs) are being considered for control of a range of pests including the cotton bollworm, tussock moth, gypsy moth, alfalfa looper, and European pine sawfly. A granulosis virus has been identified that controls the codling moth.

Several insecticidal fungi are in use in various countries. It is necessary to remember, though, that some chemical fungicides kill insecticidal fungi unless applications are timed to avoid this.

Historically, biological control of weeds has been successful only for uncultivated areas. Recently, however, the control of several weeds in cultivated crops by fungal pathogens has been moderately successful. Unfortunately, the elimination of a weed species results in its replacement by another weed that may be more or less damaging than the first.

Research on the biological control of plant diseases is increasing so rapidly that the American Phytopathological Society will soon start publishing a journal devoted to that topic.

Cultural Pest Control

Cultural pest control involves manipulation of the crop or soil to make it less favorable for pests. Various cultural practices have been used since agriculture's beginnings, and will continue to be used. The incorporation of cultural practices into integrated pest management programs can be expected to increase because of cost savings. These practices include tillage, selection of a planting date to avoid a specific pest, crop rotation, stripcropping, interplanting, and destruction of crop remains to reduce habitats for overwintering pests. Increased emphasis is being placed on the management of economically important pests on crops including citrus, cotton, tomatoes, and alfalfa. Although integrated pest management programs can be highly effective, they frequently can be profitably applied only in limited regions. Nonetheless, in the future, more opportunities to combine genetic, chemical, biological, and cultural control strategies will emerge, changing the control of pests.

SPECIAL CHALLENGES TO INNOVATION

The Minor-Use Issue

Factors that determine the minor-use status of a particular crop or crop and pest combination include gross sales from the crop's potential pesticide market (generally a function of total crop acreage); relative value of the crop per unit area; susceptibility of the crop to pest damage throughout the season; and availability of nonpesticide controls.

Production of most minor crops typically requires several pesticides. However, there is little incentive for pesticide manufacturers to pursue registration of their products for uncommon pests and crops grown on limited acreage except as a step in establishing a share in a larger market. The volume of pesticides used is often so low that a manufacturer's costs to obtain and maintain registration are not compensated by revenues from pesticide sales. This fact has important consequences, because all vegetable, fruit, and ornamental crops are in the minor use category. Vegetables and fruits currently constitute about 20 percent of consumer diets, and the percentage is increasing.

Minor-use tolerances for many pesticides are not supported by studies meeting current data requirements for oncogenicity, environmental effects, and residue chemistry. For some minor-use pesticides not registered for a major crop, particularly those no longer protected by patents, the cost of meeting the EPA's data requirements may make it uneconomical for manufacturers to pursue reregistration. Nearly all important minor-use pesticides are also registered for some major uses, however, and are less likely to encounter this problem. In these cases, registration for minor crop uses often is obtained as a label expansion after the product generates revenue from its major crop uses.

LIABILITY

The threat of liability suits is a cost that must be considered in entering any market. Liability for crop failures or crop injury resulting from product use is another impediment to pesticide registration for minor crop uses. The problem can be especially serious for many vegetable, fruit, and ornamental crops. These crops tend to have relatively high values per acre, have low pesticide sales potential relative to possible liabilities, and are expected to meet high-quality standards. Even when these considerations do not impede registration, if the acceptable daily intake for a pesticide is used fully by other tolerances involving larger markets, the minor-use tolerance generally will not be sought because it would necessitate restriction of use in a larger market.

The minor-use problem is a product of the 1972 amendments to FIFRA, which among other things made it unlawful to use any registered pesticide in a manner inconsistent with its label. These amendments banned the application of registered pesticides for uses not specified on the label, which meant that each crop and pest combination had to appear on the label. In addition to the costs of obtaining specific registrations for each crop and pest combination, the registrant was liable for phytotoxicity and other product-related failures.

Later amendments to FIFRA in 1978 and the EPA's announcement of new policies in 1986 have helped to ease the minor-use problem. The agency has announced a new definition of "use inconsistent with labeling," which permits application of a pesticide to control an unnamed target pest as long as the pesticide is registered for use on the crop. The EPA's new policies allow the agency to adjust its data demands and registration fees for minor-use registrations in light of the anticipated extent of use, degree of human and environmental exposure, toxicity of the compound, volume of use, geographic distribution of potential use, and cost of data requirements for registration.

INTERREGIONAL PROJECT 4

Another important factor in dealing with the minor-use issue is the U.S. Department of Agriculture's Cooperative State Research Service Inter-Regional Project 4 (IR-4). IR-4 provides a mechanism for state agricultural research and extension workers to identify specific pesticides that will meet particular needs on minor crops. These workers will be able to cooperate with others in research and extension to develop the efficacy and residue data necessary to obtain tolerances and secure registrations for minor uses. In all cases, the company developing or marketing the pesticide or a third party must agree to serve as the registrant before the IR-4 will develop data needed to support a minor crop use registration. Although its financial resources are limited, IR-4 efforts at the federal and state levels can relieve companies of some of the financial burden of obtaining minor-use tolerances. The IR-4 has helped to obtain tolerances and registrations for pesticide uses on many minor crops, which otherwise would not have been pursued by the pesticide companies.

Although policy changes are addressing the problem of obtaining new pesticide registrations for minor crops, the problem of liability remains. Also remaining is the lack of incentive for manufacturers to develop pesticide products that have potential uses on a small number of minor crops and limited potential uses on any major crops. In addition, the forthcoming reregistration of currently registered pesticides will probably create serious new problems for some existing minor-use registrations. The EPA has identified a substantial number of pesticides with minor-use tolerances as animal oncogens. Some tolerances and registrations for these pesticides will probably be lost during reregistration. The impact will be greatest on fungicides, which are essential for commercial fruit and vegetable production in humid production areas, and for which there are virtually no registered alternatives. Moreover, there are few potential replacements under investigation or development. The impact on minor-use insecticides and herbicides is likely to be less severe.

So far the Delaney Clause has had little impact on the registration and reregistration of minor-use pesticides. This is because the EPA has not yet applied the clause to tolerances established before contemporary oncogenicity data requirements were established. Only a small percentage of all minor crops with processed food forms are currently included in the residue chemistry guidelines (Subsection O of the Pesticide Assessment Guidelines; see Table 3-11) listing crops for which the EPA requires processing studies or in the National Food Processors Association's list of proposed additions to Subsection O (see Table 3-13). If the number of minor crops listed in Subsection O is expanded, the effects of the Delaney Clause will become proportionately larger.

The Pesticide Resistance Problem

Pesticide resistance is an increasingly serious problem. In 1984, 447 species of insects and mites, 100 species of plant pathogens, 55 species of weeds, 2 species of nematodes, and 5 species of rodents were known to be resistant in some location to one or more pesticides used for their control.[14] Combining pesticides having different modes of action, reducing application frequencies, and rotating pesticide types are important tactics of pesticide resistance management requiring the availability of several effective pesticides. To the extent that pesticide cancellations limit the number and spectrum of available pesticides, the crop producer's ability to manage pesticide resistance will be hampered.

The problem of managing pesticide resistance is likely to be acute in the case of fungicides, because many of the protectants in use for many years without causing resistance are under regulatory review at the EPA. Loss of these fungicides would lead to greater reliance on newer systemic, site-specific, eradicant fungicides, such as metalaxyl and benomyl. The long-term viability of relying on such fungicides is suspect, because plant pathogens commonly develop resistance to these types of fungicides. If the older oncogenic protectant fungicides are lost as a result of regulatory actions, innovation in integrated disease management will become not only valuable but necessary.

To slow the selection of resistant pathogens, the use of site-specific fungicides must be precisely managed. A major feature of resistance management in crop diseases is the mixing of eradicant site-specific fungicides with older, protectant fungicides. Such mixtures combined with fungicide rotation help prevent resistance. Pesticide companies and land-grant universities are developing disease resistance management schemes to prolong the effectiveness of fungicides such as triadimenol, metalaxyl, and benomyl, because resistance has developed in high-use areas. Disease-resistant crop varieties are also being introduced to reduce fungicide use and resistance. Tolerance reductions that encourage more judicious use of protectant fungicides would enhance disease management innovation and reduce the oncogenic risk associated with residues of these fungicides.

NOTES

1. National Agricultural Chemicals Association. 1986. Industry Profile Survey. Washington, D.C., p. 9.
2. *Ibid.*
3. Council on Agricultural Science and Technology. 1981. Impact of Government Regulation on the Development of Chemical Pesticides for Agriculture and Forestry. Report No. 87. Ames, Iowa: Council on Agricultural Science and Technology.
4. Office of Technology Assessment. 1981. Technological Innovation and Health, Safety, and Environmental Regulation. Washington, D.C.: Office of Technology Assessment.
5. Hatch, U. 1983. The Impact of Regulatory Delay on R&D Productivity and Costs in the Pesticide Industry. Ph.D. dissertation. University of Minnesota, St. Paul.
6. Grawbowski, H. G., and W. K. Viscusi. 1984. EPA Regulation and Pesticide Innovation: An Exploratory Analysis. Washington, D.C.
7. Grawbowski, H. G., and J. M. Vernon. 1983. The Regulation of Pharmaceuticals: Balancing the Benefits and Risks. Washington, D.C.: American Enterprise Institute.
8. National Agricultural Chemicals Association, p. 13.
9. U.S. Environmental Protection Agency. 1980. Guidelines for Contents of Economic Impact Analysis. Washington, D.C.: U.S. Environmental Protection Agency.
10. Brent, K. J. 1985. One hundred years of fungicide use. In Fungicides for Crop Protection: 100 Years of Progress. BCPC Monograph No. 31. Bordeaux, France.
11. York, A. C., ed. Insecticide and Acaricide Tests. 1984. Vol. 9. College Park, Md.: Entomological Society of America.
12. National Research Council. 1987. Agricultural Biotechnology: Strategies for National Competitiveness. Washington, D.C.: National Academy Press.
13. Reichelderfer, K. H., G. A. Carlson, and G. A. Norton. 1984. Economic Guidelines for Crop Pest Control. Food and Agriculture Organization Plant Production and Protection Paper No. 58. Rome: Food and Agriculture Organization.
14. National Research Council. 1986. Pesticide Resistance: Strategies and Tactics for Management. Washington, D.C.: National Academy Press.

APPENDIXES

A

Legislative History of the Pesticide Residues Amendment of 1954 and the Delaney Clause of the Food Additives Amendment of 1958

BRUCE S. WILSON

STATEMENT OF PROBLEMS

Section 402 of the Food, Drug and Cosmetic Act (FDC Act) includes a "flow-through" provision under which approval of a tolerance for pesticide residue in a raw agricultural commodity under the terms of section 408 serves as substitute approval of the residue in processed food under section 409. If the concentration of the residue in the processed food is still below section 408 tolerances, then no independent section 409 approval is required.

The standards for approval under sections 408 and 409 are markedly different, however. Section 408 uses a type of risk/benefit balancing—weighing the need for an adequate food supply against the need to protect the consumer's health. Section 409 includes the "Delaney Clause," which flatly prohibits approval of a food additive found to induce cancer in humans or animals.

The combination of the section 402 "flow-through" provision and the different standards in sections 408 and 409 creates an anomalous situation whereby a potentially carcinogenic pesticide residue can become a lawful additive to food in spite of the Delaney Clause. As long as the residue does not exceed the section 408 tolerance, the pesticide need not meet the more exacting Delaney standard found in section 409. This anomaly has become increasingly significant in recent years, because some previously approved pesticides have proved carcinogenic in animal studies.

161

QUESTION PRESENTED

Was Congress aware of the implications of the different approval standards in sections 408 and 409?

CONCLUSION

Three factors in the legislative history appear to have a bearing on the anomaly created by the relationship between the Delaney Clause and the section 402 "flow-through" provision. First, Congress dealt separately, both conceptually and chronologically, with food additives and pesticide residues. In considering the 1958 Food Additives Amendments, Congress appeared anxious to avoid reopening the pesticide residues debate settled in the 1954 Pesticide Residues Amendments. Hence, bill drafters and witnesses at hearings universally limited, or even precluded, applicability of the proposed food additive standards to pesticide residues.

Congress appeared willing to accept this conceptual distinction between consideration of supposedly nontoxic substances (intentionally added to food during processing), and consideration of residues from highly toxic pesticides. Congress readily accepted the necessity of using at least some pesticides to maintain an adequate food supply. In contrast, hearing testimony during consideration of the food additives legislation reveals a perception that many food additives were optional, applied either to make food appear more appealing or to provide some other marketing advantage for the food processor. Hence, this factor suggests that Congress did not view separate treatment as presenting a significant inconsistency.

A second factor suggests that Congress may have simply missed the inconsistency between the standards. This factor is the unique procedure used in the enactment of the Delaney Clause. As reported by the House Committee on Interstate and Foreign Commerce, the Food Additive Amendment did not include a Delaney Clause. However, the committee apparently wanted the support of Congressman James Delaney (D-N.Y.) badly enough to make a significant last-minute amendment to the bill. Subsequent to the publication of the report on the bill produced in committee, Congressman Delaney convinced the committee to adopt an amendment inserting his carcinogens clause into the new section 409 approval standard. The haste with which the committee added this amendment probably obscured both the contrast that the clause provided to the section 408 standard and the anomaly potentially created by the "flow-through" provision.

Finally, the FDA's own position on the food additive and pesticide residues legislation helps to explain the presence of the potentially inconsistent provisions. Shortly after passage of the 1954 Pesticide Residues Amendments, the FDA promulgated a regulation providing for automatic section 406 approval of pesticide residues remaining in processed food. Whenever the remaining residues did not exceed the section 408 tolerances for raw commodities, the FDA would approve the residues under the then-applicable criteria of section 406. When food additive legislation was later proposed, the FDA modified this regulation into the present statutory "flow-through" provision applicable to section 409.

Hence, in the case of pesticide residues in processed food, the FDA had already substituted the more flexible risk/benefit standard embodied in section 408 for the "required" or "unavoidable" standard of section 406. These circumstances suggest that the FDA believed, or succeeded in convincing Congress, that the more flexible standard contained in section 408 adequately addressed the pesticides issue even in the case of residues in processed food.

These factors—the separate consideration of pesticides and food additives legislation, the last-minute inclusion of the Delaney Clause, and the FDA's desire to use a risk/benefit standard whenever dealing with pesticide residues—all suggest that Congress was not overly concerned by the potential anomaly created by the distinctions between sections 408 and 409. The different standards resulted primarily from Congress' willingness to view pesticide issues as distinct from food additive concerns. Accordingly, the "anomaly" was, to the members who discerned it, not particularly striking. The addition of the Delaney Clause sharpened the contrast between the provisions, but most likely was the product of a necessary compromise between the different standards for food additives advocated by the FDA and by Congressman Delaney.

DISCUSSION OF AUTHORITY

The Delaney Committee Report

On June 30, 1952, the House Select Committee to Investigate the Use of Chemicals in Foods and Cosmetics (Delaney Committee) culminated its two-year investigation into the "nature, extent and effect of the use of chemicals" in food and food production.[1] The committee recommended that the House pass legislation to control the flow of chemical substances into the nation's food supply.[1] Chairman Delaney included in the report testimony from the National Cancer Institute (NCI). The testimony noted that "a large number of chemical compounds induce cancer in animals," and concluded that "any estimate of the possible injurious properties of chemicals added to nutrients consumed by men should include careful testimony for their carcinogenic properties in several species of animals prior to approving their use in food."[2] The committee report also criticized existing legislation directed at pesticide residue control, and concluded that new, more effective legislation was necessary.[3]

The discussion of pesticides and food additives in that report presaged the later development of the different standards used in two distinct pieces of legislation, the Pesticide Residues Amendments of 1954 and the Food Additives Amendments of 1958.[4] The committee report noted that some witnesses had advocated separate treatment for agricultural pesticides and those "chemicals which are added to a food product after harvesting."[5] However, the report took the position that the presence of pesticide residues even in processed food warranted strict scrutiny of potential hazards.[5] The report concluded that questions "regarding [the long- and short-term health effects of] *any alien material* which may find its way, *in any amount,* into our food supply" had to be answered to ensure the continued health of the nation (emphasis added).[5]

Although this language appears to advocate a single strict standard for pesticide residues and food additives, the report did note the committee's belief "that with proper care, and by taking reasonable precautions, it is possible to utilize the poisonous properties of [pesticide] chemicals in destroying insects and controlling diseases which attack many crops, without endangering the health of the people who consume the products."[5] Hence, the Delaney Committee's own report language exposes some tension between the desire for absolute safety in the use of chemicals and the recognition that highly toxic pesticides play a necessary role in the maintenance of the nation's food supply. The assumption that most pesticides could be used without significantly endangering health resolved this tension. However, under a standard like the Delaney Clause, or one as strict as that implied by the Delaney Committee report, few pesticides would receive approval.

Recognizing this underlying problem, the minority report submitted by Congressman Thomas G. Abernethy (D-Miss.) recommended separate treatment for pesticides and food additives.[6] The distinction suggested by Congressman Abernethy between pesticides and food additives was founded on the perceived distinction between the nature of their use. "Their [pesticides'] use is from necessity and not by choice."[7] Abernethy's distinction may lack strong factual support, but it has an intuitive appeal that may partially explain the subsequent enactment of apparently inconsistent provisions. If agricultural interest successfully characterized pesticides as "necessary" to the preservation of the nation's food supply, while food processing interests failed to dispel completely the perception that many food additives were optional (for example, used for marketing enhancement or cost savings for the manufacturer), then the distinction in the standards seems less surprising.

The Pesticide Residues Amendments

In response to the Delaney Committee report, a number of members introduced bills at the beginning of the 83d Congress designed to address the concern over pesticides. Congressman A. L. Miller (R-Neb.), one of the members of the former Delaney Committee, introduced H. No. 4277, 83d Cong., 1st sess., reprinted in XII *Legislative History* at 546. The Miller bill, which eventually became the Pesticide Residues Amendments of 1954,[8] included standards under which the FDA commissioner would evaluate pesticide chemicals. The commissioner was to establish tolerances "to the extent necessary to protect the public health."[9] Significantly, the bill also directed the commissioner to "give appropriate consideration to the necessity for the production of an adequate and wholesome food supply."[9]

During House hearings on Congressman Miller's bill and on the clean bill (which incorporated the changes made at a committee "mark-up") subsequently reported by the Committee on Interstate and Foreign Commerce,[10] the risk/benefit balancing standard took on its present form. The final version of the bill included various factors to be considered in establishing pesticide residue tolerances.[11]

In his own analysis of the final bill, Congressman Miller noted that the factors were specifically "designed to assure a proper balance between the need for protecting the consumer from unsafe pesticide chemicals in or on food, and the need for assuring an adequate, wholesome, and economical food supply."[12] Miller's risk/benefit balancing standard had found support from a number of groups interested in the legislation. Agricultural interests,[13] the pesticides industry,[14] and the FDA[15] all appeared comfortable with the balancing standard. Indeed, Congressman Miller claimed universal support for the legislation.[16]

The House report on the committee bill clearly described the balancing of factors employed in establishing pesticide tolerances.[17] Significantly, the report also includes a disclaimer regarding pesticide residues in processed food: "[T]his bill does not attempt to regulate the residue from pesticide chemicals which may remain in or on processed, fabricated, or manufactured food. . . ."[18] The bill passed without debate in the House,[19] and after brief consideration before the Senate Committee on Labor and Public Welfare,[20] the Senate also passed the bill.[21]

The Food Additives Amendment

During the same Congress, members introduced a number of bills purporting to deal with food additives.[22] The later bills, introduced after May 1954, accounted for the new pesticide legislation by exempting pesticide residues on *raw* agricultural products in the definition of food additives.

1956 HEARINGS

The House Interstate and Foreign Commerce Committee first held hearings on the proposed food additives legislation during the early part of 1956.[23] These early hearings, although less extensive than those held during the subsequent Congress, contained some significant testimony with respect to the interaction between sections 408 and 409.

First, the National Agricultural Chemicals Association suggested an amendment to the proposed bills that would have totally excluded pesticide chemicals from the definition of food additives.[24] The effect of this definitional change was to avoid subjecting pesticide residues, either on raw *or* in processed foods, to the new section 409 standards. The executive secretary of the association, Leo S. Hitchner, observed that such a definitional exclusion merely maintained the status quo with respect to pesticide residues remaining in processed food (which were not covered by section 408). Subsequent to passage of the Pesticide Residues Amendments, the FDA adopted a regulation that provided for automatic approval (for purposes of sections 402 and 406) of pesticides for which section 408 tolerances had been established.[25] Hence, in the absence of specific food additives legislation, the FDA has already adopted, by regulation, the section 408 "flow-through" provision for section 406 approval of pesticide residues in processed food.

FDA officials testifying before the subcommittee surprisingly made no reference to the existing "flow-through" regulation, nor did they advocate exemption of pesticide residues in processed food from the scope of the proposed additives legislation. To the contrary, Sunkist Growers Cooperative was the first to suggest, on the record, legislation containing the combination of both a broad definition of food additives (that is, including pesticide residues in processed food), and a "flow-through" provision granting section 409 approval where the residues remaining in processed food did not exceed section 408 tolerances.[26]

Why the FDA ignored the "flow-through" issue in its own testimony is not altogether clear. The bills before the subcommittee all clearly included in the definition of food additives any pesticide residues remaining in processed food. These bills, therefore, would have vitiated the existing "flow-through" regulation. Even though the various bills contained standards less exacting than the subsequently enacted Delaney Clause, the standards were generally stricter than those for section 408 tolerances. These stricter standards may have required the FDA to reevaluate pesticide residues in processed food.

1958 HEARINGS

Whatever the reason for the FDA silence in 1956, circumstances apparently changed, and a "flow-through" provision appeared in legislation introduced on behalf of the FDA in the following year. H. No. 6747, the U.S. Department of Health, Education, and Welfare's (HEW) own draft,[27] along with a number of the other new bills considered in the committee, included legislative versions of the "flow-through" regulation being applied to proposed section 409.[28]

Obviously, interest in and support for the "flow-through" provision had increased considerably since the 1956 hearings. The FDA may have assumed that passage of food additives legislation in 1956 was unlikely, and so avoided submitting a bill of its own or discussing more technical provisions in which it had an interest. In any case, circumstances changed between 1956 and 1958. By 1958, HEW had submitted a complete draft of the bill, and the secretary was defending the "flow-through" provision as a measure "in consonance with a regulation now in force."[29]

This change in the department's approach to the legislation may have been in response to growing momentum behind the strictest approval standards, as exemplified in the bills authored by Congressman Delaney. Congressman Delaney's bill did not include a "flow-through" provision.[30] As in the bills proposed during the latter session of the 84th and in the 85th Congress, Delaney's definition of food additives excluded pesticide residues on raw agricultural products. By negative implication, the definition thereby included pesticide residues remaining in processed foods. However, Delaney's bill, H. 7798, also included the provision regarding carcinogens, now known as the Delaney Clause.[31]

The FDA opposed the Delaney Clause. H. No. 6747 actually provided for a relaxation of existing law through a "functional value" provision. The "functional value" standard did not require that the additive be absolutely necessary to production before approval could be granted.[32] Citing consumer correspondence in the FDA files, FDA's assistant general counsel argued that consumers supported "the rational use of chemicals" in food processing.[33] Rational use could include the employment of certain poisonous chemicals as long as "there . . . [was] a good reason for the addition of the chemical and . . . [its presence] in the diet . . . [was] safe."[33] The Delaney Clause quite obviously conflicts with this approach, because it establishes a per se rule prohibiting approval of carcinogens in even the most minute concentrations.

The FDA did not couch its opposition to the bill in terms of an objection to a per se rule. Rather, the agency objected by claiming that the Delaney Clause unnecessarily singled out cancer production for specific mention.[34] The FDA claimed that its own version of the legislation without the

Delaney Clause still prohibited "the use of an additive unless it is established that [the additive] is without hazard to health."[35]

In addition to the FDA's opposition to a rigid standard, a conceptual distinction between pesticides and food additives contributed to the committee's development of distinct approval standards. In contrast to the generally accepted view that farmers had to use some toxic pesticides, testimony regarding food additives occasionally reflected a view that many potentially toxic chemicals were added to processed food without sufficient justification.[36] This distinction between the perceived value, to the nation's food supply, of pesticides and other food additives was further enhanced by the existence of legislation already addressing pesticides. Witnesses often gave the impression that the control of pesticide residues on raw agricultural commodities constituted a sufficient response to the entire pesticide residues issue.

In testimony before the House Health and Science Subcommittee, Congressman Miller, a member of the original Delaney Committee and primary sponsor of the Pesticide Residues Amendments, opined that "Congress intended to regulate the pesticide chemicals entirely separate [sic] and apart from the so-called food additive amendment. The pesticide chemicals are now classified and regulated. The public is protected."[37]

Miller added, "If people follow the directions in the use of different pesticides in the development of food, the amount [getting into processed food] is small, very small, and I think not harmful to the food supply, and that is protected now by the Agriculture Department and Food and Drug Administration."[38] Accordingly, Miller's bill (H. No. 8112) included a "flow-through" provision.[39]

Agricultural interests also supported the distinction between pesticide residues and other chemicals in food. The National Agricultural Chemicals Association reiterated the position it took during the 1956 hearings, claiming that the pesticide "legislation already enacted assures the public of a safe food supply insofar as the use of agricultural pesticides is concerned. It eliminates the need of any further regulation of these products."[40]

Given the FDA's underlying objection to the Delaney provision, the concurrent enactment of the "flow-through" provision for pesticide residues is not surprising. The FDA successfully capitalized on the conceptual distinction raised by agricultural interests and certain members of Congress between "necessary" pesticides—already addressed by the 1954 amendments—and "optional" food additives.

The "flow-through" provision, therefore, had four sources of political momentum: (1) The FDA's own support for the provision, (2) support from influential members such as Congressman Miller, (3) an implicit distinction between "necessary" pesticides and "optional" food additives, and (4) the insistence by the agricultural lobby that the pesticides issue had been fully resolved by the 1954 amendments. These factors combined to make the "flow-through" provision a palatable solution to the issue of pesticide residues in processed food.

The addition of the Delaney Clause made that solution potentially more anomalous. The sparse legislative history regarding the Delaney Clause gives no indication that Congress noticed the effect that the addition of the Delaney Clause had on the "flow-through" provision. As discussed above, the FDA opposed the Delaney Clause and supported the more flexible overall standard. When the clause was added at the last minute, the FDA could hardly be expected to draw attention to the "loophole" for pesticide residues afforded by the "flow-through" provision.

Little else in the legislative history indicates what Congress intended to accomplish in creating the anomalous combination. Witnesses advocating the Delaney Clause focused primarily on the argument that medical science could establish no safe dosage for carcinogenic substances.[41] However, some of the same witnesses expressed doubts regarding the reliability of tests on animals as a basis for concluding that a substance was carcinogenic when ingested by humans.[42] Commissioner Larrick stated in the House hearings that the HEW-drafted bill "would prohibit the addition of any chemical additive to the food supply until adequate evidence . . . shows that it will not produce cancer in man *under the conditions of use proposed* [emphasis added]."[43] This statement of the FDA-proposed standard certainly does not appear as rigid as the Delaney Clause, but the FDA made no significant attempt to distinguish the two standards.

The committee may have accepted the FDA's argument that the clause was redundant. Similarly, it may have rejected testimony regarding the impossibility of setting a safe dosage for carcinogens, and responded to doubts about the reliability of cancer tests on animals. In any event, the extensive hearing testimony eventually led to the markup and reporting of a bill *without* any Delaney Clause.[44]

ADDITION OF THE DELANEY CLAUSE

Sometime between the publication of the House report on July 28, 1958, and floor consideration on August 13, 1958, Delaney convinced the committee to amend the bill to include the Delaney Clause. Congressman Oren Harris (D-Ark.), chairman of the House Interstate and Foreign Commerce Committee, managed the bill on the floor. He inserted into the *Congressional Record* a letter from HEW Assistant Secretary Elliot

Richardson. In that letter, Richardson withdrew the department's objections to the Delaney Clause with the following statement:

To single out one class of diseases for special mention would be anomalous and could be misinterpreted. Hence, in drafting the Department's bill, (H.R. 6747) we chose general language that would restrain any use of an additive that would have any adverse effect on public health. . . .

At the same time, if it would serve to allay any lingering apprehension on the part of those who desire any explicit statutory mandate on this point, the Department would interpose no objection to appropriate mention of cancer in food additives legislation.[45]

Richardson's letter then suggested a slightly modified version of the clause proposed by Delaney in the committee hearings.[46] The modified version became the committee amendment.

Chairman Harris's own prepared remarks reflect the haste with which the committee approved the amendment. In his prepared analysis of the principal provisions in the bill, Chairman Harris describes the operation of the approval standards in the bill as reported, rather than as amended by the Delaney Clause.[47] Congressman Delaney, after noting his "deep disappointment" that the bill reported from the committee contained no specific carcinogen prohibition, observed that "prolonged consultation with representatives of the Food and Drug Administration" eventually resulted in the FDA's agreement to the modified clause. Only Congressman Miller openly opposed the clause, noting that "it would be impossible to administer."[48] The House and Senate passed the bill by substantial margins.

The procedure employed to insert the Delaney Clause into the House bill indicates that Delaney had substantial personal influence on the committee. His chairmanship of the 1950 Select Committee probably played a significant role in establishing this influence. Delaney's own bill did not include a "flow-through" clause,[49] but since the primary deliberations concerning insertion of the Delaney Clause occurred off-the-record, it is impossible to determine whether Delaney recognized the anomalous relationship between the two clauses.

This combination of factors—FDA support for a flexible standard, and, consequently for the "flow-through" provision; congressional willingness to view pesticide residues and food additives as conceptually distinct issues; and the "ex parte" procedure by which the Delaney Clause became part of the House bill—all combined to create an inconsistent approach to food additives approval in the case of pesticide residues. The first two factors suggest that Congress did not view the separate standards as presenting a particularly disturbing inconsistency. The third suggests that most members were either unaware of the inconsistency, or at least tolerated it as an accommodation to Congressman Delaney.

NOTES

1. H. Rept. No. 2356, 82d Cong., 2d sess. 1 (1952), *reprinted in A Legislative History of the Federal Food, Drug and Cosmetic Act and Its Amendments* 499 (hereinafter *Legislative History*).
2. XII *Legislative History* at 503. Here, as elsewhere in the legislative history, proponents of strict controls on cancer-inducing substances did not adequately address the connection between cancer induction in animals and cancer induction in humans. Although some witnesses opposed to a flat ban on carcinogenic substances observed that tolerances varied considerably between some species, Delaney and others supporting his bill seemed to assume the connection. There was also no indication of a willingness to use a risk/benefit or other standard that accounted for the potential benefits foregone by the ban of a given chemical. From this first report and throughout the legislative history of the Delaney Clause, proponents categorically assumed that a finding of carcinogenicity warranted a total ban of the substance from the food supply.
3. XII *Legislative History* at 520.
4. The Pesticide Residues Amendment of 1954, Pub. L. No. 83-518, ch. 559, 68 Stat. 511 [codified at 21 USC § 346a (1981)]; and the Food Additives Amendments of 1958, Pub. L. No. 85-529, ch. 4, 72 Stat. 1785 [codified at 21 USC § 348 (1981)], respectively.
5. XII *Legislative History* at 524.
6. H. Rept. No. 2356, pt. 2, 82d Cong., 2d sess. 5 (1952), *reprinted in* XII *Legislative History* at 539, 542.
7. XII *Legislative History* at 542.
8. See note 3, *supra*.
9. XII *Legislative History* at 548.
10. *Federal Food, Drug and Cosmetic Act (Pesticides): Hearing on H. 4277 Before a Subcomm. of the House Comm. on Interstate and Foreign Commerce*, 83d Cong., 1st sess. (1953), *reprinted in* XII *Legislative History* at 577; and *Federal Food, Drug and Cosmetic Act (Residues of Pesticide Chemicals—Agricultural Commodities: Hearing on H. 7175 Before the House Comm. on Interstate and Foreign Commerce*, 83d Cong., 2d sess. (1954), *reprinted in* XII *Legislative History* at 770.
11. *See* 21 USC § 346a(b) (1981). The factors included in the determination of that tolerance level "necessary to protect the public health" are, "among other relevant factors,"

    (a) "the necessity for the production of an adequate, wholesome, and economic food supply";
    (b) "the other ways in which the consumer may be affected by the same pesticide chemical or by other related substances that are poisonous or deleterious"; and
    (c) an opinion submitted by the Secretary of Agriculture regarding the agricultural usefulness of the pesticide in question.

12. XII *Legislative History* at 787.
13. *See, e.g.,* XII *Legislative History* at 592 (statement of Ernest Falk, Northwest Horticultural Council).
14. *See, e.g., id.* at 641 (statement of L. S. Hitchner, National Agricultural Chemicals Association).
15. *See Residues of Pesticide Chemicals: Hearing on S. 2868 and H. 7125 Before the Subcomm. on Health of the Senate Comm. on Labor and Public Welfare*, 83d Cong., 2d sess. 920 (1954) (statement of Dr. Charles Crawford, FDA commissioner), *reprinted in* XII *Legislative History* at 882.
16. XII *Legislative History* at 793.
17. *See* H. Rept. No. 1385, 83d Cong., 2d sess. 3 (1954), *reprinted in* XII *Legislative History* at 833, 835.

18. XII *Legislative History* at 838.
19. 100 Cong. Rec. H4604 (daily ed. April 5, 1954), *reprinted in* XII *Legislative History* at 858. See note 12, *supra.*
20. *See Residues of Pesticide Chemicals: Hearing on S. 2868 and H. 7125 Before the Subcomm. on Health of the Senate Comm. on Labor and Public Welfare,* 83d Cong., 2d Sess. (1954), *reprinted in* XII *Legislative History* at 882. Senate consideration adds nothing relevant to the legislative history with respect to this particular question, since witnesses essentially repeated earlier testimony given before the House committee.
21. 100 Cong. Rec. S9727 (daily ed. July 6, 1954), *reprinted in* XII *Legislative History* at 1028. The Senate added a minor amendment to the bill providing for fee charges for establishing tolerances under the new section. The House agreed to this amendment without debate. 100 Cong. Rec. H10095 (daily ed. July 8, 1954), *reprinted in* XII *Legislative History* at 1030.
22. The various bills from the 83d and 84th Congresses are reprinted in XII *Legislative History* at 349-510.
23. *Federal Food, Drug and Cosmetic Act (Chemical Additives in Food): Hearings on H. 4475 and H. 8275 Before the Subcomm. on Health and Science of the House Comm. on Interstate and Foreign Commerce,* 84th Cong., 2d sess. (1956), *reprinted in* XIII *Legislative History* at 510.
24. XIII *Legislative History* at 660.
25. 20 Fed. Reg. 750 (1955) [codified until repealed at 21 CFR § 120.1(f) (1956)]. The regulation read:

> (f) Where raw agricultural commodities bearing residues that have been exempted from the requirement of a tolerance, or which are within a tolerance permitted under section 408 are used, the processed foods will not be considered unsafe within the meaning of section 406 if:
>
> > (a) the poisonous or deleterious pesticide residues have been removed to the extent possible in good manufacturing practice; and
> > (b) the concentration of the pesticide in the preserved or processed food when ready to eat is not greater than the tolerance permitted on the raw agricultural commodity.

26. XIII *Legislative History* at 751 (letter from M. J. McDonald, Sunkist Growers Cooperative).
27. *See Food Additives: Hearings Before the Subcomm. on Health and Science of the House Comm. on Interstate and Foreign Commerce on Bills to Amend the Federal Food, Drug and Cosmetic Act with Respect to Chemical Additives in Food,* 85th Cong., 1st sess. 28 (1958), *reprinted in* XIV *Legislative History* at 163, 169.
28. *See, e.g.,* H. 6747, XIV *Legislative History* at 40; H. 8112, XIV *Legislative History* at 118; H. 8629, XIV *Legislative History* at 139.
29. XIV *Legislative History* at 203 (materials submitted by M. B. Folsom, secretary of HEW).
30. H. 7798, XIV *Legislative History* at 91.
31. *Id.* at 91, 95.
32. *See* XIV *Legislative History* at 610-615 (statement of George Larrick, FDA commissioner).
33. *Id.* at 615 (statement of William Goodrick, FDA general counsel).
34. *Id.* at 616 (statement of George Larrick, FDA commissioner).
35. *Id.* at 615.
36. *See* H. Rept. No. 2356, pt. 2, 82d Cong., 2d sess. 5 (1952), *reprinted in* XII *Legislative History* at 539, 542; XIV *Legislative History* at 412-422 (testimony of George Faunce,

American Bakers Association); *id.* at 462 (statement of Mrs. R. I. C. Prout, Federation of Women's Clubs); *but see id.* at 329 (statement of Congressman Miller) (noting that certain food additives are essential to maintenance of the food supply).

37. XIV *Legislative History* at 318.
38. *Id.* at 325.
39. *See id.* at 118. *See also* XIV *Legislative History* at 322 (statement by Congressman Miller). Here, Miller indicated that pesticide residues in processed food should be controlled by food additives legislation. However, he also added in testimony that any pesticide should "be under strict supervision, as it is now in the Pesticide Act," and he saw that pesticide residues could effectively become food additives, but he believed that their control under the terms of the Pesticide Act was sufficient. *But see id.* at 325, in which Miller states, "[i]f there is any question about [pesticides] getting in [to processed food] then they ought to be subject to the same approval as any other additive in food." The "flow-through" provision in Miller's own bill would have exempted many pesticides from the additives standard.
40. XIV *Legislative History* at 277 (statement of L. S. Hitchner, National Agricultural Chemicals Association).
41. *See,* e.g., XIV *Legislative History* at 336, 366, 534.
42. *See* XVI *Legislative History* at 368-370, 516, 532-533, 539.
43. XIV *Legislative History* at 615-616.
44. *See* H. Rept. No. 2284, 85th Cong., 2d sess. 24 (1958), *reprinted in* XIV *Legislative History* at 822, 845.
45. 104 Cong. Rec. H17415 (daily ed. August 13, 1958), *reprinted in* XIV *Legislative History* at 869.
46. The modified language reflected the FDA's concern that the original language of the clause would "forbid the approval for use in food of any substance that causes any type of cancer in any test animal by any route of administration." 104 Cong. Rec. H17415 (daily ed. August 3, 1958), *reprinted in* XIV *Legislative History* at 869.
47. *Id.* at 870; *see also id.* at 873 (statement of Congressman Richard H. Poff (R-Va.)) (reflecting a similar omission).
48. *Id.* at 875.
49. H. 7798, 85th Cong., 1st sess., 103 Cong. Rec. H7918 (1957), *reprinted in* XIV *Legislative History* at 91.

B

Analytical Methodology for Estimating Oncogenic Risks of Human Exposure to Agricultural Chemicals in Food Crops

JOHN P. WARGO

The charge to this committee required the ability to characterize and analyze dietary oncogenic risk associated with exposure to pesticides through food crops, totaled by individual pesticide, by crop, and by pesticide-crop combinations. The capability of responding to various assumptions and questions was also necessary; for example,

- How many pesticide residue tolerances would be affected if a regulatory threshold of 10^{-6} were established for a specific pesticide-crop combination?
- What if the risk threshold were changed, or if the threshold were applied only to risk from residues in processed foods?
- What if regulatory thresholds were established by setting a limit based on total allowable risk by crop, or by pesticide?
- How is risk distributed among types of pesticides—for example, apple fungicides or corn herbicides—and how might risk be reduced as a result of alternative regulatory scenarios?

DATA MANAGEMENT SYSTEM

No computerized data management system existed prior to this study that could respond to these questions. The conceptual framework for this effort was derived in part from the U.S. Environmental Protection Agency's (EPA's) Tolerance Assessment System (TAS), which is main-frame based. The TAS joins pesticide-commodity tolerance data with

174

food consumption data to estimate possible chemical intake levels. Pesticide intake levels can then be converted into oncogenic risk estimates if reliable oncogenic potency estimates are available. Also, the TAS permits the comparison of possible daily pesticide intake levels with Acceptable Daily Intakes.

The TAS represents a remarkable breakthrough in analytical capability by the EPA, yet it is difficult and expensive to operate and update. And because it is mainframe based, it is accessible only to those with the computers and the expertise in mainframe operating systems and data analysis software.

The microcomputer-based system designed for this committee report incorporates TAS food consumption estimates and tolerance data, but it differs radically from the TAS in several critical respects. It operates on IBM-compatible microcomputers and uses common statistical (SAS), data-base management (dBASE III), and spreadsheet (Lotus) software. Not only does this dramatically increase the types of analyses that can be conducted, it substantially reduces the cost, time, and expertise required to perform the analyses.

The new system also contains simulation models that permit the user to change assumptions regarding tolerances, commodity consumption levels, percentage of acres treated, and oncogenic potency factors, instantly recalculating risks while graphing the results. In other words, these variables are linked by formulas in the system so that if any component in the risk equation is changed, the net effect on oncogenic risk is instantly demonstrated. The effects of as many as a dozen different tolerance-setting strategies can be forecast and graphed in 15 minutes.

The structure of the new system differs significantly from the TAS in the variety of new data fields. For example, the most recent EPA oncogenic potency estimates are incorporated into the system, permitting the transformation of estimates of chemical intake into estimates of oncogenic risk. Raw commodities, processed commodities, and specific pesticide-crop combinations are uniquely coded for separation into fields, enabling the calculation of risk by each field. Economic and pesticide-use data fields were added so that economic effects of different regulatory scenarios could be forecast.

Also, new fields were created by mathematically transforming existing fields. For example, the chemical intake field is calculated as the product of the *Code of Federal Regulations* (CFR) published tolerance field and the mean consumption field, and adjusted by the standard error field in a manner dependent on the desired confidence interval. If desired, the risk field could be adjusted by the percentage of acres treated. Total risks by pesticide, by crop, and by pesticide-crop combination also exist in separate data fields, having been calculated from the individual pesticide and commodity risk fields.

The new system can be updated easily. Tolerance, toxicological, ecological, and residue data are constantly being submitted to the EPA. These new data can be added to the system simply by typing the data into appropriate boxes on the screen.

Finally, a system for rapid electronic transfer of data between the mainframes and the IBM-compatible microcomputers was designed.

DATA BASE CONSTRUCTION

Tape-to-Mainframe Transfer and Data Transformations

Several transformations of data files were necessary to conduct the analyses presented within this report. First, several TAS files formatted in SAS (Statistical Analysis System) were transferred from magnetic tapes to an IBM 4043 disk, using IBM's Job Control Language. They included the Mean Consumption file, containing estimates of consumption of the 376 distinct food types by 23 population groups along with associated standard errors, and similar mean consumption data broken into 691 separate food forms.

Two additional files—the TAS Tolerance file and the TAS Preamble file—were transferred to the mainframe disk in raw (rather than SAS) format. The commodity codes in the TAS Tolerance file match the commodity codes in the TAS Mean Consumption file, but the commodity codes in the CFR Published Tolerance file do not match commodity codes in the Mean Consumption file. A code conversion was therefore necessary to relate current CFR tolerances to TAS-formatted consumption statistics. Once on the mainframe, these files were transformed into a SAS data set.

The Mean Consumption file, the Preamble file, and the TAS Tolerance file were then merged so that individual records included pesticide names and codes, commodity names and codes, published tolerance levels, mean consumption estimates, standard errors of these estimates, and a summary of toxicological data. This merged file was then sorted, first by commodity code and second by pesticide code, and transformed into raw (ASCII) format to prepare it for transfer to a microcomputer.

Mainframe-to-Microcomputer Transfer

The ASCII data files were then electronically transferred to a micro-computer that is hardwired to the mainframe. A utility called YTERM was used to transfer the files and to compare the original data and the copied version, highlighting any transfer errors. The data were stored in the directory containing the analytical software. (However, they can be stored in any desired subdirectory on the microcomputer hard drive.)

Raw–to–dBASE III Format

dBASE III was used to analyze the master data file. It not only stores data within individual records but contains its own programming language which permits mathematical operations such as sums of risks only for specified criteria, and other operations such as merging, rapid sorting, and indexing of large files.

Before the raw data set could be loaded into a dBASE file, the dBASE file structure had to be created. Field names, types (numeric, character, date, or memo), and lengths had to be specified to precisely match the location of the data in the stream of numbers and characters lying in raw data files. When the dBASE file format was established, the raw data set was appended to the dBASE file "shell." (The only limitation to the size of the data base is the available disk memory, since dBASE files do not reside in Random Access Memory [RAM]. A 20-megabyte hard drive was sufficient for the analyses performed for this study.)

dBASE III–to–Lotus 1-2-3 Transfer

One of the major limitations of dBASE III is the fact that mathematical transformations of entire data fields must be accomplished within the context of programs. dBASE is not interactive in a way that allows the user to change a set of assumptions and to immediately see the effects on the mathematically related fields.

Lotus 1-2-3 is similar to dBASE III in that data are aligned within records and fields in a matrix format. The major difference between the two systems lies in the ability of Lotus to establish formulaic relationships between cells of the data matrix. For example, if column 1 contains data on pesticide type, column 2 contains data on commodity names, column 3 contains data on published tolerances, and column 4 contains data on mean food consumption adjusted by standard errors, it would be possible to place a formula in column 5 that tells Lotus to multiply the value in column 3 by the value in column 4 to obtain an estimate of pesticide intake (Theoretical Maximum Residue Contribution, or TMRC). Once this relationship is established by formula, any change in one of the cells on which the formula is dependent will change the visible value or result of the formula.

Lotus was therefore ideal for analyzing the sensitivity of pesticide-crop risk to changes in assumptions regarding variables such as tolerances, residues, consumption estimates, potency factors, and acres treated. Once the risk formulas were established within the spreadsheet, any changes in assumptions were instantly converted into changes in estimated risk.

The primary limitation of Lotus lies in the fact that the entire package resides in RAM, which is generally limited to 640 kilobytes (kb) by IBM's Disk Operating System (DOS) unless a special expansion board is installed to increase memory. This memory constraint limits the size of analytical spreadsheets. For example, the master dBASE file used in this study was too large to fit within a single Lotus spreadsheet and, therefore, had to be broken into smaller units—commonly, groups of pesticides or crops. For the analyses conducted for this report, the RAM residency of Lotus was not a problem, since most analyses were performed on relatively small files.

DATA DESCRIPTION AND SOURCES

Diverse types of data are contained in the microcomputer-based system used to calculate oncogenic risks for this study. These data, their sources, and their relevance to the analyses presented are briefly described below.

For clarity, a data file can be thought of as a simple electronic matrix, with data being stored within individual "cells," defined by the horizontal and vertical location of the data. The horizontal rows of the file are known as "records," and the vertical columns are known as "fields." Data can be entered in character format (e.g., "BENOMYL") or numeric format (e.g., ".0000435"). Most computer-based analyses are performed on data within the cells, through such operations as sorting or merging based upon specified criteria, statistical analyses, or mathematical transformations dependent upon user-specified formulas.

Chemical Identification Data

Chemicals are identified by various codes and names. Each chemical considered in this study was assigned three different alphanumeric codes: (1) a Chemical Abstracts Service code; (2) a Caswell code (CASWL); and (3) a Shaughnessy code. Pesticides are also identified by preferred name, and by as many as five alternate names. These data were derived almost exclusively from the Preamble file from the EPA's Tolerance Assessment System. Additional data fields were added to these identification codes to indicate the primary uses of each pesticide—for example, fungicide, herbicide, or insecticide.

Chemical Tolerance Data

Tolerance data were derived from two sources: the TAS Tolerance file and the CFR Published Tolerance file, which lists all tolerances in the *Code of Federal Regulations*.[1]

The TAS Tolerance file contains essentially the same data as the CFR

Published Tolerance file, but there are several important distinctions. The TAS file contains 16,526 pesticide-commodity records, as contrasted with 8,477 records in the CFR file. This difference in file size can be explained as follows. In the CFR file, for example, one tolerance might be listed for captan on fresh tomatoes and another for captan in processed tomato products. In the TAS file, however, each possible processed-food form—catsup, juice, puree, and paste, for example—is listed as a separate record. This expansion was accomplished to more accurately represent dietary exposure to the various food forms and to enable the estimation of average daily pesticide intakes by food form.

The TAS Tolerance file contains 342 different pesticides (each assigned a CASWL code by the EPA) and 434 different commodity or food forms (each assigned a Raw Agricultural Code—called an EPARAC—by the EPA). (See Pesticide-Commodity Codes, below, for a description of these codes.) All tolerances are expressed in parts per million. For this study, use cancellations or suspensions were identified by adding a new data field to each record. Canceled or suspended uses were deleted before any risk calculations were performed.

The CFR Published Tolerance file mirrors the data contained in the *Code of Federal Regulations*. The 1985 file includes 351 distinct chemicals, 32 of which are listed as "Exempt" (40 CFR Part 180, Subpart D), and 19 of which are listed as Generally Regarded As Safe (GRAS) (40 CFR § 180.2). Together, the Exempt and GRAS categories account for 97 of the 8,477 records.[2] Each record contains the pesticide name and unique pesticide code, the commodity name and unique code, the 1985 tolerance, the CFR citation, and an EPA-assigned petition number.

Food Consumption Data

The food consumption (Mean Consumption) file was transferred directly from the TAS, and was based on a survey conducted during 1977–1978 by the Nutrition Monitoring Division of the Human Nutrition Information Service (HNIS) of the U.S. Department of Agriculture (USDA).[3] Data were collected from 30,770 individuals who were asked to recall food eaten the previous day and to record food eaten during the day of the interview and the day that followed. Each individual reported the food ingested, an estimate of the amount, the eating "event" (such as breakfast or lunch), water consumption, general health status, height and weight, and socioeconomic and geographic characteristics.[4] The primary sample was a multistage, stratified probability sample of all households in the coterminous United States. Within this sample, four independent, interpenetrating samples were drawn in four successive seasonal quarters between April 1, 1977, and March 31, 1978. A similar survey is currently being conducted by the HNIS; however, its results will not be available until 1989 (Bruce Gray, personal communication, 1986).

The Research Triangle Institute (RTI) transformed the USDA consumption survey into a Raw Agricultural Commodity Data Base, defining 376 unique food types.[5] These foods included commodities for which the EPA would be most likely to establish pesticide residue tolerances, thereby permitting the estimation of pesticide intake by commodity. It was not intended to include all edible foods. The list was developed from various sources, including the EPA's Food Factor list, the CFR listing of then-current tolerances, and the USDA food consumption survey codebook. Although the list includes 376 unique food types, only 273 of these foods were mentioned by the USDA survey respondents.

That survey did not include food components such as spices, estimated to constitute less than 0.1 percent of a given food consumed. Estimates of consumption for the 103 food types not reported by survey respondents were derived from studies by the USDA,[6] Magness et al.,[7] the National Academy of Sciences,[8] and the International Tariff Commission.[9] Finally, an "arbitrary consumption value" (10^{-6} g/kg body weight/day) was assigned to foods for which tolerances do not exist, or in cases where information could not be obtained.[10]

RTI also developed a set of "food form" codes that distinguish between raw, cooked, fresh, frozen, canned, dried, baked, broiled, fried, pickled, corned, or salt-cured forms of the 376 food types.[11] The Food Form file includes 691 records, yet does not include any new food types. Four records exist in the Food Form file for each of the 30,770 survey respondents. The first record contains descriptive information (such as age, sex, weight, census region); the second, third, and fourth records for each respondent indicate food consumption for each of the three days surveyed. Consumption is recorded in grams of food form per day.

Basic transformations of data conducted by RTI include

• Converting consumption from grams/day to grams/kilogram of body weight/day;
• Aggregating consumption over foods; and
• Averaging consumption over days and/or individuals.

The USDA Average Food Consumption file was used as the primary basis of this analysis. It was derived from the 90,000-record Person-Day Food Consumption file which was then averaged over the three days to produce a 30,000-record Average Daily Individual Food Consumption file. This file was then averaged over individuals to provide mean consumption estimates for the 273 food types reported by survey respondents.[12]

Since this mean consumption estimate is essentially an arithmetic mean derived from the sample, it was adjusted, or weighted, on the basis of sample size to derive an estimate of the population mean consumption for each food type.[13]

Standard errors of the mean consumption estimates for each of the commodities were computed by RTI using a first-order Taylor-series approximation of the deviations of the estimates from their expected values. (Formulas used by SESUDAAN, a statistical package developed by RTI, have also been reported by RTI.[14]) These data were used to calculate various confidence intervals that bound the estimated population mean consumption.

For this study the high end of the 95 percent confidence interval, or two standard errors above the population mean consumption, was chosen by the committee to represent the U.S. average commodity consumption for each food type. Thus, if a similar-sized sample were taken from the population of the contiguous United States, there is a 95 percent probability that the population mean consumption estimate derived from the second sample would lie within the same confidence interval as the first.

This does not mean, by contrast, that 95 percent of all individuals will consume less than the computed estimate, since the statistic was calculated from the standard error of the population mean consumption estimate, not from the standard deviations of individual consumption data.

Pesticide Residue Data

In an ideal world, accurate estimates of pesticide residues in foods and in water would be available as the basis for predicting average chemical intake (commonly described by the EPA as a chemical's Theoretical Maximum Residue Contribution, or TMRC). The FDA is responsible for enforcing tolerances for all pesticides used in food. To do this, it samples 7,000 domestic and 5,000 imported shipments of food each year.

There are several potential problems with relying on the FDA's sampling results to estimate food residues, most of which are associated with the agency's declining budgetary resources. First, the number of samples tested for each pesticide-crop combination is not large enough to develop population consumption estimates with meaningful confidence intervals. Second, detection of residues in raw agricultural commodities is often a meaningful indicator of residues in processed-food forms. Drying, oil extraction, cooking, and other processing techniques can dramatically alter pesticide residue levels. Third, the EPA is currently requiring a battery of residue tests prior to pesticide reregistration. Complete residue data are available for only a small percentage of the pesticides that are currently registered, leading to gaps and significant variation in quality of data on pesticides. Fourth, the multichemical detection technology used by the FDA cannot detect residues of all registered pesticides. Fifth, this multichemical detection technology is not sufficiently sensitive to *simultaneously* detect residues of all the chemicals that can be detected individually.

Together, these conditions led the committee to base its estimate of the human pesticide intake (TMRC) on the assumption that the chemical is in or on the food at the current tolerance level. This choice was made to standardize the quality of data on chemicals, even though it will likely overestimate chemical TMRCs since most FDA samples contained residues at levels substantially below established tolerances.[15]

Toxicological Data

The pesticide oncogenic potency factors in this study were estimated by the EPA's Hazard Evaluation Division. In no instance did the staff of the Board on Agriculture or the authors of this report interpret the EPA potency estimates.

The potential for tumor induction is indicated by a "potency factor" or Q^*. The Q^* is an estimate of the number of additional tumors that can be expected to develop within a human population, based upon the dose response results of animal bioassays. Laboratory animals are generally exposed at much higher doses over their lifetimes than the average human would normally encounter in his or her lifetime. Because animal life-spans are much shorter than human life-spans, dose response data must be extrapolated to predict human tumor incidence at the lower doses that humans are likely to encounter in food or water.

With only several exceptions, the 28 potency estimates used in these analyses were derived from the linearized multistage model of low-dose extrapolation. The potency factor used by the EPA is the slope of the line at the 95 percent upper confidence limit representing the dose response relationship—(change in lifetime probability of extra tumor incidence)/ (unit of exposure of dose). The expression of the oncogenic potency factor as a linear extra tumor incidence/dose ratio enables the prediction of tumor incidence based on estimates of human chemical exposure. The potency factor (estimated extra tumor incidence/dose) is simply multiplied by the pesticide intake estimate (dose) derived from the food consumption data and assumptions regarding the pesticide residue level in the food at the time of consumption.

Regulatory Status Data

Tolerances are listed in Titles 21 and 40 of the *Code of Federal Regulations* and in the TAS Tolerance file for pesticide-commodity combinations. A separate data field was created in the data base to indicate the status of tolerances. However, risk calculations were based only on active tolerances, under the assumption that residues of canceled or suspended pesticides would not be relevant to analyses designed to measure the impact of theoretical regulatory policies. These data were provided by the EPA in January 1986.[16]

Food Processing Data

The TAS Tolerance file is an expanded version of the CFR Published Tolerance file, as described above. Risk estimates based solely on the CFR file would underestimate the risk for commodities for which tolerances are listed only for the raw form, even though residues could also be expected in processed forms. The expansion program was developed by the EPA to more acurately reflect probable sources of exposure to chemicals in processed-food forms. When the TAS expansion program is run on the CFR Published Tolerance file, a record listing a tolerance for raw tomatoes, for example, is automatically expanded to separate consumption records for tomato paste, juice, catsup, and puree. Each food form carries with it the tolerance and CFR code from the original raw commodity. Where processed-food tolerances existed in the CFR file, the correct tolerance and CFR citation are carried into the TAS Tolerance file. Duplicates created by the expansion are automatically deleted.

Since neither the TAS nor the CFR Tolerance files code individual commodities by their raw or processed state, a new data field had to be created. A new code—Phantom—was designed to distinguish CFR tolerances from TAS tolerances and to distinguish between processed forms of commodities (where residue concentration might occur) and raw agricultural commodities. The following Phantom codes were assigned to each chemical-commodity record that existed in the TAS Tolerance file:

0 = New TAS raw-commodity tolerance created by TAS expansion;
1 = New TAS processed-commodity tolerance created by TAS expansion;
2 = Old CFR processed-commodity tolerance;
3 = Old CFR raw-commodity tolerance.

The Phantom codes were assigned to the food type codes known as EPARACs, which are uniquely assigned to all food types contained in the food consumption survey (see Pesticide-Commodity Codes, below, for more information). The proper form (raw or processed) of each of the 376 commodities listed within the survey was determined by matching EPARAC codes (explained below) in the CFR Tolerance file with EPARAC codes in the TAS Tolerance file and through information provided by the Residue Chemistry Branch of the Office of Pesticide Programs (OPP).

The development and assignment of the Phantom code made possible the estimation of oncogenic risk based on the raw or processed form of the commodity. The code also made possible the distinction between risk associated with processed-commodity tolerances in the current CFR Published Tolerance file and risk associated with processed-commodity tolerances in the expanded TAS Tolerance file.

Chemical Use and Cost Data

For eight distinct crop-pesticide combinations, data on acre treatments, percentage of planted acres treated, and expenditures per acre were entered as new fields. These combinations are corn- and soybean-herbicides, cotton-insecticides, and apple-, tomato-, potato-, peanut-, and grape-fungicides. The primary sources for these data included the Economic Analysis Branch of the Office of Pesticide Programs and the USDA Economic Research Service.

The addition of these data fields facilitates the analysis of pesticide-commodity risk by acres treated, acre treatments, and expenditures. Comparison of expenditures per acre for likely substitute pesticides allows the development of analyses that estimate the cost per unit risk reduction, assuming various patterns of pesticide substitution.

Pesticide-Commodity Codes

The TAS data sets include unique codes assigned to unique pesticides (CASWL codes) and to unique commodities (EPARAC codes). Because most analyses relevant to this study involved calculation of risk by pesticide-commodity combination, it was necessary to develop a code that was also unique to pesticide-commodity combinations. The CASRAC code was designed for this purpose and is a combination of the CASWL code (for unique pesticides) and the EPARAC code (for unique commodities).

The EPA-designed EPARAC code was not suitable for the committee's analyses. Each code has a five-digit numeric prefix and a two-digit character suffix. For most commodities, all numeric suffixes are identical for basic commodity forms, such as tomatoes or apples. In several cases, such as peanuts, this was not the case, and the codes were redefined so that all peanut records began with the same numeric prefix. This was absolutely crucial to the development of a methodology to sum risks by pesticide-crop combination. Now all distinct crop groups (apples, peanuts, corn, grapes, etc.) have distinct EPARAC codes (renamed

EPARAC1). The CASRAC field, which is unique to each distinct pesticide-crop combination, permitted the calculation of total pesticide-commodity risks that might be affected if, for example, tolerances for each pesticide-commodity combination exceeding a predefined risk threshold were revoked.

ANALYTICAL METHODS

Risk Calculation

The method of oncogenic risk estimation used in this study is a minor variant of the Routine Chronic Analysis used by the EPA and described in the documentation of the Tolerance Assessment System.[17] The oncogenic risk associated with any individual chemical can be calculated only if a reliable estimate of oncogenic potency (Q^*) has been developed for that chemical. The committee's risk estimates are derived from 28 of 30 compounds for which oncogenic potencies were provided by the EPA. In these cases, risk estimates were calculated for all distinctive food types in which residues could be anticipated. For example, a separate risk estimate was calculated for the residues of alachlor in raw corn as well as alachlor in corn oil. Of the 16,500 tolerances that exist in the TAS Tolerance file, risk estimates were derived for only 2,306 pesticide-commodity combinations. The limited number of potency factors reflects findings of non-oncogenicity for many compounds and the absence of valid oncogenic or chronic feeding studies for numerous other pesticides. For several of the scenario analyses presented below, calculation of the number of pesticides and crops that would be affected by different regulatory thresholds was based on a pool of 53 chemicals that the EPA believes to be oncogenic, despite the absence of potency factors for 25 of them.

The critical variables that are components of the risk calculation are briefly described below and more thoroughly described under Data Description and Sources, above, and Uncertainty in Oncogenic Risk Estimates, below.

CHEMICAL RESIDUES

The current tolerances and the residue estimates obtained through the TAS expansion of the CFR Published Tolerance file were used as the basis for estimating "worst-case" pesticide residues in the commodities. Although a far more accurate representation of likely exposure might be developed through statistically valid commodity and residue sampling techniques, these data were not available for this study. Tolerances are expressed in parts per million.

CONSUMPTION ESTIMATES

Commodity consumption estimates were based on the mean consumption data developed from the 1977-1978 food consumption survey of individuals within the 48 contiguous states. The consumption estimate is a U.S. average statistic and could vary significantly beyond the mean for individuals. This estimate was used to calculate the high end of the 95 percent confidence interval. Consumption estimates are expressed in grams of commodity per kilogram of body weight per day.

ESTIMATE OF CHEMICAL INTAKE

An estimate of mean pesticide intake was developed by multiplying the tolerance and the mean consumption estimate for each pesticide-commodity record. This exposure estimate is called the Theoretical Maximum Residue Contribution. The TMRC assumes that residues are present at the tolerance level on every crop that has a tolerance, and that all acres of all crops with tolerances are treated. Exposure to these residues is expressed in milligrams of chemical per kilogram of body weight per day. This method of calculating exposure to residues overestimates actual dietary exposure across the whole population, but it is preferred by the EPA as an initial step in risk assessment because it incorporates a prudent safety factor into the risk assessment process.

POTENCY FACTOR OR Q*

The potency factor, as calculated by the EPA, is the slope of the dose response curve or line from animal oncogenic tests. This slope represents the change in Y (tumor incidence) over the change in X (dose). Potency therefore increases with the steepness of the slope. The units of the potency factor are tumors per milligram of pesticide per kilogram of body weight per day. The potency factor assumes that this average level of exposure over a 70-year human life span is necessary for tumor induction. The Q* used by the EPA represents the upper bound of the 95 percent confidence interval surrounding the potency estimates.

RISK ESTIMATES

The estimate of risk is derived as the product of the estimate of pesticide intake and the estimate of the potency factor. Thus,

$$\text{TMRC} \quad \times \quad Q^* \textit{ or } \text{potency factor} \quad = \quad \frac{\text{excess tumor}}{\text{incidence/unit dose}}$$

$$\begin{array}{ccc} \text{(mg pesticide/} & \text{(excess tumor} & \text{excess tumor} \\ \text{kg body wt/day)} & \times \text{ incidence/mg pesticide/} & = \frac{}{} \frac{\text{excess tumor}}{\text{incidence/unit dose.}} \\ & \text{kg body wt/day)} & \end{array}$$

This amount is commonly very small, i.e., 0.000001 or 10^{-6}, assuming daily exposure at this level for a 70-year period. This number means that an individual would have a 1 in 1 million risk of additional tumor induction above normal probability, assuming lifetime exposure to pesticide residues at the level indicated.

PERCENTAGE OF ACRES TREATED

In the crop-level analyses in the scenarios below, these risk estimates were adjusted by an additional estimate of the percentage of total acres of any single crop treated with a pesticide. The percentage of acres treated represents a national average which does not take into account regional and local pesticide application and food distribution patterns. Ideally, critical components of exposure analysis would include where the pesticide is applied as well as the distributional pattern of produce within the country.

Scenario Analyses

The analysis of changes in the distributions of risks and benefits associated with alternative regulatory scenarios is a critical component of this report. Four scenarios are considered and distinguished by various risk levels that trigger regulatory prohibitive action. The threshold risk level may vary between tolerances for raw and processed foods within any scenario. The scenario analyses were performed using dBASE files containing all pesticide-commodity combinations for the 53 compounds identified by the EPA as potential oncogens. Scenarios dependent on quantitative risk levels were conducted only on the 28 compounds with Q^*'s.

As noted in Chapters 2 and 3 of the report, it is virtually impossible to distinguish which portion of the raw commodity will be sent to the fresh produce market and which portion will be processed. In designing these scenarios, the committee adopted the EPA's assumption that a regulatory strategy is impractical if it denies processed-food tolerances while allowing raw-commodity tolerances, in the expectation that residues in the raw foods will somehow *not* make their way into the processed-food forms.

Scenario 1 revokes all tolerances for all oncogenic pesticides. Scenarios 2, 3, and 4 require the identification of combined raw- and processed-commodity risks associated with any individual pesticide under carefully defined conditions that vary among scenarios. For example, Scenario 2 requires the cancellation of all processed-commodity tolerances with a risk greater than zero, along with the cancellation of all raw commodity tolerances that are associated with the canceled processed-commodity tolerances. In this case, if the risk from pesticide X in apple juice exceeded zero, then all tolerances for pesticide X in all apple products would be canceled.

Scenario 3, by contrast, requires the cancellation of both raw- and processed-commodity tolerances for any individual pesticide, if the combination of raw-commodity and processed-commodity risks exceeds a threshold probability of 1×10^{-6}. Finally, Scenario 4 requires the revocation of both raw- and processed-commodity tolerances for any individual pesticide if and only if the risk associated with the processed commodity tolerances exceeds the threshold probability of 1×10^{-6}.

The ultimate purpose of these scenarios is to estimate and compare the amount of risk; the number of pesticides, crops, and tolerances; and the percentage of total pesticide expenditures that would be affected by the application of the regulatory thresholds described above for each scenario.

The calculation of these estimates required the development of several new data fields in the dBASE files:

- *Chemical-Crop Risk (RISKCCA),* which is the summation of tolerance-specific risks for all raw- and processed-commodity tolerances associated with any specific pesticide-commodity combination (for example, all tolerances for captafol on apple products);
- *Chemical-Crop Processed Risk (RISKCCP),* which is the summation of tolerance-specific risks for all processed-commodity tolerances for any specific pesticide-commodity combination;
- *Tolerances Affected (TOLAFF),* which is the summation of tolerances affected by applying the regulatory standard in each scenario; and
- *Crops Affected (CROPAFF),* which is the summation of crops affected by applying the regulatory standard of each scenario.

The creation of these data fields required the design of a new uniquely defined chemical-commodity code (CASRAC), which is a combination of the unique chemical code CASWL and the commodity code EPARAC. An example of the file structure is shown in Table B-1.

To perform the scenario analyses, the file is sorted on the CASRAC field and the records affected by a particular scenario are displayed. Affected risks, tolerances, and crops are summed within this file, based

TABLE B-1 Sample of Fields Created to Analyze Distribution of Risks Associated with Alternative Regulatory Scenarios

File structure used to determine effects of regulatory threshold changes

CASRAC	CHEM	COMMODITY	TOL TYPE	RISKCCA	RISKCCP	TOL AFF	CROP AFF
04001075	CHEMX	APPL RAW	RAW	.000008	.000007	3	1
04001075	CHEMX	APPL JUI	PROC	.000008	.000007	3	1
04001075	CHEMX	APPL DRY	PROC	.000008	.000007	3	1
11004093	CHEMY	SOY RAW	RAW	.000006	.000004	2	1
11004093	CHEMY	SOY OIL	PROC	.000006	.000004	2	1

File sorted on CASRAC field

CASRAC	CHEM	COMMODITY	TOL TYPE	RISKCCA	RISKCCP	TOL AFF	CROP AFF
04001075	CHEMX	APPL RAW	RAW	.000008	.000007	3	1
11004093	CHEMY	SOY RAW	RAW	.000006	.000004	2	1

on the specific conditions defined by the scenarios. For example, scenario 2 would require RISKCCA, TOLAFF, and CROPAFF to be summed conditionally for instances where processed-commodity risk (RISKCCP) exceeds zero. In the example in Table B-1, since both cases meet the condition specified, total affected risk would be 0.000014, total number of tolerances affected would be 5, and total crops affected would be 2—apples and soybeans. Scenario 3 would require that RISKCCA, TOLAFF, and CROPAFF be summed conditionally for cases where total pesticide-commodity risk exceeds the threshold probability of 0.000001. Scenario 4 would require that RISKCCA, TOLAFF, and CROPAFF be summed conditionally for cases in which RISKCCP (processed-commodity risk) exceeds the threshold probability of 0.000001.

The scenario criteria were applied to three subsets of the master dBASE file:

1. *Chemical type analyses.* The effects of applying each regulatory scenario to types of pesticides (herbicides, fungicides, and insecticides) were estimated by performing the calculations described in the previous paragraph with the added condition that only the specific chemical class of interest be used as the basis of calculation.

2. *Individual chemical analyses.* The effects of the various regulatory scenarios on individual pesticides were estimated by first creating a file of unique pesticide-commodity records. Then, within this file, RISKCCA (total pesticide-commodity risk) was summed conditionally based on the scenario-specific criteria wherein RISKCCP > 0 (scenario 2); RISKCCA

> 0.000001 (3); RISKCCP > 0.000001 (4). Again, affected risk, affected tolerances, and affected crops were all calculated for each pesticide.

3. *Crop analyses*. Finally, the effects of applying the regulatory scenario were estimated for eight crop groups of particular interest: apples, corn, cotton, grapes, peanuts, potatoes, soybeans, and tomatoes. The scenario-specific risk thresholds were again applied to calculate affected risk and affected numbers of tolerances, as in the previous two cases. In addition, percent affected acre treatments, and percent affected total pesticide expenditures were calculated for each crop.

UNCERTAINTY IN ONCOGENIC RISK ESTIMATES

This report includes numeric estimates of dietary oncogenic risk based primarily on tolerance, consumption, oncogenic potency, and percentage of crop acres treated data. This section briefly describes the types and ranges of uncertainty that surround these estimates.

All risk estimates other than the crop-level estimates adjusted by the percentage of crop acres treated represent a conservative upper-bound calculation of the additional oncogenic risk across the U.S. population from exposure to any oncogenic agent. Conservative upper-bound estimates or "worst-case" estimates are used primarily to allow for uncertainties in the independent variables that determine the risk estimate (residues/tolerances, consumption, acres treated, and chemical potency).

Residue Estimates

All risk estimates in this report assume that chemicals exist in commodities at tolerance levels when consumed. The results of the FDA's Market Basket surveys indicate that residues very rarely occur in raw commodities at the tolerance level; they are more commonly at levels of less than 50 percent of the tolerance. Similarly, residue levels can be affected by the method of food preparation; for example, boiling certain vegetables can volatilize water-soluble chemical residues. Therefore, it seems reasonable to conclude that the assumption of exposure at full tolerance is a highly conservative, very-low-probability event. However, this is not always the case. An October 1986 report by the U.S. General Accounting Office (GAO) found that 3 to 4 percent of all foods sampled by the FDA contained violative residues.[18] Further, some pesticide metabolites and conversion products are known to increase during food storage and cooking.

One of two assumptions could have been made when calculating risks—that residues exist in commodities at a level detected by the FDA's sampling surveys, or that residues exist at the tolerance level in commodities.

If one were primarily interested in calculating probable past exposure and resulting risk, use of a residue survey, if statistically valid, would seem reasonable. A problem then arises, however, when attempting to use past residue data to project future risk, particularly for pesticides with tolerances far in excess of residues actually detected. Use of such survey data could underestimate risk in some cases; further, residues could theoretically rise to the tolerance level without triggering a regulatory response.

In contrast, the assumption that residues will exist at tolerance levels will likely overestimate risk, except for new compounds for which tolerances have been set close to anticipated residue levels. The method of risk estimation adopted for this study assumes that residues occur at the tolerance levels, which the committee deems reasonable in the absence of other comprehensive and validated data sets on actual residue levels.

Food Consumption Estimates

In all cases, the U.S. mean consumption estimate has been used to calculate risk in this report. The mean consumption estimate has been adjusted by the standard error, so that it actually represents the outer bound of the 95 percent confidence interval for the population mean consumption estimate. One can therefore conclude that there is a 95 percent probability that if a similar-sized sample were surveyed from the same population at the same time, the estimate of the population mean consumption level would not exceed the original outer-bound estimate. However, one cannot conclude that 95 percent of the individual consumption reports will fall below this level. That outer bound would likely be far higher.

It is clear that using the U.S. average consumption estimate alone will inaccurately estimate food consumption for many population subgroups. For example, infants have a low level of diversity in their diets, and their consumption of fruits and fruit juices (in grams/kilogram body weight/day) is far higher than the U.S. average consumption estimate. Table B-2 demonstrates these differences for fresh apple and apple juice consumption.

As can be seen, some population groups may consume eight times the U.S. average estimate for certain foods if measured on a milligram/kilogram body weight/day basis. The certainty that U.S. mean consumption will rarely be exceeded therefore seems quite low. Specific age group-commodity combinations may exceed the U.S. mean consumption estimate by as much as an order of magnitude.

TABLE B-2   Apple Consumption by Age Class (g/kg body weight/day)

	U.S. Average	Nursing Infants	Nonnursing Infants	Children Ages 2–6	Children Ages 7–12
Fresh apples	0.457	2.203	2.854	1.228	0.762
Apple juice	0.222	2.517	3.464	0.994	0.198

NOTE: Differences in mean consumption estimates between subpopulations will result in differences in chemical intake estimates or TMRC.

SOURCE: USDA 1977–1978 food consumption survey.

On the other hand, the exposure model used for risk assessment (the TMRC method described above) also assumes that every individual consumes some portion of every food form every day for 70 years. Benomyl, for example, has nearly 100 food tolerances, and the exposure model assumes that each individual is exposed to benomyl as a residue in each of these 100 different foods every day for an average lifetime. While it is prudent to consider this a possibility, its probability is extremely remote, since most people do not eat all these foods and most chemicals are used for far less than 70 years.

Finally, the estimate of outer-bound consumption used in this study is based on a standard error adjustment of the mean consumption data. This procedure is appropriate for estimating the 95 percent outer-bound level for population consumption means, but the estimate will be far lower than would an estimate of 95 percent outer-bound consumption based on means of individual consumption data adjusted by the standard deviations. For this reason, the consumption estimates used here for individual foods are likely close to the mean. Given a sample size of over 30,000 people, something approaching a normal distribution can be assumed, suggesting that roughly 45 percent of the population will be consuming higher levels than estimated in this study.

Acreage Treated

An additional source of uncertainty in risk estimation is the fact that pesticide exposure estimates are not adjusted for likely geographical patterns of pesticide application and food distribution. For all but the above-described analyses of chemical levels in crops, the committee assumed that all acres of all crops were treated with all pesticides for which tolerances were available. In most cases this method of risk estimation is also used by the EPA. In certain cases, however, an average percentage of total acres treated is incorporated into the risk estimate and risk assessment process. For example, there may be instances in which a particular apple fungicide is used only in one part of the country, and the apples from this area are distributed only within a several-state region surrounding the production site. By incorporating the percentage of acres treated into exposure and risk estimates and by assuming a random national distribution of these treated apples, the EPA would arrive at theoretical average exposure estimates that would tend to overestimate fungicide exposure to the portion of the population living outside the distribution region but underestimate exposure to the portion living within the distribution region.

The percentage-acres-treated statistic was used to adjust the risk estimate for the eight crop analyses described above. These percentages represent an average of three years, generally between 1981 and 1984 but occasionally including 1985 use data. For soybeans, cotton, and corn, 1983 data were not used because of acreage reductions under the Payment-in-Kind program. The following method was used for these analyses: if 500,000 acres were planted with apples and 20 percent of those acres were treated with benomyl, the apple-benomyl risk estimate would be reduced by 80 percent (that is, the risk would be multiplied by 0.2). To assume that the risk to all individuals is actually reduced by 80 percent requires an assumption that all benomyl-treated apples are evenly distributed throughout the population. This is obviously a gross oversimplification of probable exposure.

If percentage-of-acres-treated data are incorporated, a theoretical U.S. average oncogenic risk can be estimated, but it will disregard the high probability that regional populations will be exposed at far higher levels. For example, if the acres-treated estimate for an apple fungicide is 0.1 and this estimate is used to adjust the risk estimate, it is probable that risk to individuals who eat the treated apples will be underestimated by an order of magnitude. If it is assumed that all acres are treated, however, then risk will be overestimated for a large percentage of the population.

Crop-level risk estimates adjusted by the acres-treated data underestimate upper-bound risk for some percentage of the U.S. population. Individual chemical risk estimates and pesticide group risk estimates for herbicides, insecticides, and fungicides assumed that 100 percent of the acres were treated and will probably overestimate risk for some percentage of the population.

The degree of over- and underestimation will be directly related to (though only partially controlled by) the degree that pesticide use and foods are evenly distributed around the country. This dispersion will vary considerably among individual pesticide-crop combinations. In all cases, the degree of uncertainty is inversely related to the percentage of acres treated; for example, if 100 percent of all corn acres are treated with atrazine, the uncertainty associated with the percentage-acres-treated statistic is negligible.

Toxicological Certainty

Oncogenic potency factors (Q*) were used as primary indicators of toxicity in this report. They were derived primarily from the linearized multistage low-dose extrapolation procedure used by the Office of Pesticide Programs, yielding upper- and lower-bound estimates of excess tumor incidence/unit of dose statistic. In order to introduce a margin of safety into the risk assessment process that will in part compensate for (1) uncertainties in characterizing the oncogenic response, (2) the existence of sensitive individuals in the population, and (3) possible synergism of pesticides or metabolites, the upper bound of the 95 percent confidence interval, or Q*, is used as the potency factor by the EPA and in all cases for this study. Most potency factors used to estimate risk in this study are averages derived from the results of several positive oncogenicity studies. The Q*'s derived from individual studies on the same compound can vary by an order of magnitude or more.

Interspecies extrapolation modeling is a predictive device based on the best available evidence. Perhaps its greatest value lies in the ability to compare relative risks associated with individual chemicals and among clusters of possible chemical substitutes, provided the chemicals being compared were all tested in a similar manner.

Conclusion—Worst-Case Scenario

The certainty surrounding oncogenic risk estimates is directly related to the uncertainty associated with components of the risk equation:

$$\text{tolerance} \times \text{consumption factor} \times \text{potency factor}$$
$$\times \text{ percent acres treated } = \text{risk.}$$

In drawing conclusions based upon this methodology, it is useful to remember a fundamental principle of probability: the probability of any outcome is the product of probabilities of independent variables that are believed to influence that outcome. Consider the case in which we are 95 percent confident that each component of our risk equation is an upper-bound estimate (i.e., 95 percent of the cases will be less than the level cited). The resulting probability of our risk estimate is then

$$(0.95)T \times (0.95)C \times (0.95)A = (0.81)RISK.$$

In summary, of the four components of the risk estimate, the use of the tolerance rather than residue levels is the factor most likely to overestimate risk since residues are commonly far below tolerance levels. The food consumption estimates used may cause risk to be underestimated because of differences in diet among subpopulations. When acreage-treated adjustment is applied as a U.S. average, exposure of regional populations can be underestimated, depending upon chemical use and food distribution patterns. Finally, it is extremely difficult to characterize the certainty surrounding the oncogenic potency factor (Q^*) other than to recognize that it represents the conservative upper bound of the number of excess tumors per unit dose at the 95 percent confidence interval.

NOTES

1. *Code of Federal Regulations.* 1986a. Title 21, Part 193. Tolerances for pesticides in food administered by EPA. Washington, D.C.: U.S. Government Printing Office.
2. *Code of Federal Regulations.* 1986b. Title 40, Part 180. Tolerances and exemptions from tolerances for pesticide chemicals in or on raw agricultural commodities. Washington, D.C.: U.S. Government Printing Office.
3. Research Triangle Institute (RTI). 1985. Documentation of Analysis and Statistical Methods Used in the Tolerance Assessment System. RTI Publ. RTI/2751/04-09F. Research Triangle Park, N.C.
4. Rizek, Robert. 1985. Nationwide Food Consumption Survey: 1977–78. Hyattsville, Md.: U.S. Department of Agriculture.
5. White, S. B., E. Crouch, and M. Cirillo. 1983. The Construction of a Raw Agricultural Commodity Data Base. Research Triangle Institute Project 252U-2123-7. Research Triangle Park, N.C.
6. U. S. Department of Agriculture. 1981. Agricultural Statistics. Washington, D.C.: U.S. Government Printing Office.
7. Magness, J. R., G. M. Marble, and C. C. Compton. 1971. Food and Feed Crops of the United States Bulletin 828. IR-4. New Jersey Agricultural Experiment Station.
8. National Research Council. 1979. 1977 Survey of Industry on the Use of Food Additives. 3 vols. Washington, D.C.: National Academy Press.
9. International Tariff Commission. 1984. Spices and herbs. In summary of Trade and Tariff Information. Publication 288. From personal communication with John Reeder, Washington, D.C.
10. Research Triangle Institute, 1985, Appendix D.
11. Research Triangle Institute, 1985.
12. *Id.*, p. 22.
13. *Id.*, p. 25.
14. *Id.*, Appendix D.
15. U.S. Food and Drug Administration. 1986. Annual Report of Food Residues in Domestic and Imported Commodities: 1985. Washington, D.C.
16. U.S. Environmental Protection Agency. 1986a. Guidelines for estimating exposures. *Federal Register* 51:185. 9-24-86.
17. U.S. Environmental Protection Agency. 1986b. Guidelines for carcinogen risk assessment. *Federal Register* 51:185. 9-24-86; Research Triangle Institute, p. 50.
18. U.S. General Accounting Office. 1986. Pesticide Need to Enhance FDA's Ability to Protect the Public From Illegal Residues. GAO/RCED 87-7. Washington, D.C.: U.S. General Accounting Office.

C

Case Studies of the EPA's Application of the Delaney Clause in the Tolerance-Setting Process

RICHARD WILES

Case studies of nine pesticide active ingredients—fosetyl Al, benomyl, captan, chlorobenzilate, dicamba, the ethylenebisdithiocarbamates (EBDCs), metalaxyl, permethrin, and thiodicarb—are presented. Descriptions of each chemical are included along with regulatory status, special review criteria that have been triggered, oncogenic findings and risk estimation, alternative pesticides, and a discussion of issues relevant to tolerances and the Delaney Clause (section 409).

FOSETYL AL

Description of the Chemical

Common name:	Aluminum tris (ethyl phosphonate) or fosetyl Al
Trade name:	Aliette
Pesticide type:	Systemic fungicide
Chemical family:	Organophosphate
Year registered:	1983
Major producer:	Rhone-Poulenc, under patent
Volume of use:	Small
Tolerances:	Fosetyl Al has section 408 tolerances of 0.1 parts per million (ppm) for pineapples, pineapple fodder, and pineapple forage. A recent petition for sections 408 and 409 tolerances on hops was denied. An application for a section 408 tolerance on citrus is pending.

Regulatory Status

General-use pesticide

Special Review Criteria Triggered

Evidence of weak oncogenicity was dealt with in the registration process.

Summary of Oncogenic Findings and Risk Estimation

The incidence of kidney tumors was statistically significant in the high dose of one chronic feeding study. However, the high-dose feeding level was approximately 35,000 ppm, a rate equivalent to about 4 percent of the total diet of the test animal. Tumors termed by the EPA as of "questionable significance" also appeared at the mid-dose level of 8,000 ppm, about 1 percent of the diet of the test animal. Alone, the mid-dose findings would not support a finding of oncogenicity, but because of the high-dose tumors, the pesticide was classified as oncogenic. According to informal discussions with EPA staff, the data base for fosetyl Al is complete and of high caliber. In fact, the data are of such high quality that they may actually be working against further registration of the chemical.

Fosetyl Al has an extremely low acute toxicity. Thus, in complying strictly with EPA guidelines instructing registrants to study the effect of chronic feeding at the maximum tolerated dose (MTD), the registrant fed extremely high doses of the chemical to test animals. The only oncogenic effect observed was that mentioned above. The oncogenic risk from dietary exposure to fosetyl Al is calculated by the EPA at about 1×10^{-8}, or 1 in 100 million.

Tolerance and Delaney Clause Issues

A recent request for a section 3 registration on hops was denied because it was determined that the use of fosetyl Al on hops required a section 409 tolerance. This tolerance could not be granted under current law (the Delaney Clause) because residue studies showed that during drying, fosetyl Al concentrates to levels above the proposed 408 tolerances for hops. The proposed tolerance level for fosetyl Al was 10 ppm on green hops and 15 ppm on dried hops.

The registrant anticipated that fosetyl Al would make significant inroads into the U.S. fungicide market and quickly become a major product. Fosetyl Al is designed to control downy mildew in vines, as well as numerous fungi in fruits and vegetables. Its use in these areas has expanded since its introduction in Europe in 1978. It is possible that fosetyl Al could eventually command a significant share of the U.S. market currently occupied by more toxic or less-studied fungicides such as the ethylenebisdithiocarbamates (EBDCs), captan, or benomyl.

For example, currently the most widely used fungicides on hops are the EBDCs. The estimated dietary oncogenic risk from residues of EBDCs and its metabolite ethylenethiourea (ETU) in and on hops is 1×10^{-4} to 1×10^{-5}. The risk from the same use of fosetyl Al is 1×10^{-8} or less. Were fosetyl Al to have acquired any share of the EBDC market it may have lowered exposure to the more oncogenic EBDC and ETU residues.

BENOMYL

Description of the Chemical

Common name:	Benomyl
Trade name:	Benlate
Pesticide type:	Systemic fungicide
Chemical family:	Benzimidazole
Year registered:	1972
Major producer:	Du Pont, under patent
Volume of use:	Benomyl accounts for 55 percent of the $320 million worldwide benzimidazole fungicide market. In 1984, U.S. sales amounted to approximately $60 million. In 1979 about 3 million pounds were used in the United States on 43 food crops and 41 ornamentals.
Tolerances:	Benomyl has numerous section 408 tolerances and several section 409 tolerances. New sections 408 and 409 feed additive tolerances were issued for benomyl in wheat, barley, and other small grains on November 7, 1984.

Regulatory Status

A notice of Rebuttable Presumption Against Registration (RPAR, now known as a special review) of benomyl was initiated in 1977 because benomyl exceeded the risk criteria cited below; oncogenicity was not an initial risk consideration. The Position Document (PD) 1 was published December 6, 1977. Findings of oncogenicity were made subsequent to the EPA's proposed decision in the PD 2/3.

A PD 4, or Notice of Determination, was published on October 12, 1982. The notice allows continued registration of all uses with protective clothing requirements and registrant submission of field studies to identify residues that may enter aquatic sites after use on rice. A registration standard for benomyl was completed in 1986.

Special Review Criteria Triggered

Reduction in nontarget species
Mutagenicity
Teratogenicity
Reproductive effects
Hazard to wildlife

Summary of Oncogenic Findings and Risk Estimation

In tests with benomyl, hepatocellular carcinomas or combined hepato-cellular neoplasms in both male and female mice were observed at all doses (the low dose was 500 ppm). Similar tests with a metabolite of benomyl, methyl-2-benzimidazole carbamate (MBC), revealed combined hepatocellular neoplasms in male mice and hepatocellular adenomas, carcinomas, and combined hepatocellular neoplasms in female mice. These data were received subsequent to the EPA's proposed regulatory decision (PD 2/3) but prior to the final Notice of Determination (PD 4).

Based on findings of oncogencity for benomyl and MBC, an oncogenic potency factor (Q^*, or extra incidence of tumors/unit dose) of 2.065×10^{-3} was determined. Multiplying projected human exposure by Q^* will estimate the 95 percent upper bound on cancer risks to humans from lifetime exposures. Using the multistage model and residues at the tolerance level, the upper limit of oncogenic risk to the general public via dietary exposure to benomyl was estimated as 6.8×10^{-5}. On the basis of residue analyses, the lifetime oncogenic risk from dietary exposure to benomyl at average expected residue levels was calculated at 7.2×10^{-6}.[1]

Tolerance and Delaney Clause Issues

The case of benomyl illustrates the relationship between the reregistration process, tolerance reassessments, and the Delaney Clause. Benomyl currently has section 409 feed additive tolerances on apple pomace, grape pomace, citrus pulp, rice hulls, and tomato products.

Benomyl was granted these tolerances prior to knowledge of its oncogenicity. There is also evidence (contained in data submitted by Du Pont to the EPA) that benomyl concentrates in orange juice, dried apricots, plums, and grape juice. On the basis of current studies indicating oncogencity, section 409 tolerance applications for these uses would probably be denied under the Delaney Clause.[2]

Benomyl is the first pesticide registered before 1972 for which the EPA will have residue data sufficient to support tolerance actions pursuant to the Delaney Clause at the time of a major regulatory action (registration standard). If the Delaney Clause is strictly applied, benomyl could lose section 409 and possibly section 408 tolerances for apples, grapes, citrus, rice, and tomatoes. These uses account for around 1.1 million pounds of benomyl applications, or approximately one-third of all benomyl sales. Reduction in estimated dietary oncogenic risk from revocation of these tolerances would largely be a function of the oncogenic risk associated with benomyl's replacements. (See Chapter 5 for further discussion of this issue.)

Pest Resistance

A distinct feature of benomyl is that it acts systemically. Because of this, benomyl has many more uses and does not have to be applied as often, in as high rates, or prophylactically, as do nonsystemic fungicides such as captan and the EBDCs. However, this characteristic has led to the development of resistance in target fungi. According to Dr. George Georghiou of the University of California at Riverside, of the 70 species of fungi reported as resistant to fungicides by 1979, 69 species (84 percent) were resistant to one material—benomyl. Du Pont has recommended lower doses per application and more precisely timed use of benomyl in order to control the exacerbation of this problem.

To retain the advantages of benomyl use and to retard the spread of resistance, growers often curtail use or apply benomyl in combination with captan and/or the EBDCs. For example, Pacific Northwest apple and pear growers use benomyl only for post-harvest disease control to reduce the possibility of tolerant fungi strains.

Alternatives

For several pests and diseases, there are no registered substitutes for benomyl. For example, benomyl is the only pesticide registered to control rice blast and stem rot, which cause approximately a 12 to 15 percent loss in rice production annually. And according to the EPA, neither cultural practices, crop rotations, nor water management are effective in controlling these diseases.

The principal replacements for benomyl in fruit and vegetable production are captan, the EBDCs, captafol, or newer systemic fungicides such as metalaxyl or fosetyl Al. However, both captan and the EBDCs are under special review for oncogenic, mutagenic, and teratogenic effects, pending the receipt of data. Although a weak oncogen, fosetyl Al has been denied tolerances due to the Delaney Clause.

CAPTAN

Description of the Chemical

Common name: Captan
Trade names: Merpan, Orthocide, Vondcaptan, Vancide-89, and SR-46
Pesticide type: Nonsystemic fungicide
Chemical family: Dicarboximides
Year registered: 1951
Major producers: Stauffer Chemical and Chevron Chemical produce the technical material. There are over 600 registered products containing captan, with registrations held by 139 formulators and producers.
Volume of use: Approximately 9 to 10 million pounds are applied annually.
Tolerances: Captan has more than 70 section 408 tolerances ranging from 0.25 to 100 ppm. One section 409 food additive tolerance is established for raisins and one feed additive tolerance is in place for corn seed used as animal feed.

Regulatory Status

An RPAR and PD 1 were issued on August 18, 1980. At that time the EPA sought information on the oncogenic, mutagenic, teratogenic, and other reproductive effects of captan.

PD 2/3 was issued June 21, 1985, in which the EPA proposed to cancel all uses of captan on food crops unless "data are submitted that demonstrate that actual residues are sufficiently lower than current tolerances or that modification to application practices will sufficiently reduce dietary risk."

Special Review Criteria Triggered

Oncogenicity
Mutagenicity

Summary of Oncogenic Findings

At the time of PD 1, the strongest evidence of captan's oncogenicity was in studies by the National Cancer Institute (NCI) and Innes et al.[3] These studies showed that captan can induce adenocarcinomas, adenomatous polyps, and mucosal hyperplasia in both sexes of mice. Two subsequent studies for Chevron, one a high-dose (6,000 to 16,000 ppm) and one a low-dose study (0 to 6,000 ppm), replicated the positive finding of adenocarcinomas of the digestive tract in both sexes in mice. A concurrent rat study, cosponsored by Stauffer and Chevron, found statistically significant increases in combined malignant and benign kidney tumors. The determination of oncogenicity has been contested by captan's registrants. In support of its finding of oncogenicity for captan, the EPA cites the rarity and replication of intestinal tumors in mice, and the fact that captan is structurally similar to captafol and folpet, both of which have demonstrated oncogenic effects in laboratory animals. Of particular significance is the occurrence of rare intestinal tumors, including adenocarcinomas, in chronic feeding studies of both captan and folpet.

On the basis of this information, the EPA has assigned captan to category B2 in their modification of the International Agency for Research on Cancer (IARC) classification "probable human carcinogen." The EPA calculated the Q* (potency) factor for captan as 2.3 × 10⁻³.

The EPA is also requesting chronic data on tetrahydrophthalimide (THPI), a metabolite of captan. There is some concern within the agency that THPI may also cause tumors in laboratory animals.

Estimate of Dietary Oncogenic Risk

Using the multistage model for risk assessment, the EPA has calculated two estimates of dietary oncogenic risk. One is based on residues of captan at tolerance levels; the other is based on data from market basket surveys conducted by Chevron, Stauffer, the FDA, and the Canadian government.[4]

Using Food Factor consumption estimates assuming that 100 percent of all crops with tolerances for captan are treated and that residues are at the tolerance level, the agency estimates a dietary upper-bound oncogenic risk of 10^{-3} to 10^{-4}.

When market basket survey residue figures are used, the risk is calculated at 10^{-6} to 10^{-7}. Although calculations using tolerances probably overstate exposure and risk, the use of market basket data may underestimate exposure and risk because the frequency of treatment was not stated and because both treated and untreated foods were examined.

Tolerance and Delaney Clause Issues

Captan illustrates the difficulty of conducting risk assessments using raw agricultural commodity (section 408) tolerances based on little or no data. These tolerances are generally high and in many cases not supported with valid data. They are often estimates set to accommodate the greatest conceivable residue of the chemical. Thus, they tend to inflate risk estimates. For example, the tolerance for apples—the major use of captan—is 25 ppm, whereas the highest residue detected in the studies cited above[5] was 0.08 ppm. The difference in these exposure estimates could alter risk estimates for consumption of captan-treated apples by three or four orders of magnitude.

Further, in many cases, pesticides registered in the 1950s and 1960s (such as captan) have been subjected to few if any of the studies necessary to determine whether residues concentrate in processed foods or animal feeds. Although the residue data cited above[6] indicate that captan residues generally decline with the processing of foods, it is possible that residues could concentrate in animal feed portions of many crops, thus necessitating section 409 feed additive tolerances for these crops. If tolerances were denied or revoked because of the concentration of residues in animal feeds, significant adjustments would be required of growers highly dependent on captan.

Other Chronic Health Risks

Captan illustrates the limitations of the Delaney Clause in reducing a non-oncogenic dietary risk—in this case a reproductive risk. The No Observable Effect Level (NOEL) for toxic effects in reproductive studies using captan is 12.5 mg/kg body weight/day. Using a safety factor of 100, the allowable daily intake of captan would be 0.125 mg/kg body weight/day. For a 60-kg person this translates into a maximum allowable intake of 7.5 mg/day. However, using the EPA theoretical maximum residue contributions (TMRCs) based on dietary exposure to captan residues at the tolerance level, a person would consume 12.2 mg/kg body weight/day of captan residues, or 63 percent more than the estimated safe daily dose. In the absence of concurrent oncogenicity, these risks could not be reduced by the Delaney Clause.

CHLOROBENZILATE

Description of the Chemical

Common name:	Chlorobenzilate, or ethyl-4,4'-dichlorobenzilate
Trade name:	Chlorobenzilate
Pesticide type:	Acaricide
Chemical family:	Organochlorine
Year registered:	1956
Major producer:	Ciba-Geigy
Volume of use:	Approximately 1.5 million pounds per year are applied on citrus.
Tolerances:	Chlorobenzilate has a section 408 tolerance of 5.0 ppm in citrus. There are no section 409 tolerances.

Regulatory Status

An RPAR against the registration of pesticide products containing chlorobenzilate was issued May 26, 1976, on the basis of findings of oncogenicity in mice.

A PD 4, Notice of Intent to Cancel Registrations of pesticide products containing chlorobenzilate, was issued February 13, 1979. This notice canceled all uses except on citrus in Florida, Texas, California, and Arizona. These remaining uses are classified as restricted and require protective clothing during application. A registration standard was completed in 1984.

Special Review Criteria Triggered

Oncogenicity

Summary of Oncogenic Findings and Risk Estimation

Evidence of oncogenicity was found in an 18-month feeding study in which male mice exhibited a statistically significant increase in liver tumors when fed chlorobenzilate. An NCI study also found statistically significant increases in total tumors and hepatocellular carcinomas in mice. The EPA's Cancer Assessment Group classified chlorobenzilate as a class C "possible human carcinogen."

For most foods with tolerances, tests revealed no detectable chlorobenzilate residues. In these cases, a residue level of 0.1 ppm (the level of detection) was used in calculating dietary exposure. Exceptions were made for apples and pears because the whole fruit is consumed; residues in these cases were set at 5.0 ppm. Because residues of 0.01–0.02

ppm were detected in milk and beef, a 0.04-ppm residue level was used. Using the one-hit model and these residue levels, the oncogenic risk from dietary exposure to chlorobenzilate was calculated at 0.4×10^{-6} to 2.1×10^{-6} throughout the U.S. population.

Tolerance and Delaney Clause Issues

A potential conflict with the Delaney Clause arose during the review of residue chemistry data for the preparation of the registration standard. Residue studies reveal that chlorobenzilate concentrates by a factor of 5 in citrus oil. Because of the Delaney Clause, agency findings of oncogenicity would normally block the issuance of a section 409 tolerance and, moreover, would draw into question the section 408 tolerance for use in citrus. Were chlorobenzilate a new product, it would most likely have been denied both section 408 and section 409 tolerances on citrus (see Chapter 3). However, in this case the section 409 tolerance for citrus oil was not issued, and the section 408 tolerance for use on citrus remains in effect. The EPA has taken the position in this case that the oncogenic potential of chlorobenzilate is so weak, and the consumption of citrus oil so small, that a quantitative assessment of the oncogenic risk from consumption of citrus oil cannot be supported by the available data.

Benefits and Alternatives

At the time of the RPAR, the EPA estimated the increased total cost to citrus growers from the cancellation of chlorobenzilate at $57 million. Other benefits of retaining chlorobenzilate use are its application in integrated pest management (IPM) programs and its effectiveness for control of mites. However, some experts have argued that the EPA's analysis exaggerated the value of chlorobenzilate in citrus production.

A 1980 study by the National Research Council[7] (NRC) used chlorobenzilate as a case study of the RPAR process. The NRC analysis concluded that "the evidence indicates that the yield and quality of citrus crops will not be diminished appreciably, if at all, if farmers are required to replace chlorobenzilate treatments with some alternative" (p. 196). Further, the NRC calculated the added cost of these alternatives to be in the $0–$3 million range, rather than the $57 million cited by the EPA.

The principal alternative pesticides are ethion, carbophenthion, sulfur, and dicofol. Dicofol is currently under special review and the remaining are in the registration standard process with no evidence of oncogenic effects. Ethion and carbophenthion are potent organophosphate insecticides which present other types of risks to applicators and the environment.

DICAMBA

Description of the Chemical

Common name:	Dicamba
Trade name:	Banvel
Pesticide type:	Broadleaf herbicide
Chemical family:	Benzoic acid
Major producer:	Velsicol
Year registered:	1967
Volume of use:	3 million pounds annually
Tolerances:	Dicamba has numerous section 408 tolerances. The establishment of a section 409 tolerance for dicamba residues in sugarcane molasses involved the application of the FDA "constituents policy" as discussed below.

Regulatory Status

General-use pesticide. Registration standard was completed in 1983. Oncogencity data are due in October 1987.

Special Review Criteria Triggered

None

Oncogenic Contaminants and the Delaney Clause

Animal studies submitted to the EPA do not show dicamba to be oncogenic. However, these experiments were conducted at Industrial Biotest Laboratories (IBT) and are considered invalid. Replacement tests are scheduled for submission to the EPA in October 1987.

Studies with a contaminant of dicamba—dimethylnitrosamine (DMNA)—have shown it to be an animal oncogen. The presence of an oncogenic contaminant in a non-oncogenic food or feed additive (pesticide residue) could in theory trigger the Delaney Clause. However, because dicamba as a whole is considered non-oncogenic in spite of the presence of an oncogenic contaminant, the EPA employed the "constituents policy" articulated by the FDA in D&C Green No. 6[8] to issue a section 409 tolerance.

The FDA's constituents argument states that the safety of undesired (oncogenic) nonfunctional constituents (in non-oncogenic substances) should be judged under the general safety provisions of the FDC Act (not the Delaney Clause), using risk assessment as one of the decision-making tools. In this case the additional oncogenic risk from exposure to DMNA residues in sugarcane molasses, with expected residue levels of 8–16 parts per trillion (ppt), was calculated as 2.9×10^{-8}. This level of risk was deemed acceptable in lieu of losing the benefits, and the section 409 tolerance was granted.

Discussion

There are at least three basic issues involved in the issuance of a section 409 tolerance for dicamba. One centers on the regulation of oncogens under the general safety clause of the FDC Act, the second involves the FDA's so-called "constituents policy," and the third entails the consideration of comparative risks and benefits under the FDC Act.

GENERAL SAFETY CLAUSE

Several comments on the rule establishing a section 409 tolerance for dicamba argued against the use of the general safety clause of the FDC Act on the grounds that it is generally established in the scientific and regulatory literature that there is no safe level of exposure to a carcinogenic substance. In other words, there is no threshold level below which tumors are known to not be induced. This argument contends that because residues in the diet at tolerance levels must be shown to be safe (in section 409 of the FDC Act and in the FDA's constituents policy), and because there is presently no known safe level of exposure to an oncogen, then section 409 tolerances for dicamba cannot legally be issued under the general safety clause.

On the other hand, the FDA argues that, using a set of conservative assumptions, exposures that create an additional oncogenic risk of less than 1 in 1 million (1×10^{-6}) throughout the lifetime of the population shall be considered safe. The oncogenic risk from exposure to DMNA in dicamba residues is estimated to fall in the 1 in 100 million (1×10^{-8}) range.

THE CONSTITUENTS POLICY

Regarding the definition of a constituent and the future use of the constituents policy for the issuance of section 409 tolerances for pesticides, the EPA stated its policy as follows:

EPA does not regard deliberately added active or inert ingredients, or metabolites thereof, as potential candidates for clearance under the constituents policy rationale. . . . Rather, EPA will only consider applying this rationale to impurities arising from the manufacture of the pesticide (residual reactants, intermediates, and products of side reactions and chemical degradates). Furthermore the Agency will consider using this rationale in issuing a food additive regulation only where the potential risk from the impurity is extremely low.[9]

(How low was not specified in the *Federal Register* notice; however, 1 × 10⁻⁶ has been the criteria used by the FDA.) The EPA has not subsequently invoked the constituents policy to grant any food or feed tolerance.

BENEFITS OF DICAMBA

Dicamba is one of several products available to replace the suspended and eventually voluntarily withdrawn herbicides 2,4,5-T and silvex. Other alternatives in sugar production include paraquat, glyphosate, and 2,4-D.

It is likely that the EPA's desire to find a replacement for the suspended herbicide 2,4,5-T played a part in the use of the constituents policy in this case. Although the comparative risks of these two compounds were not discussed in the *Federal Register* notice establishing this tolerance, the EPA's fact sheet and the registration standard document both note that "The performance of dicamba containing herbicides is such that they are viable alternatives to the suspended uses of silvex and 2,4,5-T."

One result of this use of the constituents policy was to provide an alternative to 2,4,5-T and silvex which, although not risk free, clearly presented less risk. In this way the constituents policy provided a mechanism to move toward the use of safer pesticides. On the other hand, the constituents policy does allow small amounts of theoretical risk (generally less than 1 × 10⁻⁶) from residues of oncogenic pesticide contaminants in food *if the product when tested as a whole is non-oncogenic*.

ETHYLENEBISDITHIOCARBAMATES (EBDCs)

Description of the Chemical

Trade names:	Major products include maneb, zineb, mancozeb, and metiram
Pesticide type:	Nonsystemic fungicide
Chemical family:	Dithiocarbamate
Years registered:	Introduced from the 1930s through the 1960s
Major producers:	There are over 40 manufacturers worldwide. In the United States, EBDCs are produced by Rohm and Haas, Du Pont, FMC, Stauffer Chemical, and seven

	other corporations. Major foreign producers are Montedison (Italy) and Rhone-Poulenc (France).
Volume of use:	EBDCs are the most widely used group of fungicides in the world. The global market was estimated at $525 million in 1984. In the United States, more than 30 million pounds are used annually to control a wide variety of fungal diseases on fruits, vegetables, field crops, seeds, and ornamentals. Approximately one-third of all fruits and vegetables in the United States are treated with EBDCs. They are also used as industrial slimicides. No other commercial fungicides have as broad a spectrum of activity on as many crops as the EBDCs.
Tolerances:	There are more than 150 section 408 tolerances for EBDC fungicides. Mancozeb has been granted section 409 tolerances for raisins, cereal grain, and bran, as well as animal feed tolerances for barley, oats, rye, and wheat. No meat, milk, or egg tolerances have been established, although EBDC fungicides are applied to numerous commodities used as animal feed. No feed additive tolerances have been established for the many EBDC-treated vegetable and fruit byproducts that are used as animal feed. No tolerances have been established for ETU—a contaminant conversion product and metabolite of the EBDCs.

Regulatory Status

An RPAR against the EBDCs was initiated in August 1977, on the basis of oncogenicity, teratogenicity, and acute toxicity to aquatic organisms.

The PD 4 was completed on October 14, 1982. None of the presumptions of risk were rebutted, yet all registrations were continued contingent on label modifications to include requirements for protective clothing for mixers and loaders, an aquatic toxicity warning statement, and the completion of specified chronic toxicology, metabolism, and dermal absorption studies. The EBDCs have extremely low acute toxicities.

The EPA was sued by the Natural Resources Defense Council (NRDC) on this and 12 other RPAR decisions. NRDC charged that the RPAR process was not sufficiently open and that industry had an unfair influence on the resolution of these RPAR proceedings. In a consent decree agreement with the NRDC, the EPA agreed to review its decision on the EBDCs during the registration standard for the chemicals originally scheduled for FY 1986.[10] The EPA recently proposed to postpone the completion of the registration standard to 1990.

Special Review Criteria Triggered

EBDCs

Oncogenicity
Teratogenicity
Acute aquatic toxicity
Thyroid toxicity

ETU

Oncogenicity
Teratogenicity
Acute aquatic toxicity
Mutagenicity
Thyroid toxicity

Summary of Oncogenic Findings

An RPAR was initiated against the EBDCs largely on the basis of studies indicating the oncogenic potential of EBDCs and their contaminant and conversion product ETU. These studies found

- Increased lung adenomas in three short-term (6- to 11-week) single-dose EBDC feeding studies with mice;
- Increased liver and lung tumors and lymphomas in mice fed a single dose of ETU for 80 weeks;
- Thyroid carcinomas in both doses of an 18-month ETU feeding study of rats; and
- Dose-related thyroid carcinomas, thyroid adenomas, and thyroid hyperplasia during a 2-year ETU feeding study of rats.

The agency agreed with rebutters that the EBDC feeding studies could not be used for quantitative risk assessment purposes. Several registrants argued that the liver and thyroid tumors found in these studies could have been indirectly induced. The EPA recognized this possibility and requested more data on the subject. The agency rejected epidemiological evidence provided by registrants claiming to show that EBDCs and ETU are not oncogenic. The EPA has requested new chronic feeding studies from the registrants.

Dietary Exposure

Because ETU is a metabolite of the EBDCs and because the chronic data on ETU are of higher quality and generally indicate that ETU is a more potent oncogen, teratogen, and thyrotoxin than the EBDCs, the EPA conducted its risk assessment on the basis of exposure to ETU resulting from EBDC usage. ETU is also a contaminant and degradation product of the EBDC fungicides and is thus present on raw agricultural commodities prior to processing.

In estimating dietary exposure to ETU, the agency made several assumptions. First, it factored the percentage of each crop treated with EBDCs in estimating a high and a low dietary exposure level. Although 11 to 48 percent of EBDCs have been shown to convert to ETU during cooking, the agency assumed a one-to-one conversion rate for the purpose of an upper-bound dietary exposure calculation. This was justified by the general uncertainty in estimating overall exposure, as well as the exclusion of major exposure factors from sources such as drinking water, and meat and dairy products, for which there are no tolerances, but where residues have been detected in the past. (The EPA expects to find ETU residues in meat and dairy products. These ETU residues are produced by animals during metabolism of feeds such as apple and tomato pomace and citrus pulp, known and suspected to have EBDC and ETU residues.)

The worst-case ETU dietary exposure for a 60-kg person—when estimating EBDC residues at the tolerance levels, a one-to-one EBDC-to-ETU conversion rate, commonly used food factors, the percentage of food treated, and residues at the level of detection (0.02 ppm) for milk and meat—is 3.65×10^{-3} mg/kg body weight/day.

The lowest-case estimate for ETU dietary exposure—calculated using the same food factors, the level-of-detection residues for milk and meat and all other foods except spinach and tomatoes (where residue survey data were utilized), the percentages of crops treated, and a mean averaging of positive residue samples for raw and processed foods—is 2.4×10^{-4} mg/kg body weight/day for a 60-kg person. When exposure to ETU residues through metabolism of EBDC residues calculated at survey levels or the level of detection were added to the lowest-case estimate, the dietary exposure level was calculated as 3.4×10^{-4}, or an additional 0.00010 mg/kg body weight/day.

Risk Assessment

Using the one-hit model, oncogenic risks from dietary exposure were calculated for both a worst-case and a lowest-case estimate. The worst case assumed residues at the tolerance level and a 38 percent conversion of EBDC to ETU (not one-to-one as with the worst-case exposure assessment), whereas the lowest case used the 38 percent conversion and residues based on survey data or the level of detection. Both assumed exposure over 70 years. The lifetime worst-case estimate of oncogenic risk through dietary exposure was calculated as 4.9×10^{-4}, whereas the lowest-case estimate was calculated as 4.8×10^{-5}. The agency has stated that it may have underestimated the upper limit on risk because of inadequate data on animal metabolism, ETU in processed foods, residues on raw agricultural commodities, and residue in drinking water, meat, milk, eggs, and animal feeds.

Tolerance and Delaney Clause Issues

Specific issues include

- Prior sanctioned tolerances;
- Readjustment of section 408 tolerances in 1972;
- Conversion of EBDCs to ETU, and thus ETU concentration during cooking, canning, and other processing;
- Absence of sections 408 and 409 tolerances for ETU;
- Absence of section 409 feed additive tolerances for many vegetable and fruit by-products; and
- Absence of tolerances for milk, meat, and eggs, even though EBDCs are applied to numerous commodities used as animal feed, and ETU has been detected in those foods.

HISTORY

In 1955, section 408 tolerances for Zineb (the first EBDC to receive tolerances) were set at 7 ppm for fruits and vegetables on "very little data showing residues from actual commercial use."[11] In 1957, section 408 tolerances for Zineb in spinach, lettuce, and six other related crops were increased from 7 to 25 ppm. For some of these uses, there may be approved residues in processed foods sanctioned prior to the Food Additive Amendments of 1958 which includes the Delaney Clause.

Other EBDC tolerances were established throughout the 1960s, ranging from 7 to 15 ppm. However, in 1970, final action on a petition for a 1-ppm section 408 tolerance for Zineb in potatoes was never taken because the FDA notified the EPA that an FDA rat feeding study confirmed findings of ETU carcinogenicity. In October 1971, the EPA and the FDA tolerance-setting staffs recommended the revocation of all

EBDC tolerances except those where no residues were detected. According to EPA staff, no tolerances were revoked, however, because of insufficient data on ETU residues on crops. Representatives of Du Pont, FMC, and Rohm and Haas met with the EPA in early 1972 and agreed to lower tolerances on major-use crops. Because many of these tolerances had been previously raised, these current (lowered) tolerances remain in the 5- to 15-ppm range. Further, the residue chemistry and toxicological data to support EBDC tolerances are generally not complete.[12]

CONVERSION TO ETU

In addition to the presence of ETU in EBDC fungicides as applied to raw agricultural commodities, EDBC residues are known to degrade readily to ETU during the commercial processing or home cooking of various foods—in particular, during the cooking or canning of spinach, carrots, potatoes, snap beans, and apples. A study of processed foods by Du Pont found ETU in 23 percent of the samples.[13] A 1978 FDA study found ETU in 100 percent of both raw and canned spinach samples.[14]

Although ETU's presence as a contaminant and a degradation product could necessitate tolerances for ETU, to date no section 408 or 409 tolerances have been established. For enforcement purposes, ETU is considered to be covered by EBDC tolerances and to be present at levels equivalent to a 100 percent conversion of EBDC residues.

There are problems, however, with this enforcement system in relation to the Delaney Clause. Although the accepted average rate of EBDC-to-ETU conversion of 38 percent indicates that ETU residues per se concentrate during cooking and processing, it is unlikely that ETU residues in a processed food will exceed the EBDC residues in the raw agricultural commodity. However, where conversion takes place, the ETU residues in processed foods will be greater than the ETU levels in the raw agricultural commodity. In other words, ETU is an oncogenic by-product of an oncogenic pesticide, concentrating to levels in processed foods that are not likely to exceed the relatively high section 408 tolerances for the EBDCs that for enforcement purposes are applied to ETU; but ETU residues are potentially higher in processed foods than they are in raw agricultural commodities.

Available metabolism studies, although not complete, show that EBDCs are metabolized to ETU in animals. An adequate understanding of this problem is further complicated by the dearth of residue studies and the absence of EBDC or ETU tolerances for meat, milk, and eggs, even though EBDCs are applied to numerous commodities used as animal feed. Both EBDCs and ETU have been detected in milk and butter.

Alternatives

EBDC fungicides control nearly all foliar pathogens of vegetables found in the United States. The EBDCs are desirable to growers because they are inexpensive, have few phytotoxic effects, have no problem with pest resistance, can be used in some integrated programs, control a wide spectrum of diseases, and are compatible for tank mixing with other pesticides. Effective alternatives are registered for nearly all registered uses of EBDCs, but they are generally more expensive.

In some cases the increase in cost to achieve equivalent control would be quite significant, particularly in humid areas such as the Southeast. For example, with the currently available fungicides, Florida growers use an average of 20.2 EBDC applications to control early and late blight in celery, whereas in California the average number of applications is around 7. According to a USDA/State/EPA assessment team, the cost per acre is the only real difference in controlling early- and late-season blight with the following fungicides: $3.00 for EBDCs, $3.80 for captafol, and $5.80 for chlorothalonil. If the EBDC registrations were canceled, southeastern vegetable growers would suffer the greatest economic losses. Indeed, it is the use of these fungicides that has permitted the expansion of the production of certain vegetables into the humid areas of the Southeast. It is noteworthy, however, that many of these crops have no processed form, and thus remain beyond the scope of the tolerance-setting limitations of the Delaney Clause.

METALAXYL

Description of the Chemical

Common name: Metalaxyl
Trade name: Ridomil
Pesticide type: Systemic fungicide
Chemical family: Benzenoid
Year registered: 1979, conditional registration
Major producer: Ciba-Geigy, under patent
Volume of use: Approximately 400,000 pounds were used on tobacco in 1982. Other uses include vines, potatoes, and vegetable crops.

Tolerances: Metalaxyl has numerous permanent section 408 tolerances on vegetables as well as section 409 tolerances on potato and tomato products, and feed additive tolerances for tomato and potato by-products.

Regulatory Status

General-use pesticide with a section 3 registration. Evidence of potential oncogenicity was reviewed extensively for several years. The final EPA decision was that metalaxyl is not an oncogen.

Special Review Criteria Triggered

Issues of oncogenicity were dealt with in the registration process.

Summary of Oncogenic Findings

Chronic rat feeding studies to support the registration of metalaxyl were initially accepted, and the determination was made that the fungicide was not an oncogen. However, questions later arose regarding the possibility that the EPA staff had "cut and pasted" Ciba-Geigy's analysis onto EPA letterhead to expedite their review of the chemical. Subsequently, a reevaluation of the data and a lab audit were ordered.

During the data reevaluation, concerns arose surrounding the appearance of statistically significant parafollicular adenomas of the thyroid in female rats at the low and middle dose, but *not* at the high dose, of a two-year rat feeding study. Concurrently, the lab audit team could not validate that the chronic feeding studies were in fact done using metalaxyl. At this point, December 1983, all actions on metalaxyl were halted, including tolerance approvals and emergency exemptions.

Under instructions from the registrant, the test samples were unsealed and results showed that the studies were in fact conducted with metalaxyl. However, upon further investigation, the EPA staff found evidence of pheochromocytomas of the adrenal gland medulla in male rats. Questions also appeared regarding whether the maximum tolerated dose had been administered during the teratology and chronic feeding studies. The toxicology branch turned the oncogenic evaluation over to the EPA's Cancer Assessment Group which, in conjunction with other agency staff, decided in early 1986 that metalaxyl should not be classified as an oncogen.

Estimation of Risk

There was a difference of opinion among the EPA staff as to whether metalaxyl is an oncogen. One statistical analysis of the data submitted by Ciba-Geigy concluded that when the upper-dose finding of thyroid adenomas in females rats was excluded, a significant dose response relationship emerges. Using a risk estimation derived from this statistical analysis, the EPA staff have calculated eight upper limits of oncogenic risk from dietary exposure ranging from 2.41 per 10,000 (2.41×10^{-4}) to 2.27 per 1,000 (2.27×10^{-3}).

However, the validity of this interpretation is disputed within the agency. Several staff have argued, in agreement with Ciba-Geigy, that when the upper-dose finding is included in a calculation of oncogenic potential, there is no dose response relationship and the incidence of this tumor in this species in comparison to the control group is not statistically significant.

Tolerance and Delaney Clause Issues

This example illustrates the importance of data interpretation and the far-reaching consequences of a borderline decision on oncogenicity. The EPA staff interpretation of data on metalaxyl ranged from classifying it as non-oncogenic, to characterizing the dietary risk at 2.27×10^{-3}.

If metalaxyl had been declared an oncogen, the Delaney Clause would have been invoked, and metalaxyl would have been denied permanent section 408 and section 409 tolerances in cases where residues concentrate in processed foods or feeds. However, because it has been declared non-oncogenic, it will retain current tolerances and will presumably be granted permanent tolerances for pending petitions.

Potential Uses and Alternatives

In 1979, metalaxyl was granted a conditional registration based on its potential economic benefits to tobacco farmers in controlling blue mold and downy mildew. Temporary tolerances exist for many other uses, but the economic benefits of its use are not well quantified. However, metalaxyl is generally more expensive than currently used compounds. Pest resistance has also been a problem in isolated areas.

Currently registered alternatives to metalaxyl include the EBDCs, captan, benomyl, captafol, and chlorothalonil. Although all of these have chronic toxicity data indicating adverse effects usually more severe than those associated with metalaxyl, the agency has yet to apply Delaney to section 409 tolerances for old chemicals found to be oncogenic. Theoretically, metalaxyl could replace some percentage of uses of the currently used fungicides.

In the absence of use cancellations or tolerance revocations for these compounds, however, metalaxyl is expected to complement rather than replace older fungicides for most crops.

PERMETHRIN

Description of the Chemical

Common name:	Permethrin
Trade names:	Pounce, Ambush
Pesticide type:	Pyrethroid insecticide
Chemical family:	Synthetic pyrethroid
Major producers:	Imperial Chemicals Industries and FMC
Year registered:	Conditional registration in 1978
Volume of use:	Used on cotton, corn, soybeans, fruits, and vegetables. As a family, synthethic pyrethroids are the fastest growing sector of the insecticide market, with projected annual sales growth rate of 30 percent. Permethrin, however, has experienced a recent decline in use, partially due to pest resistance.
Tolerances:	Numerous section 408 tolerances are established. No section 409 tolerances have been issued because of oncogenicity and the Delaney Clause.

Regulatory Status

General-use pesticide

Special Review Criteria Triggered

Positive findings of oncogenicity in mice were dealt with in the registration process.

Summary of Oncogenic Findings and Risk Estimation

Among six long-term mouse and rat oncogenicity studies, an increase in malignant tumors was evident only in the lungs of female mice from one test. For total tumors, dose response relationships were established in two mice studies. No evidence of mutagenicity was observed in a battery of tests including a test for DNA damage. All other oncogenicity and mutagenicity tests were negative. After an evaluation of the weight of toxicological evidence, the EPA concluded that at doses above 250 mg/kg body weight/day, permethrin exhibits low oncogenic potential in mice.

The EPA concluded that although permethrin is a possible human oncogen, the potential for oncogenic effects in humans at expected exposure levels is "extremely low."

Delaney Clause Issues

As a result of these findings, permethrin is being regulated as an oncogen. Most section 408 tolerances were finalized in a rule published October 13, 1982, in the *Federal Register*.[15] However, the same *Federal Register* notice identified tomatoes, corn, soybeans, and apples as commodities in need of section 409 tolerances that would be acted upon separately "because the results of the mouse oncogenicity studies raise questions under the Delaney Clause." Because residues of permethrin concentrate during processes associated with these commodities (that is, because section 409 tolerances are required), final *section 408* tolerances for corn, soybeans, and tomatoes were delayed. No section 409 tolerances have been issued for these crops. All 409 tolerances have also been denied for apples.

For tomatoes, corn, and soybeans, three different methods were used to grant section 408 tolerances. Each case involved eliminating the need to promulgate the associated section 409 tolerances which could not be set because of the Delaney Clause.

TOMATOES

During processing of tomatoes, permethrin residues concentrate about 230-fold, clearly necessitating section 409 tolerances for processed tomato products. Because of positive findings of oncogenicity in mice, the Delaney Clause prohibits the granting of section 409 tolerances.

Prior to the issuance of section 408 tolerances for tomatoes, no section 408 tolerance had been granted for any oncogenic pesticide in a commodity where any portion of that commodity would be processed and need a section 409 tolerance. For enforcement purposes, it was deemed impossible to determine whether any portion of the treated raw agricultural commodity would be present in any processed food or animal feed. Permethrin was granted a section 408 tolerance, however, for use only on "Tomatoes Grown in Florida for Final Marketing as Fresh Tomatoes." By prohibiting the use of permethrin on tomatoes for processing, the Delaney Clause was not invoked. Three factors were cited by the EPA to support this decision:

1. Approximately 98 percent of all tomatoes grown in Florida are for the fresh market.

2. All Florida canneries (a total of four that process tomatoes) have signed agreements that no cannery waste from the canning of whole (not processed) tomatoes will be used as animal feed.

3. Shipping to canneries in adjoining states is economically unfeasible.

Because no waste will be fed to animals, no section 408 tolerances for meat, milk, or eggs were deemed necessary.

CORN

Tolerances were initially proposed for residues of permethrin and its metabolites in or on the following raw agricultural commodities: corn fodder at 5 ppm, corn forage at 12 ppm, and corn grain at 0.05 ppm. The petition for corn fodder was subsequently raised to 12 ppm, whereupon applications for both forage and fodder tolerances were dropped after section 408 forage and fodder tolerances were granted on sweet corn. These section 408 tolerances for sweet-corn forage and fodder carry over to field-corn forage and fodder.

The initial tolerance petition for residues of permethrin in corn proposed a use pattern for permethrin that would have allowed application of permethrin *after ears had formed* and included a 30-day preharvest interval (PHI) and a prohibition on cutting for silage within seven days of the last application. However, residues resulting from this practice necessitated section 409 tolerances for corn oil and soap stock.

Because the Delaney Clause will not allow section 409 tolerances for permethrin, section 408 tolerances for permethrin in corn were denied. In order to avoid the application of the Delaney Clause to these uses, label restrictions were developed, supported by residue data that show that if permethrin were *not applied after ear formation*, no detectable residues (at 0.02-ppm level of detection) would remain at harvest. Lowering residues below the level of detection (or theoretically eliminating these residues) eliminated the need for section 409 tolerances; thus a section 408 tolerance of 0.02 ppm for permethrin in or on the raw agricultural commodity, corn grain, was granted. Subsequently, data were submitted to support a label change allowing application after ear formation but prior to brown silking.

This policy also prevented the need for section 408 tolerances to cover residues in eggs, milk, fat, and meat by-products of cattle, goats, hogs, horses, poultry, and sheep.

SOYBEANS

Section 408 tolerances for permethrin on soybeans were also denied pending resolution of similar Delaney issues. The need for section 409 tolerances were obviated and section 408 tolerances were ultimately granted, when residues were lowered below the level of detection through the application of a 60-day PHI.

Discussion

One major criticism of the tolerance-setting system is that the process is generally devoid of incentives to drive tolerances to the lowest levels necessary for efficacious use of the product. Usually, it is only when the Theoretical Maximum Residue Contribution (TMRC) approaches the Acceptable Daily Intake that registrants seek to lower existing tolerances to allow for new uses. Presumably, a tolerance lowered in this fashion could have been lower at the time it was granted.

In the case of permethrin, the Delaney Clause provided this incentive and clearly forced a reduction (in theory an elimination) of residues on two major food crops—corn and soybeans—while at the same time allowing these uses, and providing agriculture with new insecticides that are generally less toxic and provide significant benefits when compared with their major alternatives. However, where the elimination of residues cannot be achieved, the Delaney Clause does not allow the use of permethrin when processing will necessitate a section 409 tolerance for that crop.

THIODICARB

Description of the Chemical

Common name:	Thiodicarb
Trade name:	Larvin
Pesticide type:	Insecticide
Chemical family:	Carbamate
Year registered:	1979
Major producer:	Union Carbide, under patent
Volume of use:	Not available
Tolerances:	A section 408 tolerance of 2.0 ppm for thiodicarb residues in sweet corn was established in 1984. Sections 408 and 409 tolerances for thiodicarb and its metabolite methomyl in or on cotton, cottonseed, soybeans, and soybean hulls were initially denied under the Delaney Clause. Using the FDA's sensitivity-of-the-method approach, these tolerances were finalized on October 10, 1985.

Regulatory Status

General-use pesticide

Special Review Criteria Triggered

Positive findings of oncogenicity for acetamide, a metabolite of thiodicarb, were dealt with in the registration process.

Summary of Oncogenic Findings and Risk Estimation

Thiodicarb has a complete data base of acceptable grade. All thiodicarb oncogenicity studies have been submitted, and all are negative. However, animal metabolism studies show that acetamide, an animal oncogen, is a metabolite of thiodicarb. Four tests performed from 1955 to 1980 show that at doses ranging from 12,500 to 80,000 ppm, acetamide is oncogenic in test animals. Although none of these studies meet current standards for oncogenicity testing, it is the conclusion of the agency that "the studies collectively demonstrate that, at least under certain conditions, long-term dietary administration of acetamide at high doses is associated with the occurrence of liver tumors in rats." Further, "the agency believes it is prudent to assume for present purposes that acetamide is a possible human carcinogen."[16]

Using the positive results in male rats from the most recent study, the EPA calculated a level of risk from acetamide in the human diet as a result of thiodicarb residues. This exercise employed a set of conservative principles in which, among other things, the agency assumed that

• The metabolic pathway of thiodicarb is the same as that found in test animals, and the highest value of risk obtainable from the animal data is applicable to humans;

• All consumed residues of thiodicarb are converted to acetamide (which the EPA states is unlikely as suggested by the available data); and

• All cotton and soybeans grown in the United States will be treated with thiodicarb.

On the basis of this body of evidence and these presumptions, the EPA calculated an upper-bound estimate of total dietary oncogenic risk from acetamide in the diet as a result of thiodicarb residues on cotton and soybeans, of approximately 1×10^{-6}. Yet, it is clear that the agency does not believe that the dietary risks are this high. In concluding comments discussing these finds in the *Federal Register,* the EPA states that because of the extremely conservative methodology employed in the risk estimation, it "believes that the actual risk is less than 10^{-6}."[17]

For purposes of the committee's work, it is noteworthy that the risks involved here were insufficient to trigger a special review of thiodicarb. As stated by the EPA in the proposed final rule:

There are no regulatory actions pending against the registration of thiodicarb. On the basis of the available studies on acetamide and the chronic oncogenicity studies for thiodicarb, the Agency has concluded that the human risks posed by the use of thiodicarb on cotton and soybeans does [sic] not raise prudent concerns of unreasonable adverse effects and that a special review under 40 CFR 162.11 is not warranted.[18]

Put another way, this statement means that in the opinion of the agency, the regulatory actions surrounding thiodicarb arise entirely from the Delaney Clause, and concern the issuance of tolerances rather than the granting of product registration, in a case where the risk involved would not otherwise warrant review or a delay in the issuance of such tolerances.

THIODICARB AND METHOMYL

Thiodicarb breaks down to methomyl soon after application. In fact, the tolerances at issue here are for "thiodicarb and its metabolite methomyl." Methomyl itself is a registered pesticide with two valid studies showing no oncogenicity. Even though it is very likely that acetamide is also a metabolite of methomyl, it has not yet been detected in animal metabolism or residue studies accepted by the EPA in support of methomyl registrations. To date, methomyl and its metabolites have not been regulated as oncogens, nor has the Delaney Clause been invoked against any tolerances for methomyl.

The available data do not show methomyl to concentrate during the processing of food or animal feeds. Therefore, although section 409 tolerances have been a major issue for thiodicarb, section 409 tolerances have not been required for methomyl. Until *concentrating oncogenic* residues of methomyl and/or its metabolites are detected, the Delaney Clause will not apply to methomyl, regardless of its chemical similarity to thiodicarb.

Tolerance and Delaney Clause Issues

Because thiodicarb is known to concentrate in cotton seed and soybean hulls, its use on soybeans and cotton requires section 409 feed additive tolerances. These tolerances were initially denied because of acetamide oncogenicity and the Delaney Clause. As stated in the *Federal Register*, the additional cancer risk from the proposed uses of thiodicarb is less than 1×10^{-6}.[19]

According to agency sources, thiodicarb is, in a sense, a victim of the high quality of its supporting studies. In particular, the animal metabolism studies that detected acetamide pursued thiodicarb metabolites to an exceptional level of detail. Had these studies not traced the metabolism of thiodicarb so thoroughly, they might have met the EPA requirements but not have detected acetamide as a thiodicarb metabolite. Data supporting methomyl—the major metabolite of thiodicarb and itself a registered pesticide active ingredient—have been reviewed and accepted by the EPA, yet acetamide was not detected as a metabolite. Were acetamide not detected as a metabolite, thiodicarb would have received section 409 tolerances and section 3 registrations on the basis of its negative oncogenicity.

To summarize, thiodicarb needs a section 409 tolerance because it concentrates in cottonseed and soybean hulls used as animal feed. Thiodicarb is non-oncogenic and regardless of its concentration in feed, in the absence of an oncogenic metabolite, the Delaney Clause would not apply. However, thiodicarb is metabolized by livestock into acetamide, an oncogen, which is present in meat, milk, and eggs. Thus, the EPA interprets the Delaney Clause to prohibit the use of thiodicarb on crops fed to animals that produce these foods.

Sensitivity-of-the-Method Procedure

Because acetamide is an animal metabolite of thiodicarb, and not present in *foods* derived from soybeans and cotton treated with thiodicarb, the setting of animal *feed* additive tolerances under section 409 of the FDC Act is the focal point of this exercise. Within section 409(c)(3)(A) of the FDC Act is the so-called "DES proviso" which states that the Delaney Clause

shall not apply with respect to the use of a substance as an ingredient of feed for animals which are raised for food production, if the [Administrator] finds . . . (ii) that no residue of the additive will be found (by methods of examination prescribed and approved by the [Administrator] by regulation) in any edible portion of the animal after slaughter or in any food yielded by or derived from the living animal.

The FDA has extensively analyzed the meaning of this exception in a document published in the March 20, 1979, *Federal Register*.[20] Therein, the FDA concludes that the proviso should be implemented by requiring that residues of an oncogenic compound should not be allowed in the total diet of humans unless it can be verified analytically that they occur at levels less than those that, as determined by prescribed methods of extrapolation based on animal bioassay data and a series of conservative assumptions, yield an insignificant excess cancer risk (which the FDA sets at 1 in 1 million or 1×10^{-6}).

Although this analysis of the DES proviso has not yet been formally adopted through a final rule, the EPA employed this rationale in issuing section 409 tolerances for thiodicarb: "For the purposes of this action, EPA adopts the reasoning and methodology of the FDA document."[21] Several comments on the issuance of these tolerances criticize the EPA's use of a procedure that has not been finalized through a formal rule making.

Using the FDA's methodology as explained in the July 3, 1985, proposed rulemaking for thiodicarb tolerances, the EPA calculated that meat and poultry could contain 90 ppb acetamide residues, and the excess lifetime cancer risk would not exceed 1×10^{-6}. The agency further estimates that at the proposed tolerance levels for thiodicarb, maximum concentrations of acetamide residues in beef and poultry *liver*, which on average contain 17 and 6 times the residues found in muscle tissue, would be 1.8 and 0.6 ppb, respectively. For enforcement purposes (the liver will be monitored to detect violative residues in meat) one should multiply 17 times 90 ppb to get 1,530 ppb, the maximum level of acetamide residues allowed in liver.

The lowest levels of reliable measurement for acetamide in beef and poultry liver, using the analytical method submitted by Union Carbide, are 700 and 400 ppb, respectively. In the EPA's judgment, this method is sufficient to detect violative residues in beef and poultry. Clearly, both the level of detection and the allowable level of residues of acetamide are far above levels expected to result from residues of thiodicarb at the tolerances, 1.8 and 0.6 ppb.

In the cases of milk and eggs, allowable levels of acetamide of 30 and 90 ppb, respectively, were determined. In contrast, the maximum expected acetamide levels in milk and eggs resulting from thiodicarb residues on cottonseed and soybean hulls are 0.3 and 0.07 ppb, respectively. Union Carbide requested a waiver from the requirement for an analytical method of detection because milk and egg samples purchased at grocery stores in 11 states contained levels of 275–500 ppb acetamide for milk, and 75–350 ppb acetamide for eggs—far above anticipated maximum residues from use of thiodicarb as well as those equivalent to a risk of 1×10^{-6} (30 and 90 ppb). Because EPA tests also found acetamide residues to be ubiquitous, the requirement for an analytical method was waived.

NOTES

1. U.S. Environmental Protection Agency. 1982. Benomyl Fact Sheet. Washington, D.C.
2. Holder, J. A. 1980. Memorandum to C. Chaisson, U.S. Environmental Protection Agency, regarding correction of worst-case dietary exposure to benomyl in the United States for percent crop tracked and direct sampling of selected crops in a Du Pont market booklet survey. U.S. Environmental Protection Agency, Washington, D.C.
3. Environmental Protection Agency Rebuttable Presumption Against Continued Registration of Products Containing Captan. 1980. *Federal Register* 45(No. 161, August 18): 54938–54985.
4. U.S. Environmental Protection Agency. 1985. Captan Special Review Position Document 2/3. Washington, D.C.: U.S. Environmental Protection Agency. Sec. 2, pp. 91–92.
5. *Ibid.*
6. *Ibid.*
7. National Research Council. 1980. Regulating Pesticides. Washington, D.C.: National Academy Press.
8. *Federal Register* 47(April 2, 1982):14136.
9. *Federal Register* 49(December 5, 1984):47482.
10. Environmental Forum. December 1984. Pesticides—Changing the Way EPA Does Business, pp. 17–18.
11. U.S. Environmental Protection Agency. 1982. Ethylenebisdithiocarbamates. Decision Document, Office of Pesticides and Toxic Substances. Washington, D.C., p. I-11.
12. *Ibid.*
13. *Ibid.*, p. I-38.
14. *Ibid.*, p. I-39.
15. *Federal Register* 47(October 13, 1982):45008.
16. *Federal Register* 50(No. 128):27453.
17. *Federal Register* 50(No. 197):41342.
18. *Federal Register* 50(July 3, 1985):27464.
19. *Federal Register* 50(No. 197):41342.
20. *Federal Register* 44(March 20, 1979):17020.
21. *Ibid.*

D

Pesticide Innovation

TRENDS IN INNOVATION

EARL R. SWANSON

The role of innovation in a pesticide regulatory action depends on the scope of the benefit analysis. Neither FIFRA nor the FDC Act (section 408) prescribes in detail the nature of the benefit analysis.[1] For example, there is no legal requirement for a formal benefit-cost analysis and no specification of the future time period to be considered. Benefit assessments performed by the EPA usually focus on short-run economic impacts (three to five years) and consider only currently registered chemical and nonchemical controls as alternatives. There are cases, however, in which the EPA risk/benefit decision process has taken into account pending registrations. For example, in the Rebuttable Presumption Against Registration (RPAR) process on trifluralin (Treflan), the pending registrations of pendimethalin (Prowl) were considered.[2]

One of the reasons for the focus on short-run impacts in the EPA benefit analyses is the difficulty of forecasting the rates of innovation in pest control methods. Nevertheless, the committee believes that the EPA should give added emphasis in benefit analysis to alternative pest control technologies under development. The methodology for such evaluation, however, is not well developed at present. Ideally, information at each stage of the development of a pesticide would be useful. Although there is considerable firm-to-firm and compound-to-compound variation in the discovery and development process, the stages suggested by Goring[3] are informative. In terms of sequence, these five components may overlap and some are performed simultaneously:

1. Synthesis, screening, and preliminary field research;
2. Expanded field research, field development, and sales support;

226

3. Metabolism, environment, residues, and toxicology;
4. Formulation, process, and pilot plant; and
5. Registration.

In this appendix, broad perspectives of the changes that are occurring in methods for control of insects and weeds are presented.

The partial inventory of compounds undergoing testing presented in Chapter 6 illustrates one type of data that might be used in expanded risk/benefit analyses. Other sources of information include examination of chemical patents and applications to the EPA for registration. Searches of the trade literature may also provide an indication of particular pest control innovations at various stages of development. Certain limitations in the data sources should be noted. The field testing done under the auspices of public agencies and reported, for example, in the *Fungicide and Nematicide Tests* published by the American Phytopathological Society may underestimate the actual level of testing activity for new compounds. Universities and experiment stations are becoming less willing to perform tests on experimental pesticides, and an increasing amount of such testing is now conducted in the private sector and thus not reported. Nevertheless, the efficacy data on experimental compounds available in the reports of professional associations provide evidence of possible replacements for compounds presently used. Clearly, a systematic methodology needs to be developed for assessing the innovation process at its various stages and integrating such assessments into the benefit analysis.

If the EPA were to emphasize the prospects for new pest control technologies in its benefit analyses, such a shift to a wider range of alternatives would decrease the long-run benefits of the pesticide under consideration, but not necessarily the more immediate impacts of its withdrawal. In principle, the broadened scope of benefit analysis would increase the risk/benefit ratio and the probability of cancellation of a registered pesticide or the rejection of the application of an unregistered pesticide. If this expanded benefit analysis by the EPA is perceived by industry to be reasonably stable, pesticide manufacturers may be expected to respond by increasing production of registered substitutes and/or developing new pesticides for a changed market.

NOTES

1. 7 USC § 136 (1978) and 21 USC § 346(b) (1984).
2. U.S. Environmental Protection Agency. 1982. Trifluralin (Treflan). Position Document 4. Office of Pesticides and Toxic Substances. Washington, D.C., pp. 59–60.
3. Goring, C.A.I. 1977. The costs of commercializing pesticides. Pp. 1–33 in Pesticide Management and Insect Resistance, David L. Watson and A.W.A. Brown, eds. New York: Academic Press.

WEED CONTROL

Fred H. Tschirley

HERBICIDES

During the past 15 years, the use of herbicides on crops in the United States has increased dramatically. Farm use of herbicides totaled 215 million pounds in 1971, 376 million pounds in 1976, 445 million pounds in 1982, and 435 million pounds in 1984.[1] Herbicides now account for about 65 percent of the total pesticide use on farms. This increase occurred because their use produces an economic benefit for growers.

Although cultivation is still practiced for the control of weeds, and crop rotation provides some weed control, synthetic organic herbicides have become the predominant technology. Led by the discovery of the herbicidal properties of the phenoxy alkanoic acids in the early 1940s, chemistry soon followed that provided different mechanisms of action, a wider range of herbicidal activity on weeds, and differing selectivities to crops.

Modern herbicides represent a large number of chemical classes, many of which have only one or a few herbicides in the entire class. Important classes include the phenoxy alkanoic acids, *s*-triazines, substituted amides, carbamates and thiocarbamates, substituted ureas, and nitroanilines. Herbicides in other classes are also important, including amitrole, paraquat and diquat, bensulide, chloramben, DCPA, endothall, picloram, and nitrofen. Herbicides used for weed control on corn and soybean crops, which represent 93 percent of the farm use of herbicides, are listed in Table D-1.

Certainly, the past rate of increase of use will not continue. In fact, there are indications that use has already leveled off. Ninety-three percent or more of the acreage planted to corn, soybeans, cotton, peanuts, and rice was treated with herbicides in 1982. In addition, 71 percent of the tobacco acreage; 59 percent of grain sorghum; and 40 to 45 percent of the wheat, barley, and oat acreage was treated with herbicides. Although marked increases in herbicide usage are not expected in the foreseeable future, neither is a marked decrease expected, and herbicides will surely continue to be the predominant technology for weed control.

NEW CHEMISTRY

Manufacturers have become more sophisticated in designing new molecules with a reasonable expectation that they will have herbicidal activity. Researchers can target a specific enzyme system that is known to

TABLE D-1 Herbicidal Active Ingredients Used on Corn and Soybeans During 1982

	Active Ingredient (million lbs.)	
Herbicide	Corn	Soybeans
Single applications		
Acifluorfen		0.9
Alachlor	19.7	10.3
Atrazine	22.4	
Bentazon		6.7
Butylate	22.4	
Chloramben		2.7
Cyanazine	4.9	
2,4-D	3.3	
Dicamba	0.9	
Fluchloralin		2.6
Glyphosate		2.2
Linuron		1.3
Metolachlor	3.2	6.9
Metribuzin		2.2
Trifluralin		20.4
Other	9.5	5.5
Total	86.3	61.7
Tank mixes		
Acifluorfen + bentazon		0.3 + 0.7
Alachlor + metribuzin		6.9 + 1.7
Alachlor + linuron		8.1 + 3.2
Alachlor + naptalam + dinoseb		1.5 + 1.3 + 0.6
Atrazine + alachlor	16.4 + 21.2	
Atrazine + butylate	8.7 + 23.7	
Atrazine + cyanazine	2.7 + 3.6	
Atrazine + metolachlor	8.7 + 10.7	
Atrazine + simazine	1.3 + 1.2	
Bentazon + 2,4-D		0.4 + *
Chloramben + alachlor		1.5 + 1.8
Chloramben + trifluralin		0.9 + 0.5
Cyanazine + alachlor	6.1 + 7.6	
Cyanazine + butylate	2.7 + 4.9	
Cyanazine + metolachlor	0.9 + 1.2	
Dicamba + 2,4-D	1.0 + 1.6	
Dinoseb + naptalam		1.2 + 2.4
Metolachlor + metribuzin		4.2 + 1.6
Metolachlor + atrazine + simazine	3.2 + 2.6 + 1.3	
Metolachlor + cyanazine + atrazine	1.4 + 0.6 + 0.6	
Oryzalin + linuron		0.4 + 0.3
Paraquat + others		0.4 + 1.7
Trifluralin + metribuzin		8.8 + 3.8
Other	8.9	11.1
Total	142.8	65.3
Total herbicides	229.1	127.0

*Less than 100,000 pounds.

SOURCE: Adapted from Delvo, H. W. November 1984. Inputs: Outlook and Situation Report. Washington, D.C.: U.S. Department of Agriculture, Economic Research Service.

be affected by one or more functional groups. Unfortunately, mechanisms of action are not completely known for all active ingredients. For example, the mechanism of action of the phenoxy herbicides is still unknown, even after 40 years of use. Nevertheless, the discovery of new herbicides has a firmer scientific base today than 10 years ago.

Several compounds representing new chemistry have been commercially introduced in the past several years, and others, now being tested under experimental permits, can be expected to reach commercial use in the next few years. An exciting aspect of this new chemistry is the remarkably low rates needed for weed control. Older herbicides were applied in pounds per acre; some of the new materials are effective at ounces per acre. For example, control of annual and perennial grass weeds is accomplished with 4 to 8 ounces of fluazifop per acre, 3 to 7.5 ounces of sethoxydim per acre, 1 to 5 ounces of sulfometuron methyl per acre, and 0.17 to 0.5 ounce of chlorsulfuron per acre.

Such herbicidal activity is remarkable. One-sixth of an ounce per acre is only 0.09 mg per square foot. Ten or more other herbicides for which rates of fractions of an ounce or a few ounces per acre are needed are in various stages of development. Moreover, they are being developed by several manufacturers, and their chemistry varies, rather than being mere analogs of one basic molecule.

An increase in the use of the potent (low-application-rate) herbicides would significantly decrease the quantity of herbicides being applied, and presumably, lower residues in raw agricultural commodities. At present, the crops on which these potent materials are registered is limited. Chlorsulfuron is registered only on wheat, spring oats, and barley; fluazifop on cotton and soybeans; and sethoxydim on soybeans, cotton, sugar beets, and nonbearing food crops. Sulfometuron methyl is not yet registered on any crops. Thus, registration of these herbicides is required on a far greater number of crops before herbicide use will significantly decrease. Herbicidal activity at such low rates requires cautious appraisal, however. If a material with high biological activity is resistant to degradation, its use would have to be limited to avoid carryover damage to other crops. In fact, carryover potential for the new classes of soybean herbicides is a matter of growing concern for weed scientists.

BIOLOGICAL CONTROL

Weed control by insects has been studied by a few scientists for a long time, and successful control has been accomplished for numerous weeds occurring in noncrop areas. However, it has not been successful in cropland, because crops are planted in fallowed land, which is ideal for the germination of weed seeds, phytophagous insects must have a specific host or a narrow host range so that weeds are destroyed without danger to crops, and there is usually a complex of weed species in cultivated crops, so controlling one will simply provide a ,competitive edge to the remaining weeds. At best, the control of weeds by phytophagous insects might be feasible in perennial crops, such as orchards, or for particularly troublesome weeds, such as nutgrass (*Cypercus* sp.) or downy bromegrass (*Bromus tectorum*). Nutgrass and other sedges, however, are important beneficial plants in other habitats, and downy bromegrass provides forage for animals on rangelands.[2]

Recently, interest in plant pathogens to control weeds has increased, and several notable successes have occurred. Northern jointvetch in rice can be controlled with an endemic fungal disease,[3] and milkweed vine in citrus is now controlled by a pathotype of *Phytophthora*.[4] More recently, Walker[5-8] reported the successful control by pathogens of spurred anoda, prickly sida, velvetleaf, and sicklepod. For this technology, spores are produced in the laboratory, incorporated into an appropriate carrier, and then distributed in a selected area at the appropriate time. Combining spores of different fungi, Boyette and coworkers[9] applied pathogens for the simultaneous control of winged waterprimrose and northern jointvetch.

The limited number of scientists pursuing research in this field may impede its rapid advance. Control by pathogens has the promise of contributing to the development of integrated weed control systems. Further success requires the discovery of more pathogens so that weed complexes can be controlled rather than just a single species. Moreover, for sustained success, farmers must be weaned away from the synthetic organic herbicides that ensure effective weed control.

In a similar vein, increased emphasis has recently been given to natural phytotoxins from pathogens that might be formulated and applied to weeds. This bypasses the problem of introducing a living organism into the environment, which, through mutation, could persist and become destructive rather than beneficial. There is no assurance, however, that a natural phytotoxin would be any less hazardous to human health and the environment than the synthetic molecules now in use.

ALLELOPATHY

Allelopathy, coined by Hans Molisch in 1937, refers to the release of chemical inhibitors by certain plants, which adversely affect other plant species. Specific cases of allelopathy have been observed in crops, forests, grasslands, deserts, and even aquatic systems.[10] The inhibiting chemicals may be released from living plants via exudation from roots, from litter on the soil surface, or from decomposing organic matter.

Although, theoretically, allelopathy seems to offer a direct impact on weed control technology, the greatest benefits may come from spin-offs of allelopathic research. Although genotypes of some crops, such as cucumber, inhibited some important weeds in the laboratory and greenhouse, the results were less dramatic and consistent in the field, perhaps because the concentrations of the allelopathic chemicals in the soil were too low to inhibit the weeds. Allelopathy could be effective in crops such as turfgrass, cereal grains, and forage legumes, because of a higher concentration and more even distribution of the inhibitory chemicals. Developing the technique requires the identification of allelopathic properties and their incorporation into crops.

Once allelopathic chemicals are identified, they might be synthesized as herbicides. That route engenders the same problems that now beset organic herbicides synthesized de novo. As with phytotoxins, natural products may be no less hazardous to humans and the environment than ones first synthesized by man.

GENETIC ENGINEERING

Conceivably, crop varieties could be developed for allelopathic control of weeds. For example, Putnam[10] reported that some wild progenitors of modern crop varieties demonstrate greater allelopathy than the varieties now in use. Attention has also been given to breeding varieties that have greater tolerance for herbicides, so that rates to control weeds can be used without endangering the crop.[11]

Incorporation of herbicide resistance in the crop has been achieved in three ways:[12]

1. By the transfer of a metabolic detoxification mechanism (in which an enzyme inactivates the herbicide) from a resistant plant to a susceptible one. A good example is the herbicide atrazine, which is used widely in corn. Weeds lack the rapid detoxification pathway of corn that replaces the chlorine atom with a peptide via a conjugation reaction. Several laboratories have shown that the enzyme is glutathione-S-transferase. In principle, it should be possible to transfer the glutathione-S-transferase gene into, for example, soybeans, to make it herbicide resistant. Research is still needed, however, before application is practical.

2. By the transfer of a restricted uptake or translocation trait. A new plant variety has emerged in Egypt that is resistant to paraquat. The phytotoxicity of paraquat results from its chemical reductions in the chloroplasts, which generates free radicals that destroy the plant. In the Egyptian biotype, an unknown process restricts the paraquat to the veins of the leaves, preventing it from entering the cells that contain the chloroplasts. Today, however, the probability of genetically transferring this sort of trait from one crop to another is low.

3. By modification of the target of the herbicide. In the short term, target site modification looks promising. A herbicide translocated to a

specific target in the plant interacts with that target, blocking some metabolic event and killing the plant. If, through genetic manipulation, the target site could be altered so that it no longer recognizes the herbicide, the plant would be resistant. An example is pigweed, which is resistant to atrazine because a natural mutation occurred that changed the protein that normally binds the atrazine. The protein in susceptible plants contains the amino acid serine, which is required for hydrogen bonding of · the triazine molecule to the protein. In resistant plants, this amino acid had been replaced by glycine, with which triazine cannot bond. This mechanism of resistance has been exploited to develop a triazine-resistant tobacco plant.

Another example comes from scientists of Calgene, Inc., who incorporated a mutant EPSP synthase gene, isolated from glyphosate-resistant *Salmonella,* into tobacco. Other scientists from Monsanto Chemical Company achieved greater glyphosate resistance in petunia plants by inducing them to make 20 to 40 times the usual amount of normal petunia EPSP synthase.

DuPont researchers used both chemical and random mutations to isolate mutant plants that varied in response to chlorosulfuron and sulfometuron methyl. Various tests and correlations established the site of action as acetolacetate synthase. Production of an insensitive form of the enzyme is the basis for resistance.

CONCLUSIONS

Since their introduction in the early 1940s, synthetic organic herbicides have dominated weed control. Although alternative weed control technologies hold some promise and may become more important, synthetic organic herbicides seem certain to be the preferred technology until the end of the century. Development of alternative technologies will require not only time and research, but also practical demonstrations to convince farmers that the alternatives will be as economical and dependable as synthetic organic herbicides.

NOTES

1. Delvo, H. W. November 1984. Inputs: Outlook and Situation Report. Washington, D.C.: Department of Agriculture, Economic Research Service.
2. Morrow, L. A., and P. W. Stahlman. 1984. The history and distribution of downy brome (*Bromus tectorum*) in North America. Weed Sci. 32(Suppl. 1):2– 6.
3. Daniel, J. T., G. E. Templeton, R. J. Smith, Jr., and W. T. Fox. 1973. Biological control of northern jointvetch in rice with an endemic fungal disease. Weed Sci. 21:303–307.

4. Ridings, W. H., D. J. Mitchell, C. J. Shoulties, and N. E. El-Ghell. 1976. Biological control of milkweed vine in Florida citrus groves with a pathotype of *Phytophthora citrophthora*. Pp. 224–240 in T. E. Freeman, ed., Proceedings of the IV International Symposium on Biological Control of Weeds.

5. Walker, H. L. 1980. *Alternaria macrospora* as a potential biocontrol agent for spurred anoda: Production of spores for field studies. U.S. Science Education Administration, Advanced Agricultural Technology, South. Ser. (ISSN 0193-3728), No. 12, 5 pp.

6. Walker, H. L. 1981. Granular formulation of *Alternaria macrospora* for control of spurred anoda (*Anoda cristata*). Weed Sci. 29:342–345.

7. Walker, H. L. 1981. *Fusarium lateritium:* A pathogen of spurred anoda *(Anoda cristata)*, prickly sida (*Sida spinosa*), and velvetleaf (*Abutilon theophrasti*). Weed Sci. 29:629–631.

8. Walker, H. L., and J. A. Riley. 1982. Evaluation of *Alternaria cassiae* for the biocontrol of sicklepod (*Cassia obtusifolia*). Weed Sci. 30(6):651–654.

9. Boyette, C. D., G. E. Templeton, and R. J. Smith, Jr. 1979. Control of winged waterprimrose (*Jussiaea decurrens*) and northern jointvetch (*Aeschynomene virginica*) with fungal pathogens. Weed Sci. 27:497–501.

10. Putnam, A. 1983. Allelopathic chemicals: Nature's herbicides in action. Chem. & Eng. News April 4, 1983, pp. 34–45.

11. Marx, J. L. 1985. Plant gene transfer becomes a fertile field. Science 230(4730): 1148–1150.

12. Chemical and Engineering News, October 29, 1984, p. 16.

INSECT CONTROL

T. Roy Fukuto

INTRODUCTION

Because they are effective, economical, and fast-acting, insecticides and acaricides are unique tools for relegating damaging insect and mite populations to subeconomic levels. Thus, despite problems such as the development of insecticide-resistant pest populations and undesirable nontarget effects, they will remain one of the basic tools for managing insects and mites in crops.

Virtually all major insecticides that are widely used on crops, except organochlorines, are acute neurotoxins and fall into the chemical classes of organophosphates, carbamates, and pyrethroids. Owing to their persistence in the environment and unfavorable toxicological properties, most of the organochlorine insecticides either have been banned or are used only in special situations. Pyrethroids are now receiving the greatest attention from industry. These broad-spectrum insecticides are highly effective at application rates measured in ounces and fractions of an ounce instead of the 0.5 to 2 pounds applied per acre of most compounds in the other classes.

Advances in insect physiology, toxicology, and analytical chemistry are responsible for discoveries of new compounds with novel modes of action that disrupt the normal growth of insects. The juvenile hormone analogs, for example, prevent the insect from molting to the adult stage. Unfortunately, because the larval stages typically are most damaging to crops, these compounds appear to have limited use in crop protection. They will, however, control such insects as fleas and biting flies, which are pests in the adult stage. Antijuvenile hormones causing insects to molt prematurely to adults have been discovered and offer more promise for managing agricultural insect pests. The relatively recent discovery of compounds that disrupt the molting process of insects by interfering with the synthesis and deposition of chitin (a principal component of the exoskeleton of insects) also holds promise. One such chitin inhibitor, Diflubenzuron (Dimilin) is registered for control of cotton boll weevils and gypsy moths.

Similarly, advances in natural products chemistry and the study of plant defenses against insects are leading to the identification of numerous, naturally occurring, insecticidal and acaricidal compounds with novel modes of action. To date, biologically active, natural products have been looked to by the agrochemical industry as leads for the chemical synthesis of structurally related compounds with improved biological and physical properties that are amenable to large-scale chemical synthesis. This latter requirement may ultimately become less important with advances in genetic engineering, since even complex molecules can be produced on a large scale, using fermentation processes with genetically engineered microorganisms.

NEW CHEMISTRY

Motivation for the discovery of new pest control agents by the chemical industry originates from the ongoing desire to develop a proprietary agent with superior pesticidal activity and favorable environmental and toxicological properties. Although a significant amount of effort is still being devoted to research on organophosphates, carbamates, and pyrethroids, the chemical industry is turning to other classes of compounds in seeking new control agents. Increased attention to unconventional chemicals has been hastened by the prospect of the development of insect resistance to present-day insecticides.[1]

During the past decade, novel insecticides with different modes of action have been discovered. With the elucidation of their modes of action, the way has been paved for further search within these classes for new insect control agents. Areas that have been or are currently being explored for new insect control agents are described below.

Octopamine Agonists

Chlordimeform (Fundal, Galecron) and amitraz are formamidine derivatives that effectively control phytophagus mites, ticks, and a limited range of insects, for example, many Lepidoptera, Hemiptera, and some Homoptera.[2] The formamidine derivatives are most effective as ovicides although they are also toxic to nymphs and adults. In addition to mortality, the formamidines also cause unusual behavioral effects, for example, on locomotion, flight, dispersal, and oviposition. Due to adverse human health effects, chlordimeform is registered for use only on cotton.

Evidence accumulated over the past decade supports an octopaminomimetic mechanism of action for chlordimeform and related compounds. The elucidation of the mechanism of action of this compound has stimulated work on the design and synthesis of compounds with octopaminomimetic activity. Octopamine, a biogenic amine that serves as neurotransmitter and neuromodulator, is found primarily in invertebrates and, therefore, compounds mimicking its action are expected to be selectively toxic to insects and acarines.

Avermectins and Milbemycines

The avermectins and milbemycins are natural products obtained by fermentation of the soil fungus species *Streptomyces*, which have demonstrated potent anthelmintic, acaricidal, and insecticidal activities.[3,4] For example, the avermectins are highly effective against common veterinary ectoparasites, phytophagus mites, nematodes, and various insect species of Lepidoptera, Coleoptera, and Homoptera. They are highly complex molecules consisting of eight major components. Ivermectin, a commercial product currently under development, is a hydrogenated derivative of avermectin B^1, the most active of the eight components. The avermectins behave as agonists or cause the release of the inhibitory neurotransmitter γ-aminobutyric acid (GABA).

Avermectins and milbemycins exhibit unusually potent insecticidal and acaricidal activities, but have highly complicated structures. Therefore, work has been started on the synthesis and evaluation of analogs of less structural complexity.[5,6] This work is expected to result in new analogs with similar modes of action.

A new class of insecticide, the 1,4-disubstituted-2,6,7-trioxabicyclo-[2,2,2]octanes, has recently been discovered.[7] These compounds appear to act at the neuromuscular junction by inhibiting GABAergic synaptic transmission, possibly by closing off chloride channels. The high insecticidal potency of the avermectins, milbemycins, and trioxabicyclo[2,2,2]-

octanes warrants further exploitation of the GABA system for new insecticides.

Amidinohydrazones

New amidinohydrazone insecticides have recently been registered under the trade names Amdro for control of imported red fire ants and Combat and Maxforce for use against cockroaches. The compound is a slow-acting stomach insecticide whose mode of action appears to be inhibition of electron transport and oxidative phosphorylation.[8] The amidinohydrazones represent a novel structure for an insecticide, and other compounds of similar mode of action are presently being sought. However, Amdro is unstable in light and therefore is not useful for agricultural purposes.

Benzoylphenylureas

The benzoylphenylureas represent a new class of insecticides that are effective as larvicides and ovicides by either contact or as a stomach poison.[9] The most prominent of the benzoylphenylureas is diflubenzuron (Dimilin) and BAY SIR 8514. As indicated earlier, diflubenzuron inhibits chitin synthesis and is widely regarded as an insect growth regulator.[10] Because of chitin-inhibiting action, diflubenzuron and related analogs should affect insects in all cuticle-forming stages. In view of the favorable selectivity and effectiveness of diflubenzuron, a great deal of interest has developed in the search for other insect growth regulators.

Pyrethroids

Owing to the outstanding insecticidal properties of the synthetic pyrethroids, much effort is still being devoted to the synthesis and evaluation of new compounds.[11] Since the stereochemical structure of the pyrethroid molecule has such a profound effect on insecticidal activity, work is being conducted on the stereospecific synthesis of the most active enantiomers. Research on new pyrethroids is expected to continue, and new compounds are likely to be developed in the future.

Proinsecticides

During the past decade, new, less toxic derivatives of methylcarbamate insecticides have been discovered, and several are now close to commercial use.[12] These carbamate derivatives are called procarbamates; that is, they are carbamate derivatives that must be transformed back to the original carbamate by a plant, animal, or microorganism in order for intoxication to occur. Thiodicarb (a derivative of the carbamate methomyl) and carbosulfan (a derivative of the carbamate carbofuran) are examples of procarbamate insecticides that have attained commercial importance. Both are highly effective insecticides and are substantially less acutely toxic to mammals than the parent carbamates. Several other procarbamate insecticides are currently undergoing commercial development.

Nereistoxin, a substance found in a poisonous marine annelid, has been derivatized to form another type of proinsecticide. Nereistoxin paralyzes insects by a blocking action on the central nervous system. Examples of nereistoxin proinsecticides are cartap and bensultap. Bensultap, a more recent discovery, has shown excellent effectiveness against the Colorado potato beetle and different lepidopterous larvae.[13]

Natural Products

Much effort is being devoted to the study of various plant products that could be used for protection against plant-feeding insects.[14] For example, pellitorine, a potent insecticidal amide recently isolated from the root of a compositae, has stimulated the synthesis and examination of structural analogs.[15] Pellitorine, although highly insecticidal, unfortunately is unstable in a field environment.

Other types of plants being sought as control agents are insect growth and behavior regulators, morphogenetic agents, insect juvenile hormones and phytochemical analogs, antijuvenile hormones, sex and alarm pheromones, and antifeedants.[14] The examination of plant products for antifeedant compounds has recently attracted much attention.[16] A number of plants are recognized for their elaborate chemical defense systems against phytophagous insects, and various naturally occurring compounds are being discovered that permanently impede feeding by specific insects. In general, natural products occurring in plants, animals, and microorganisms provide a rich source for new types of insect control agents.

Although synthetic organic chemicals remain the principal pest control materials, other types of control agents or methods are currently in use or have the potential to provide effective pest control. They may be divided into three major categories—biological control, natural products approach, and plant modification. These are briefly described below.

GENETICALLY ENGINEERED MICROORGANISMS

Strategies and methods have been proposed for the use of microorganisms for pest control. Among the microorganisms showing promise are bacteria, viruses, and fungi. The potential for microorganisms as pesticides has been increased by progress in genetic engineering, which is expected be important in the development of bacterial, viral, and fungal pesticides effective enough to displace the synthetic chemicals, which dominate the market today.[17]

Bacterial Insecticides

The sporeforming bacteria *Bacillus thuringiensus kurstaki* has been developed commercially and is registered by the EPA as a bacterial insecticide for use on field and vegetable crops, trees, ornamentals, and stored products (primarily grain and grain products) to control lepidopterous larvae.[18] However, the bacteria's effectiveness is limited to certain species of Lepidoptera.

Monsanto is attempting to engineer a microbial pesticide by taking the δ-endotoxin gene from *B. thuringiensis kurstaki* and placing this toxin gene in another kind of bacteria, for example, *Pseudomonas fluorescens*, that can colonize the roots of plants such as corn.[19] When root-eating pests ingest the genetically engineered bacteria on the plant roots, the toxin in the bacteria will get into the gut of the pests where it will be activated and will intoxicate them. Unfortunately, agricultural pests that are vulnerable to this microbial pesticide are still mainly lepidopterous species (tobacco hornworms, black cutworms, cabbage and soybean loopers, and corn earworms) that do not attack plant roots.

Discovery of other *B. thuringiensis* isolates producing proteins toxic to root-feeding species would be required for this particular strategy to work. However, the same general strategy might work using genes from presently available *B. thuringiensis* strains and bacteria that colonize plant foliage. Monsanto reasons that since these engineered strains are not toxic to beneficial insects such as honeybees, their genetically engineered bacterial pesticides will have the same attributes.

There is under way considerable research directed toward identifying strains of *B. thuringiensis* that produce more virulent toxins and are effective against a wider diversity of insect pests. Research of this type has already led to the commercial development of *B. thuringiensis* var. *israelensis*, which is an effective control agent for mosquito larvae and will very likely expand the spectrum of crop pests that can be controlled by bacterial insecticides.

RESISTANCE

Resistance is a preadaptive phenomenon, and since insects and bacteria have been together in nature for ages, it is conceivable that low levels of resistance to the bacterial toxins already exist.

Evidence has not been provided for the development of insect resistance to *B. thuringiensis* in the field although a recent report has demonstrated that resistance to *B. thuringiensis* could be selected for in the laboratory. In a microbial control program, development of pest resistance can be averted by the following strategies:

- Use of multifunctional agents (*B. thuringiensis* produces several toxins), because the greater the number of targets in the insect the less likely it is that mutations will lead to increased resistance;
- Simultaneous use of chemical and microbial agents for the same reason—more than one target is involved; and
- Use of an agent—microbiological or chemical—with a rapid toxic action, to avoid a lasting selection pressure for resistance since the number of mutants produced will be proportional to exposure time.

However, in a stable environment such as in stored grains where the bacterial toxin is stable, the insect can breed for successive generations in contact with *B. thuringiensis*. In this situation, resistance is very likely to develop.

This scenario has recently been observed with the Indian meal moth *Plodia interpunctella*, which developed a 100-fold increase in resistance after 15 generations on diets treated with bacterial toxin.[20] In this case, the resistance was inherited as a recessive trait.

Fortunately, in field crop situations, the instability of foliarly applied *B. thuringiensis* and the transitory nature of plant pest interactions decrease the possibility of resistance. The use of *B. thuringiensis* over a wide geographic area for several years would be required to expose the pests for many successive generations.

PRODUCT NAMES AND USES

A number of biological insecticides exist on the market that have *B. thuringiensis* as their active ingredient. These include

- Thuricide, having *B. thuringiensis* Berliner as the active species;
- Thuricide-HP, also derived from *B. thuringiensis* Berliner. However, unlike Thuricide, it is twice as concentrated; and
- Bactospeine, Javelin, and Dipel all contain *B. thuringiensis* Berliner var. *kurstaki* as their active ingredient. However, with regard to concentration, the ratio of active ingredients among the three is 1:2:4, respectively.

These formulations of *B . thuringiensis* are active over a broad range of lepidopterous pests in a vast array of crops, including vegetables, cotton, and various fruits. Among the disadvantages, however, is the slow killing action that allows more damage before death. These materials are also less toxic to large worms.

MUTATIONS

Dangerous mutations may be of two types: mutation to infect a mammal and mutation to produce a toxin harmful to mammals.[21] The most useful test for detecting the ability of *B. thuringiensis* to mutate is serial passage of the agent in an environment in which the mutants in question would have a selective advantage over the parent agents and so reveal their presence in the mammalian body.

TOXICITY

In Europe and North America, new *B. thuringiensis* products have been subjected to extensive toxicological tests, which confirmed their innocuity. However, regulatory agencies have not specified what tests should be required for new *B. thuringiensis* products. Recently, the toxin of *B. thuringiensis israelensis*, when dissolved and injected intravenously into mice, was found to be highly toxic (LD_{50} 1.3 mg/kg), being more so to the mouse than to the American cockroach and cabbage looper.[22]

FUTURE OF SAFETY TESTING

Work has been started on the improvement of industrial strains of *B. thuringiensis*. It is still mainly at the stage of selecting from existing strains, with a start being made toward utilization of genetic engineering to transfer and to amplify characteristics—for example, the possible use of *B. subtilis* to mediate change in *B. thuringiensis*. Unique codes of safety are being formulated worldwide for genetic engineering. Safety problems are not expected during manipulation of pest-control pathogens, because factors harmful to pests rather than to humans are being manipulated. From this viewpoint, it has been postulated that bacterial insect pathogens are ideal systems for basic work on genetic engineering. However, mediator organisms must be selected with care and a watch kept to avoid undesirable contaminants entering the systems.

B. THURINGIENSIS USAGE

Since bacterial control agents are not restricted-use materials, quantitative information on the usage of *B. thuringiensis* in agriculture is difficult to obtain. An annual report on pesticide use is published by the California Department of Food and Agriculture (CDFA). The most recent report

(1983) provides quantitative data for virtually all pesticides used in California, giving amounts used on different crops, but figures were not available for bacterial agents. Therefore, it was necessary to approach manufacturers of *B. thuringiensis* (for example, Abbott Laboratories and Sandoz-Zoecon) for this information.

T. Hsieh of Sandoz-Zoecon indicated that Javelin, a recent *B. thuringiensis* isolate developed by his company, is used primarily for the control of forest insects (gypsy moth, spruce budworm) and vegetable and alfalfa insects. He estimates that in the first two-and-one-half months on the market, 70,000 to 90,000 gallons of Javelin was sold in the United States alone. One to two quarts of Javelin are required per acre. Hsieh admitted that growth in the use of *B. thuringiensis* has been very slow, attributable mainly to the relatively low cost and effectiveness of conventional insecticides. Further, as a stomach poison, Javelin is restricted primarily to lepidopteran larvae that chew. However, recently a *B. thuringiensis* isolate has been discovered in Germany which is highly active against the Colorado potato beetle.

Hsieh's estimate of the total amount of conventional *B. thuringiensis* (not including Javelin) sold by Sandoz-Zoecon last year is around 2 million gallons. This material is sold in many developing countries to control vegetable crop pests that can no longer be controlled by conventional insecticides.

Phillip Grau of Abbott Laboratories estimates worldwide sales of Abbott's *B. thuringiensis* (Dipel) to be in the neighborhood of 3.5–4.0 million pounds. It has been sold mainly for use on vegetables (lettuce, cole crops, tomatoes, mixed vegetables) and mosquito control. More recently, it is finding increasing use against forest insects. However, use on vegetable crops is being supplanted to some degree by the pyrethroids since they are registered for use on vegetables.

B. thuringiensis is also used effectively to control mosquito larvae. According to recent annual reports of the California Mosquito and Vector Control Association, the following amounts of *B. thuringiensis* were used for mosquito control in California: 1983—5,547 $\times$ 10^9 biological units (approximately 20,350 pounds); 1984—18,630 $\times$ 10^9 biological units (approximately 68,370 pounds). For 1985, usage is expected to have doubled over that of 1984.

According to M. Mulla (University of California, Riverside) and Hsieh, approximately 1 million gallons per year of *B. thuringiensis* are being used in West Africa against black flies (vector of onchocerciasis) by the World Health Organization. Mulla stated that a new bacterium (*B. sphaericus*) is being developed for use specifically on mosquitoes. It is more persistent than *B. thuringiensis* and will be used to complement *B. thuringiensis*.

From discussion with a number of individuals, including those mentioned above, it is clear that the use of bacterial agents for insect control will increase substantially in the immediate future. However, it must be pointed out that the total amount of these materials used compared to synthetic organic chemicals is still extremely small, probably less than 0.5 percent.

Viral Insecticides

A typical nucleopolyhedrosis virus (NPV) is *Baculovirus heliothis* which produces crystal-like, irregular, proteinaceous polyhedral inclusion bodies (PIB) in nuclei of infected cells.[23] Development of the NPV of *Heliothis* sp. began in 1961, progressed through various research and development phases, and attained technical realization as the first commercial viral pesticide. An exemption from the requirement of a tolerance was granted in May 1973 by the EPA and a label was approved in December 1975. Currently, *B. heliothis* is marketed as safe and effective for use on cotton against *Heliothis zea* under the name Elcar (Sandoz, Inc.); Nutrilite products, Inc., has an equivalent experimental product called Biotrol-VHZ.

Resistance

Selection pressures of LC_{50-70} maintained for 20 and 25 generations did not yield resistance in *H. zea*. Similar results were obtained with laboratory populations of *H. armigera* selected for resistance over 22 generations.

There is no record of indisputable resistance of insects to viral agents in field trials or control programs. However, these agents have not been used for long and it is possible that low levels of resistance are present but are not readily detectable.

In one case, NPV collected from distant plantations was more effective against the wattle bagworm, *Kotochalia junodi*, than virus collected from the local plantation in which tests were performed. Resistance might have been acquired by the local insects to the local virus or the observation might reflect differing levels of virulence among virus isolates.

Stability, Sensitivity, and Persistence

Natural sunlight-ultraviolet radiation (> 290 nm) is the major environmental factor inactivating *B. heliothis* and probably most insect viruses. Although field temperatures of 15°–45°C had no effect on the stability of PIB, viral replication was inhibited at 40°C. In general, high temperatures (70°–80°C) and the presence of water completely inactivate PIB. Acids and alkalis disrupt PIB and thus presumably destroy viral activity. Early field and lab studies have indicated that most insecticides or insecticidal adjuvants are compatible with *B. heliothis*.

TOXICOLOGICAL STUDIES

· The baculovirus of *H. zea* and *Lymantria dispar* exhibited no harm to mammals, fish, birds, or beneficial insects (including parasitic insects), had no relationship to arboviruses, and had no effect on aquatic invertebrates.[24]

Extensive safety testing of *Neodiprion lecontei* NPV and *N. sertifer* NPV was undertaken; carcinogenicity tests on newborn hamsters and a two-year carcinogenicity test on rats were among the battery of tests. There was no evidence that the viral preparation has any harmful effects.

PRODUCTION

B. heliothis can be produced only in Heliothis larvae, although several sophisticated processes have been suggested. Production of sawfly (*N. sertifer*) NPV is complicated by the fact that there are no synthetic diets or established cell cultures for sawflies.[25] Hence, for virus production, larvae must be reared on their host food plant, infected with virus, and then harvested and processed.

FIELD TRIALS

Control by *B. heliothis* generally was as effective on cotton as with standard insecticides. Control was less effective on corn than with standard insecticides. Although all spray treatments were effective on soybeans, poorer results were obtained by releasing virus-infected larvae. Desired levels of control were not obtained on tobacco and tomatoes. Results on sorghum were comparable to those obtained with carbaryl and endosulfan.

With the notable exception of sawflies, little is known of viruses pathogenic for nonlepidopteran insects, and continuous cell cultures from such important groups as the Hymenoptera, Coleoptera, and Orthoptera are lacking.

FUTURE DEVELOPMENTS

Several procedures for producing baculoviruses in either homologous or nonhomologous hosts have been proposed. Although *B. heliothis* produced in cell lines was as effective as that from larvae and it will replicate in cell lines, this technology will not be commercially practical for a long time. Significant development in production of *B. heliothis* will probably come from new techniques such as production in nonhomologous hosts coupled with recombinant DNA techniques.

A key to the development of viral products is whether they can be safely released into the environment.[26] Lois Miller, University of Idaho, is studying the replication of the baculovirus DNA, which could lead to a better understanding of how to enhance the virus' pathogenicity and expand its host range as well. EPA scientist Daphne Kamely observed that the fate of the baculovirus and retroviruses in the environment is not well understood. Studies are currently going on at Harvard University and at the National Institutes of Health to develop risk assessment models that may help the EPA to evaluate the consequences of the release of viruses into the environment.

Fungal Insecticides

Although mycoses caused by the entomopathogenic Fungi Imperfecti, *Beauveria bassiana*, *Metarhizium anisopliae* var. *anisopliae* and var. *major* (the color of the spores) have been studied for about a century, it is principally during the past 15–20 years that special attention has been focused on them to develop new methods of microbial control of insects.[27] For many years they were regarded as biological agents of secondary interest, due to pessimistic conclusions from the first field trials in several countries at the end of the last century. However, in the 1950s East European countries started investigations, particularly with *B. bassiana*, as part of a general strategy to control the Colorado potato beetle, *Leptinotarsa decemlineata*.

PRODUCTION

A new stage technique for mass production of *B. bassiana* conidiospores is used in the USSR. First the biomass is produced as mycelium in a fermentor, and subsequently surface-cultured in trays of nutrient medium for sporulation. A similar technique is used for the mass production of *M. anisopliae*. The preparations have a limited viability of 2 or 3 months, a serious failure that considerably limits their industrial potential. In addition, production costs are high.

TOXICITY

In numerous safety tests, no infections have been induced in mammals with the common microbiological control fungi. These include short-term tests (feeding, inhalation, and intravenous and subcutaneous injection) and 90-day subacute inhalation and feeding studies of *B. bassiana* and *M.*

anisopoliae in rodents; two-year intraperitoneal and subcutaneous injection, lactatation and fertility tests in rats; and three-month and one-and-a-half-year studies of dusting effects on rats and mice.

RESISTANCE

Since these pathogens have been in nature for a long time, it is reasonable to presume that insects have developed low levels of resistance to them. With regard to infectivity, fungi reach their sites of action in the haemocoel through the cuticle, or possibly through the mouth parts and not via the gut wall as do bacteria and viruses. They become established only when the infective phase interacts with a susceptible host (that is, one that does not produce local reactions to ward off penetration).

These factors are sobering reminders that fungi and their products as pest control agents do not have an unlimited potential.

PRODUCTS AND USES

Boverin, the trade name under which *B. bassiana* is marketed, is not used in the United States possibly because of economic considerations, which may not have been taken into account in the USSR in evaluating effectiveness, or because of climatic considerations. The climate in the Ukraine has justified the combined use of Boverin and reduced dosages of chemical insecticides such as chlorophos or malathion. However, when summers are particularly dry and hot, results are poor.

Mycar, a preparation of *Hirsutella thompsonii,* was marketed by Abbott Laboratories until recently. The product was discontinued because it was expensive to produce and large quantities were needed for each application.

It is well established now that entomopathogenic fungi have a certain specificity. In the same species of fungus, different strains can have very different activity.

FUTURE DEVELOPMENTS IN MICROBIOLOGICAL AGENTS

The success of *B. thuringiensis* as an insecticide has initiated research to incorporate its toxin-coding genes into plant genomes in a manner that will allow them to be expressed and the toxin to occur either symplastically or apoplastically within plants.

One idea is to nick the circular *B. thuringiensis* plasmid and join it directly to a plant plasmid in vitro. Upon reintroduction of the now extended plasmid into a plant cell, it is conceivable that the *B. thuringiensis* toxin could be one of the translation products of its expression.

Since gene-incorporated traits are generally transmissible to future progenies, the *B. thuringiensis* gene might well end up in new seeds on the market. This was accomplished in tobacco by the Rohm and Haas Co. The plant did not produce enough insecticide, however, to kill insects.

Another idea is to transfer the *B. thuringiensis* plasmid through the intermediacy of gall-producing bacteria to plants. A possible plasmid carrier could be attenuated *Agrobacterium tumefasciens* or its antagonist *A. radiobacter*.

Plasmid transfer to the nitrogen-fixing bacteria in the Rhizobium genus and eventual expression inside the root system of the plant is also a possibility. Since these bacteria are already used commercially to inoculate legumes, it is only one step to incorporate an extra gene into them for *B. thuringiensis* toxin production.

One cautionary note in these ideas is whether the *B. thuringiensis* toxin-producing genes can or will be transferred through the plant plasmids to weeds, thereby having an adverse affect on the beneficial insects that suppress the proliferation of weeds.

SUMMARY

The potential of microbiological insecticides has barely been tapped. The advent of new viral, bacterial, and fungal insecticides with remarkable insect toxicity to selected target pests and negligible mammalian toxicity is possible. The pragmatic view of biological insecticides taken by regulatory agencies is likely to continue and anecdotal reports of toxicity such as that of *B. thuringiensis israelensis* to mice by intravenous administration will be placed in their proper perspective.

Viral insecticides are particularly promising for the future. Safety prospects are also good and the chances of mutation to forms that are virulent to mammals and other vertebrates are practically nonexistent.

The future is also likely to see structure-activity studies on the microbial toxins to determine if any underlying common molecular rationale exists to explain their mode of toxic action. These studies and the topographic details of the toxins derivable from them could also form the basis for a new generation of highly selective chemical insectides with high toxicity to only a very narrow spectrum of pests. These new chemicals are expected to better withstand scrutiny by the Delaney Clause.

NOTES

1. National Research Council. 1986. Pesticide Resistance: Strategies and Tactics for Management. Washington, D.C.: National Academy Press.

2. Hollingworth, R. M. and A. E. Luna. 1982. Pesticidal Mode of Action, J. R. Coats, ed., New York: Academic Press.

3. Albers-Schonberg, G., B. H. Arison, J. C. Chabala, A. W. Douglas, P. Eskola, M. H. Fisher, A. Lusi, H. Mrozik, J. L. Smith, and H. L. Tolman. 1981. J. Amer. Chem. Soc. 103:4216.

4. Fisher, M. H. 1985. Pp. 53–72 in Recent Advances in the Chemistry of Insect Control, N. F. Janes, ed. London: Burlington House.

5. Kay, I. T., and M. D. Turnbull. 1985. Pp. 229–244 in Recent Advances in the Chemistry of Insect Control.

6. Baker, R., C. J. Swain, and J. Head. 1985. Pp. 245–256 in Recent Advances in the Chemistry of Insect Control.

7. Palmer, C. J., and J. E. Casida, 1984. J. Agr. Food Chem. 33: 976.

8. Hollingshaus, J. G., and R. J. Little. 1985. Abstract. Agrochemicals Division National Meeting, American Chemical Society, Miami Beach, Fla., April 28–May 3.

9. Grosscurt, A. C. 1978. Pestic. Sci. 9:373.

10. Cohen, E., and J. E. Casida. 1982. Pestic. Biochem. Physiol. 17: 301.

11. Janes, N. F., ed. 1985. Recent Advances in the Chemistry of Insect Control. London: Burlington House.

12. Fukuto, T. R. 1984. ACS Symposium Series, No. 255. Washington, D.C.: American Chemical Society, pp. 87–101.

13. Sakai, M. 1983. Abstracts. 5th International Congress on Pesticide Chemicals, IIa-2, Kyoto, Japan.

14. Bowers, W. S. 1985. Pp. 53–72 in Recent Advances in the Chemistry of Insect Control.

15. Miyakado, M., I. Nakayama, A. Inoue, M. Hatakoshi and N. Ohno. 1985. J. Pestic. Sci. 10:11.

16. Lay, S. V. 1985. Pp.305–322 in Recent Advances in the Chemistry of Insect Control.

17. Agrios, G. N. 1978. Plant Pathology, 2nd ed. New York: Academic Press.

18. Dulmage, H. T. 1981. Insecticidal activity of isolates of Bacillus thuringiensis and their potential for pest control. P. 193 in Microbial Control of Pests and Plant Diseases (1970–1980), H. D. Burges, ed. London: Academic Press.

19. Kolata, G. 1985. Genetically engineered organisms in agriculture. Science 229 (5 July):34.

20. McGaughey, W. H. 1985. Insect resistance to the biological insecticide Bacillus thuringiensis. Science 229(12 July): 193–195.

21. Burges, H. D. 1981. Safety, safety testing and quality control of microbial pesticides. P. 737 in Microbial Control of Pests and Plant Diseases (1970–1980).

22. Roe, M. R., P. Y. K. Cheung, B. D. Hammock, D. Buster, and R. A. Alford. 1985. Endotoxin of Bacillus thuringiensis var. israelensis—broad spectrum toxicity and neural response elicited in mice and insects. Pp. 279–292 in Bioregulators for Pest Control, P. A. Hedin, ed., ACS Symposium Series 276.

23. Ignoffo, C. M., and T. L. Couch. 1981. The nucleopolyhedrosis virus of Heliothis species as a microbial insecticide. P. 330 in Microbial Control of Pests and Plant Diseases (1970–1980).

24. Lewis, F. B. 1981. Control of the gypsy moth by a Baculovirus. P. 363 in Microbial Control of Pests and Plant Diseases (1970–1980).

25. Cunningham, T. C., and P. F. Entwistle. 1981. Control of Sawflies by Baculovirus. P. 379 in Microbial Control of Pests and Plant Diseases (1970–1980).

26. Sun, M. 1985. Biotechnology—focus on viruses. Science 228 (14 June):1294–1295.

27. Ferron, P. 1981. Pest control by the Fungi Beauveria and Metarhizium. P. 465 in Microbial Control of Pests and Plant Diseases (1970–1980).

E

Survey of Pesticide R&D Directors: How Do Current Laws Affect Agricultural Pesticide Research Productivity?

Twenty research directors of major pesticide manufacturers participated in the survey below. All are involved in investment planning to accommodate changes in EPA and other regulations. Survey responses are in boxes.

I. Assume your company has a new product under development which produced an undisputed oncogenic response (statistically significant increase in the usual tumors seen in rat or mouse control populations), and the use pattern results in residues in processed products which require a section 409 (food additive) tolerance.

    A. What would be the percent reductions in R&D cost (direct and administrative) to obtain a tolerance if the Delaney Clause was *not* applicable, e.g., such tolerances could be granted on the basis of a benefit/risk analysis as is done for setting 408 (raw agricultural commodity) tolerances?

> Answers varied from 0 to 25 percent, but most responses were in the 5–15 percent range. Two remarks suggested the same studies are needed in either case, whereas one remark suggested oncogenicity tests need to be repeated.

    B. What is the probability of receiving a tolerance if:
        (1) the current law remains as is?

249

(2) the Delaney Clause was not applicable?

---

(1) Most respondents agreed the chances would be practically nonexistent.
(2) The majority of respondents agreed that the probability in the absence of the Delaney Clause would be 50 percent or greater.

C. What *reduction* in time delays from product discovery to final registration would occur if Delaney was *not* applicable? (months)

Answers varied from 0 to 48 months on this question, but there was general agreement in the range of 12–24 months.

II. With regard to oncogenicity testing requirements that the entire industry must complete under the reregistration process:

A. What percent of your currently registered product line do you estimate will trigger Delaney?

Most answers to this question were in the 10–20 percent range, but six companies responded with answers of 35 percent or above. There were also three companies who felt Delaney would not be triggered for any of their reregistration compounds.

B. What percent of the market for your products will be lost because of application of Delaney?

Answers to this question were consistently in the 5–20 percent range. One company, however, correctly observed that the agency has not yet used Delaney in the reregistration process.

C. What percent of your currently registered products in each class do you feel will be impacted substantially by Delaney (greater than 10% of sales)?
insecticides   herbicides
fungicides   other

General feelings were that currently registered fungicides would be affected significantly by the Delaney Clause with answers (when not zero) at 50 percent or greater. Insecticides were the next most likely to be affected with answers in the 10–20 percent range. The responses on herbicides varied greatly with eight answers ranging from 10 to 80 percent. There was an insignificant number of responses under the "other" category. There were 60 zero or blank answers out of a possible 80 answers to this question. The blank answers might mean the company has no reregistration candidates in the class, and the zeros could indicate either a certainty that none would be affected or that the EPA would not apply the Delaney Clause to cancel tolerances during the reregistration process.

    D. In terms of lost products and lack of substitute pesticides or other control practices, which two or three crops do you believe will be most significantly impacted by Delaney?

The crops cited most frequently were citrus, apples, tomatoes, grapes, corn, soybeans, cotton, and small grains.

III. A. Has the Delaney Clause ever been used by the EPA to deny the granting of a tolerance on a raw agricultural commodity (408) which did not involve the need for a food additive (409) tolerance?

All answers were negative.

    B. If the Delaney Clause could be cited against one of your products to deny the granting of a necessary food additive tolerance (409), would you:

(1) Abandon the pursuit of the tolerance?

(2) Investigate changes in use pattern to eliminate the residue on the crop?

(3) Other (please specify)

(4) What would be the cost of whatever action you chose to take? Specify action—
lost sales   direct testing cost
months delay

(1) Only four companies answered this question with an unqualified *yes*. Three were ambivalent and the remainder said *no*.

(2) With two exceptions, all companies said *yes* to this question. This indicates that attempts to change use patterns as a means of avoiding a Delaney Clause issue is or could be a routine or common approach in seeking a section 409 tolerance.

(3) Most companies did not respond to this part, but two companies indicated they would examine the risk/benefit aspects of the situation and a third indicated it would attempt to argue on the basis of the FDA de minimus, sensitivity of the method (SOM), or constituents policy loopholes.

(4) There was no consensus on lost sales. More than half the respondents did not answer. The responses of those who did answer varied from $0.25MM to $50MM. The delay estimates varied from one year at a minimum to a three-year maximum with two years about average. The direct testing cost ranged from $200M to $500M.

C. To your knowledge, has the EPA granted food additive tolerances for compounds when there is clear evidence that the tumor of concern is benign rather than malignant?

No evidence was cited that a tolerance was granted under these conditions, but one company reminded the committee that the EPA has not used Delaney in the reregistration process.

D. Are food processing studies for determining the declining/increasing concentration of pesticide residues part of your company's usual battery of tests for a new food use pesticide?
If yes, what are the typical costs of such studies per product?
Where are these processing studies done?
Internal ___ Universities ___ Food processing companies___

Eighteen of 20 companies answered *yes* to this question, with costs in the $25M–$50M range for each crop processed. Most of the companies used all three sources for doing these studies, but the university and food processing companies were named more frequently than internal studies.

IV. Concerns have been raised that Delaney will prevent registration of new and/or old products for minor crops and pests.

Do you view this concern as major?   average?   minimal?

Eleven of the respondents viewed the impact of Delaney on minor crops as *major* and an additional five felt the impact would be *average*. It might be concluded, therefore, that the burden on IR-4 (see Chapter 6) may be significantly increased in the future. Incentives for companies to seek minor-use registrations must also be addressed.

V. Given that our knowledge of oncogenic responses in laboratory animals and methods of risk assessment have advanced since the Delaney Clause became part of the Food, Drug and Cosmetic Act, what options would you favor for its modification (please rank in order of preference)?

A. Status quo

B. Repeal with no substitute language—make section 409 track section 408.

C. Apply Delaney to section 408—make 408 track section 409.

D. Repeal with substitute language stating approval of 409's for oncogenic substances based on benefit/risk considerations.

E. D., but specific risk criteria.

F. An amendment stating the Delaney Clause is not applicable to pesticides when they are not intentionally added to processed foods or animal feed.

G. Amendment of section 409 to state that pesticides not intentionally added to processed foods or animal feed are not subject to the 409 provisions.

H. Other (please specify)

It is difficult to summarize the responses to this question since the responses varied widely. Some statements can be made, however:

- No company rated the *status quo* higher than *5* and most rated this choice as *6* or *7*.
- Making section 409 track section 408 was a popular choice (*3* or higher) with nine companies.
- Applying Delaney to section 408 was rated no higher than *7* by any respondent.
- Repeal with substitute language was rated no lower than *3* by any company with most answers being either *1* or *2*.

• The application of specific risk criteria was rated from *1* to *6* with no consensus at all.

• The amendment stating Delaney is not applicable to pesticides when not added deliberately to food received a lot of support but there were also six companies who rated it *4* or below.

• Similarly, the amendment stating that pesticides not added intentionally to processed foods or animal feeds are not subject to section 409 provisions received mixed responses with seven answers *3* or higher and nine answers *4* or lower.

• Most companies (16) did not respond to *other*, but one response suggested that the definition of oncogen be sharpened so that only a clearly oncogenic substance (multiple species, metastasis, etc.) would trigger Delaney. The sensitivity of the method should also be considered since zero residue is approachable but not attainable.

VI. A. How would your company's total discovery activities change (% increase or decrease) if:
(1) 408 with specified risk criteria replaced 409 with Delaney?
(2) 408 with benefit-risk criteria replaced 409 with Delaney?
(3) Delaney also applied to 408?

(1) A few companies felt their discovery activities would increase, but most believed the replacement would have no impact.
(2) Similarly, a few companies felt discovery activities would increase 5–30 percent but most said no impact.
(3) About a fourth of the respondents felt no change would take place; most companies said that if Delaney was applied to section 408, discovery activities would decrease, with those listing percentages ranging from a decrease of 35 to 100 percent.
This response when compared with question **II** C indicates that possibly companies whose products are dominated by fungicide and herbicide products would anticipate the greatest decrease in discovery activities.

B. List any other regulatory components you consider to be more restrictive than Delaney for your company (e.g., drinking water, mutagenicity, special review, teratology, reproductive effects, etc.).
(1) In the past.
(2) In the future.

Special review, teratology, and reproductive effects were mentioned most frequently (by about half) as being more restrictive in the past, and groundwater and/or drinking water restrictions were listed by over half of the respondents as being more restrictive than Delaney in the future. This may indicate that Delaney is one of the most restrictive regulatory components but is not alone in its restrictive impact on companies.

C. Would your company abandon development of a promising new active ingredient if it tested positive in:
One mutagenic end point?
Two mutagenic end points?
Three mutagenic end points?

One positive mutagenic result would cause no company to abandon development. Two mutagenic end points yielded only five *yes* or "possible" yes and 12 definite *no* answers. Three positive mutagenic end points, however, prompted *14* of the respondents to answer *yes* with only a few caveats.

VII. Your company's approximate pesticides sales. Check one:
Less than $100 million $100–$400 million
More than $400 million

There were no obvious trends in the replies as a function of company size. It is possible to conclude, therefore, that issues such as impact on discovery activities, testing methodologies, approaches (for example, changing use patterns in order to acquire tolerances) may be equally significant.

Among the respondents, five companies have <$100MM in sales, nine have between $100MM and $400MM, and six have >$400MM.

Index

A

Acaricides, 52–53, 204; *see also*
  Chlorobenzilate
Acceptable Daily Intake (ADI), calculation
  of, for non-oncogenic pesticides,
  31–32
Acephate
  crop uses, 52, 68, 77
  dietary oncogenic risk from, 68, 77, 84
  Q* for, 55, 77
  risk reduced through tolerance
    revocations, 115
  TMRC, 77
  volume of use, 52
  weight-of-the-evidence classification, 67,
    77
  year of first tolerance, 52, 68
Acetamide, 88, 93–94, 222–224
Acifluorfen, 47, 52
Acre treatments
  definition, 47
  lost under policy scenarios, 107, 111,
    114, 116, 122, 124–129
  with oncogenic fungicides, 48, 122,
    125–128
  with oncogenic herbicides, 122, 124
  with oncogenic insecticides, 47–48, 122,
    124–125

Active ingredients, *see* Pesticide active
  ingredients
Alachlor
  crop uses, 52, 68, 76, 89
  dietary oncogenic risk from, 68, 76, 83,
    84, 89, 98
  herbicide market share, 98
  possible date for tolerance revocation,
    98
  potential short-term impact of Delaney
    Clause on, 98
  Q* for, 55, 76
  risk reduced through tolerance
    revocations, 110, 121
  TMRC, 76
  use cancellations, 68
  volume of use, 47, 89
  weight-of-the-evidence classification, 67,
    76
  year of first tolerance, 52, 68
Alar, *see* Daminozide
Aliette, *see* Fosetyl Al
Allelopathy, 231–232
Ambush, *see* Permethrin
Amitraz
  application of Delaney Clause to, 88, 90
  dietary oncogenic risk from, 88
  major crop uses, 52
  volume of use, 52

year of first tolerance, 52
Ammo, *see* Cypermethrin
Animal drugs, applicability of Delaney
    Clause to, 38
Animal feeds
    commodities affected by pesticide
        residues in, 74
    concentration of residues in, 37, 40, 73
    effect of loss of crop tolerances for, 120
    estimated oncogenic risk from residues
        in, 71–74
    not subject to feed-additive regulations,
        73
    problems posed by, 110
Animal products
    concentration of residues in, 37, 93–94
    Delaney Clause effect on, 73
    dietary oncogenic risk from 119–120
    effect of risk reduction strategies on,
        119
    problems posed by, 110
    sensitivity-of-the-method procedure
        applied to, 88, 93–94, 223–224
Animal studies of oncogenicity/
    carcinogenicity, relevance to humans,
        30, 33, 38, 49–50, 66, 67
Apples
    consumption estimates, 57–58
    effect of policy scenarios on, 107, 111,
        114–116, 125–126
    estimated oncogenic risk from, 78, 80,
        85, 133–134
    pesticide use levels on, 48, 52
    risk reduced by tolerance revocations,
        122
    tolerance denials for, 88, 90
    vulnerability to tolerance revocations, 10
Arsenic acid, 52
Asulam
    exclusion from this study, 51
    major crop uses, 52
    Q* for, 55
    volume of use, 52
    year of first tolerance, 52
Atrazine, 47
Azinphos-methyl
    crop uses, 52, 68, 77
    dietary oncogenic risk from, 68, 77, 84
    Q* for, 55, 77
    TMRC, 77
    volume of use, 52
    weight-of-the-evidence classification, 67,
        77
    year of first tolerance, 52, 68

B

Baam, *see* Amitraz
Bacillus thuringiensis, 153–154, 239–242,
    246–247
Baculovirus, 151–152
Beef, estimated oncogenic risk from,
    78–79, 84
Benlate, *see* Benomyl
Benomyl
    alternatives to, 201–202
    application of Delaney Clause to, 95–97,
        132, 199–200
    concentration in processed foods, 19, 95
    crop uses, 52, 68, 77, 89
    dietary oncogenic risk from, 68, 77, 85,
        89, 97, 132, 134, 199
    fungicide market share, 97, 132
    metabolite, 199
    number of tolerances, 109
    pest resistance to, 200
    possible date for tolerance revocation,
        97, 132
    Q* for, 55, 77
    regulatory status, 198
    risk reduced through tolerance
        revocation, 109–110, 113, 115,
        120–121, 132–133
    TMRC, 77
    tolerances, 198, 199–200
    volume of use, 52, 89, 95, 198
    weight-of-the-evidence classification, 67,
        77
    year of first tolerance, 52, 68
Biological pest control
    allelopathy, 231–231
    innovation prospects in, 9, 153–154
    weed control by insects, 230–231
Biotechnology, innovations in, 9
Blazer, *see* Acifluorfen
Bravo, *see* Chlorothalonil

C

Calcium arsenate, 52
Cancer
    background risk, 3
    induction, evidence of, 38
Captafol
    crop uses, 52, 68, 77
    dietary oncogenic risk from, 68, 77, 83,
        85, 97, 132–134
    fungicide market share, 97, 132
    possible date for tolerance revocation,

97, 132
potential impact of Delaney Clause on,
  97, 132
Q* for, 55, 77
TMRC, 77
volume of use, 52
weight-of-the-evidence classification, 67,
  77
year of first tolerance, 52, 68
Captan
  crop uses, 52, 68, 77, 89
  dietary oncogenic risk from, 68, 77, 83,
    85, 89, 97, 132, 134, 202–203
  fungicide market share, 97, 132
  non-oncogenic health risks, 201
  possible date for tolerance revocation,
    97, 132
  potential impact of Delaney Clause on,
    97, 132, 203
  Q* for, 55, 77
  regulatory status, 201
  risk reduced through tolerance
    revocation, 109–110, 121
  TMRC, 77
  tolerances, 201, 203
  volume of use, 52, 89, 201
  weight-of-the-evidence classification, 67,
    77
  year of first tolerance, 52, 68
Carcinogenicity
  determination of, 39
  distinction between oncogenicity and, 3,
    30–31
Carcinogens
  definition, 30, 31
  EPA classification system for, 4, 31, 66,
    67
  negligible-risk standard for, 12–14
Case studies for potential policy
    precedents
  benomyl, 95–96, 198–201
  captan, 201–204
  chlorobenzilate, 95, 204–205
  dicamba, 94–95, 206–208
  dicofol, 95
  EBDCs, 208–214
  fosetyl Al, 192, 196–198
  metalaxyl, 214–217
  new active ingredients, 95–96
  permethrin, 92–93, 217–220
  prior-sanctioned pesticides, 91–92
  thiodicarb, 93–94, 220–224
  tolerances for new active ingredients, 91
Cattle, relevant pesticide use levels, 51, 53

Chlordimeform
  crop uses, 52, 68, 77
  dietary oncogenic risk from, 68, 74, 75,
    76, 77, 83, 84, 125
  Q* for, 55, 77
  risk reduced through tolerance
    revocation, 121
  TMRC, 77
  volume of use, 52
  weight-of-the-evidence classification, 67,
    77
  year of first tolerance, 52, 68
Chlorobenzilate
  alternatives to, 205
  application of Delaney Clause to, 205
  benefits of, 205
  dietary oncogenic risk from, 89, 95,
    204–205
  major crop uses, 52, 89, 95
  regulatory status, 204
  tolerance actions on, 95, 205
  volume of use, 52, 89, 204
  year of first tolerance, 52
Chlorothalonil
  crop uses, 52, 68, 77
  dietary oncogenic risk from, 68, 77, 83,
    85, 97, 132–134
  fungicide market share, 97, 132
  possible date for tolerance revocation,
    97, 132
  potential short-term impact of Delaney
    Clause on, 97, 132
  Q* for, 55, 77
  TMRC, 77
  volume of use, 52
  weight-of-the-evidence classification, 67,
    77
  year of first tolerance, 52, 68
Citrus
  consumption estimates, 57–58
  pesticide use levels on, 48, 52–53, 89
  vulnerability to tolerance revocations, 10
Code of Federal Regulations, tolerances
    for oncogens, 19, 35, 36
Commodities, processed
  concentration of residues in, *see*
    Concentration of pesticide residues
  data sources on, 183–184
  definition of, 42, 73, 110
  dried, 37
  estimated risk associated with, 5, 75,
    85–86
  estimation of residues in, 61–63,
    185–186, 190–191

from minor crops, 10
pesticide residues as food additives in, 25–26, 35
risk standards applied to oncogenic pesticides in, 40
with section 409 tolerances for oncogenic pesticides, 4, 61–63
without section 409 tolerances for oncogenic pesticides, 5, 61–63
in TAS compared with section 409 tolerances, 64
Commodities, raw
adulterated, 25
estimated risk associated with, 5, 86
estimation of residues in, 185–186, 190–191
risk standards applied to oncogenic pesticides in, 40
with no processed form, 5, 41–42, 70–72, 108, 110, 117
Concentration of pesticide residues
in animal feeds, 37, 40, 73
in animal products, 37, 93–94
authority governing, *see* FDC Act, section 409
basis for determining, 37
Delaney Clause application to, 28
EPA tolerance-setting policy on, 2, 28, 41
examples, 19
impact on distribution and character of dietary oncogenic risk, 81–82
regulatory implications, 19–20, 27, 28, 35–37, 40
risk standards for, 40
TAS conversion factors for, 62
in tomato products, 81–82
Copper arsenate, 52, 56
Corn
consumption estimates, 57–58
effect of policy scenarios on, 107, 111, 114, 115–116, 124
estimated oncogenic risk from, 15, 78, 79
oncogenic risk associated with, 15
pesticide use levels on, 52–53, 89
risk reduced by tolerance revocations, 122
tolerances for processed forms, 64, 219
Cotton
effect of policy scenarios on, 107, 111, 114–116
pesticide use levels on, 52–53, 89
Crop-level scenario analyses

apple fungicides, 107, 111, 114–116, 122, 125–126, 147–148
citrus insecticides, 146
coding for this study, 184–185
corn herbicides, 107, 111, 114–116, 122, 124, 129, 146–147
cotton insecticides, 107, 111, 114–116, 122, 124–125, 129, 146
data sources on, 184
grape fungicides, 105, 107, 111, 114, 116, 122
peanut fungicides, 7, 105, 107, 110–111, 114, 116–117, 122, 128–129, 147–148
potato fungicides, 105, 107, 111, 114–116, 122, 126–127, 147–148
prospects for innovation in, 145–148
selection of, 102
soybean herbicides, 107, 111, 114, 116–117, 122, 124, 129, 146–147
tomato fungicides, 107, 111, 114–116, 122, 127–128, 147–148
Crops
distribution of dietary oncogenic risk by, 76, 78–83
herbicide-resistant, 152, 232–233
losing tolerances under policy scenarios, 106, 109–110, 113–116
not dependent on pesticides, 49
orchard, pesticide use levels on, 52–53
requiring processing studies under EPA guidelines, 70
see also Commodities, raw; Minor crops; specific crops
Cultural pest control, prospects for innovation in, 9, 154–155
Cymbush, *see* Cypermethrin
Cypermethrin
application rates, 47
crop uses, 52, 68, 77
dietary oncogenic risk from, 68, 77, 84
Q* for, 55, 77
risk reduced through tolerance revocation, 121, 124–125
TMRC, 77
volume of use, 52
weight-of-the-evidence classification, 67, 77
year of first tolerance, 52, 68
Cyromazine
application of Delaney Clause to, 88, 90
crop uses, 52, 68, 77
dietary oncogenic risk from, 68, 77, 88
Q* for, 55, 77
TMRC, 77

volume of use, 52
weight-of-the-evidence classification, 67, 77
year of first tolerance, 52, 68

D

2,4-D, 47, 137
Daminozide, 51, 52, 89
Delaney Clause
  constituents policy on, 39, 88, 90, 94, 207–208
  de minimis interpretation, 39–40, 89, 95
  DES Proviso, 38, 224–225
  EPA interpretation of, 20, 30, 38, 83, 85–91, 196–224
  economic effects, 136
  exemptions from, 5, 26–27, 41–42, 70–72, 91–92, 107–108
  FDA interpretation of, 30, 37–40
  general safety clause, 26, 39, 40, 41, 94–95, 207
  interpretation of, 20, 30, 37–40, 83, 85–91
  legislative history, 38, 161–173
  pest resistance and, 10–11
  problems and issues posed by, 40–43
  regulatory impacts of, 61, 69–70
  requirement for proof of carcinogenicity, 31
  responsibility for implementing and interpreting, 12
  risk standard of, 22, 26, 35
  scope of, 1–2
  worst-case impact of, 71
Delaney Clause application
  to already-registered pesticides, 35, 95–96
  to animal drugs and feed additives, 38
  case studies of, 196–224
  to concentrating residues, 28
  to fungicides, 8, 97–98
  to new pesticides, 2, 36, 86–96, 107–108
Delaney Clause effects
  on animal products, 73
  on dietary oncogenic risk, 5, 69–70
  on EPA decision making, 4
  on fungicides, 97–98
  on herbicides, 98
  on minor crops, 71, 157
  on pesticide availability, 20
  on R&D, 9–10, 137, 140, 149–150
  short-term, 97–98
Diallate, 52

Dicamba
  application of Delaney Clause to, 88, 90, 94–95, 206–208
  benefits, 208
  dietary oncogenic risk associated with, 88, 94–95, 206–207
  tolerances, 206
  volume of use, 206
Diclofop methyl
  crop uses, 52, 68, 76
  dietary oncogenic risk from, 68, 76
  Q* for, 55, 76
  TMRC, 76
  volume of use, 52
  weight-of-the-evidence classification, 67, 76
  year of first tolerance, 52, 68
Dicofol, 52, 89, 95
Dietary exposure to pesticides
  complications in determining, 61
  conservatisms in calculating, 32
  estimation of, 56–63
  sources of data on, 181–182
  variables in, 49
  see also Theoretical Maximum Residue Contribution (TMRC)
Dietary oncogenic risk
  by active ingredient, 75–77, 83–84; *see also* specific active ingredients
  analysis of estimates, 66–83
  chemical pesticide prospects relative to, 148–150
  by commodity, 5, 75–76, 78–86; *see also* specific commodities
  from concentration of residues, 81–82
  from current EPA policy, 12–13
  by date of tolerance, 85–86
  distribution in food supply, 4–6
  effect of Delaney Clause on, 5, 69–70
  expression of, 34
  extrapolation from animal studies, 30, 33, 38, 49–50, 66, 67
  increase through tolerance revocation/denial, 8, 14–15, 20, 41–42, 126, 127, 131–134
  from minor crops, 10
  negligible-risk scenarios of, 6–7, 12–14, 104, 110–114
  from old pesticides, 11, 85
  by pesticide type, 8, 69, 74–77, 79–82, 84–85
  from replacement chemicals, 76
  from residues in animal feeds, 71–74
  by tolerance type, 67–71, 85–86

zero-risk scenarios of, 6–7, 13–14,
    103–110
Dietary oncogenic risk estimation
    acreage treated in, 187, 192–194
    active ingredients included in, 4
    analytical method, 3, 15–16, 21, 50–63,
        185–195
    assumptions in, 3, 33–34, 49, 65
    balancing of benefits in, 18, 34–35, 43
    benefits characterized for, 4
    bias in, 60
    confidence limit, 34, 54
    conservatisms in, 33–34, 59, 65
    crop-level analyses, 7, 102–117, 187, 193
    data base, 4, 21, 50–55, 57–59, 176–185
    data management system, 174–176
    dietary exposure calculations in, 32,
        56–63, 186
    EPA method for, 3; *see also*
        Quantitative risk assessment
    food consumption estimates in, 57–59,
        186, 191–192
    formula, 63, 186–187
    potency factor, *see* Oncogenicity
        potency factor (Q*)
    problems, 49–50
    residues in commodities, 61–63, 185–186,
        190–191
    sources of data in, 178–185
    transfer and transformation of files for,
        176–178
    treatment of malignant and benign
        tumors in, 3, 38–39, 50, 54
    uncertainties in, 3, 4, 18, 33–34, 50,
        190–195
    weight-of-the-evidence approach, 3, 66,
        101
    see also Scenarios for regulating
        oncogenic pesticides
Dietary oncogenic risk reduction
    in crop-level analyses, 7, 102–103,
        105–107, 110, 113–117
    through cropwide tolerance reduction,
        131–134
    in negligible-risk scenario 3, 112–114,
        122
    in negligible-risk scenario 4, 115–117,
        122
    by pesticide type in scenarios, 118–120,
        124–129
    in zero-risk scenario 1, 104–105, 122
    in zero-risk scenario 2, 108–110, 122
Difolatan, *see* Captafol
Dimethoate, 188

Dimethylnitrosamine, 88, 94–95
Dithane M-45, *see* Mancozeb
Dual, *see* Metolachlor

E

EBDCs (ethylenebisdithiocarbamates)
    alternatives to, 214
    application of Delaney Clause to,
        212–214
    dietary oncogenic risk from, 68, 77, 89,
        92, 198, 210–212
    effect of cropwide tolerance reductions
        on risk from, 133–134
    major crop uses, 89
    market life, 137
    metabolite, *see* Ethylenethiourea
    regulatory status, 209–210
    tolerances, 209, 212
    volume of use, 89, 209
    see also Mancozeb; Maneb; Metiram;
        Zineb
Environmental Protection Agency (EPA)
    analytical framework recommended for,
        15–16
    classification system for carcinogens, 4,
        31, 66, 67
    Data Call-In Program, 36–37, 96–97
    definition of processed feed, 73
    definition of processed food, 42
    difficulties in reaching and defending
        regulatory decisions, 22
    food consumption data bases, *see* Food
        Factor system; Tolerance Assessment
        System (TAS)
    interpretation of the Delaney Clause, 4,
        20, 30, 38, 83, 85–91, 196–224
    regulation and review of pesticides,
        100–101
    regulatory actions scheduled for next 10
        years, 5, 85–86
    responsibilities in regulating pesticides,
        18–19, 21–22, 25–26
EPA policy
    on application of Delaney Clause to new
        pesticides, 2, 86–91, 107–108, 131
    case studies for potential precedents,
        91–96
    coordination with FDA in, 12
    current dietary oncogenic risk
        estimation, 3, 12–13, 33–35, 50; *see
        also* Quantitative risk assessment
    on suspect oncogens, 50–51
    for tolerance setting, 2, 27–36

tolerances for oncogenic pesticides, 34
Ethalfluralin
  crop uses, 52, 68
  dietary oncogenic risk from, 68, 76
  Q* for, 55, 76
  TMRC, 76
  volume of use, 52
  weight-of-the-evidence classification, 67, 76
  year of first tolerance, 52, 68
Ethylene oxide, 52, 56
Ethylenethiourea, 68, 77, 198, 209–214

F

FDC Act
  basic goals of, 18
  divergences between FIFRA and, 19
  EPA responsibilities under, 18–19, 25
  Food Additives Amendment of 1958, 162, 164–166
  Pesticide Residues Amendment of 1954, 161–162, 165–166
  tolerance setting under, 24–36
FDC Act, section 201(s), definition of food additive, 25
FDC Act, section 402, standard for pesticide residues in processed foods, 26–27, 161–163, 166–170
FDC Act, section 408
  EPA responsibilities under, 25
  scope of, 1, 25
  tolerance setting for non-oncogenic pesticides under, 31–33
  tolerance setting for oncogenic pesticides under, 33–35
  see also Tolerances, raw commodity (section 408)
FDC Act, section 409
  EPA's regulatory responsibilities under, 25–26
  FDA responsibilities under, 25
  general safety clause, 26, 39, 40, 41, 94–95, 207
  prior-sanction exception to, 91–92
  scope of, 1, 25
  tolerance setting under, 35–36
  see also Delaney Clause; Tolerances, processed commodity (section 409)
Feed additives, applicability of Delaney Clause to, 38
FIFRA
  basic goals of, 18
  divergences between FDC Act and, 19

EPA responsibilities under, 18
1972 amendments to, 139, 156
registration of pesticides under, 2, 23–24
section 3, 24
Fodders, risk standard applied to oncogenic pesticides in, 40, 73
Folpet
  crop uses, 52, 68, 77
  dietary oncogenic risk from, 68, 77, 83, 85, 97, 132, 132, 134
  fungicide market share, 97, 132
  possible date for tolerance revocation, 97, 132
  potential short-term impact of Delaney Clause on, 97, 132
  Q* for, 55, 77
  TMRC, 77
  volume of use, 52
  weight-of-the-evidence classification, 67, 77
  year of first tolerance, 52, 68
Food additives
  definition, 25, 91
  FDA interpretation of, 39
  general safety clause, 26, 39, 40, 41, 94–95
  regulation of pesticides in processed foods as, 26
  unsafe, 26
Food and Drug Administration (FDA)
  benchmark for judging safety, 39
  constituents policy, 39, 88, 90, 94, 207–208
  coordination with EPA on policy, 12
  de minimis standard, 39–40, 89, 95
  interpretation of "additives," 39
  interpretation of Delaney Clause, 30, 37–40
  responsibilities under FDC Act, section 409, 25
  sensitivity-of-the-method procedure, 38, 40, 73, 88, 90, 93–94, 223–224
Food consumption
  comparison of raw and processed crops, 58
  estimates of, 57–59, 191–192
  sources of data on, 179–181
Food Factor system, TAS contrasted with, 57–59
Fosetyl Al
  application of Delaney Clause to, 88, 92, 197–198
  crop uses, 52, 68, 77, 92
  dietary oncogenic risk from, 68, 77, 88,

92, 197
Q* for, 55, 77
TMRC, 77
tolerances, 196–198
volume of use, 52, 196, 198
weight-of-the-evidence classification, 67, 77
year of first tolerance, 52, 68
Fruits
  as animal feeds, 72
  dependency on pesticides, 49
  importance of fungicides in production of, 8
  pesticide use levels on, 52–53, 89
  see also Citrus
Fundal, *see* Chlordimeform
Fungicides
  action, 129–130
  benefits of, 7–8, 129
  Delaney Clause impacts on, 8, 97–98
  historical perspective on R&D in, 144–145
  innovation in, 8–9, 125, 128, 129, 131, 145, 147–148
  non-oncogenic, 8, 125, 127–129, 131
  number of CFR tolerances for, 19, 35, 36
  percent oncogenic, 4, 8, 14, 48
  pest resistance to, 10, 130, 200
  problems of, 130
  R&D expenditures, 129, 149–150
  sales of, 5, 14, 129
  toxicity of, 145
  use for major food commodities, 48
  volume of use, 5, 48, 49
  see also Crop-level scenario analyses; specific active ingredients
Fungicides, oncogenic
  acre treatments, 48, 122, 125–128
  active ingredients affected by policy scenarios, 106–107, 109–111, 113–114, 116
  estimated risk from, 5, 8, 69, 74–75, 77, 80, 81, 85, 120, 129–130
  expenditures, 48, 105, 107, 111, 114, 116, 122, 125–128
  forecasting applications of, 126–127
  major crop uses, 52–53
  number, 36, 56
  old, 85
  risk reductions in policy scenarios, 105, 107, 108, 111, 112, 114–117
  substitutes for, 106, 125–127, 130–131, 200–201, 214

TMRCs for, 60
tolerance revocations under policy scenarios, 105–107, 109, 111, 113–114, 116, 122, 125–128
volume of use, 48, 52–53
weak, 10, 95
worst-case impact of Delaney Clause on, 71
year of first tolerance, 52–53, 85

G

Galecron, *see* Chlordimeform
Genetic engineering
  bacterial insecticides, 239–243
  fungal insecticides, 245–246
  innovation prospects in, 151–152, 246–247
  insect control through, 238–247
  viral insecticides, 243–245
  weed control through, 232–233
Gluthion, *see* Azinphos-methyl
Glyphosate
  crop uses, 52, 68, 76
  dietary oncogenic risk from, 68, 76, 84
  Q* for, 55, 76
  risk reduced by tolerance revocations, 113, 121
  TMRC, 76
  volume of use, 47, 52
  weight-of-the-evidence classification, 67, 76
  year of first tolerance, 52, 68
Gramoxone, *see* Paraquat
Grapes
  effect of policy scenarios on, 105, 107, 111, 114, 116
  estimated oncogenic risk from, 78, 80
  pesticide use levels on, 53
  risk reduced by tolerance revocations, 122
  tolerances for processed forms, 64
  vulnerability to tolerance revocations, 10

H

Hays
  pesticide use levels on, 52
  risk standard applied to oncogenic pesticides in, 40, 73
Herbicides
  historical perspective on R&D in, 144
  innovation in, 9, 129, 146–147, 228, 230
  low-application-rate, 229

non-oncogenic, 131, 144
number of CFR tolerances for, 19, 35, 36
percent oncogenic, 4
potential short-term impact of Delaney Clause on, 98
R&D expenditures for, 149–150
volume of use, 228, 229
see also Crop-level scenario analyses; specific active ingredients
Herbicides, oncogenic
acre treatments, 122, 124
active ingredients affected by policy scenarios, 106–107, 109–111, 113–114, 116
estimated risk from, 5, 69, 74–76, 79, 82, 84, 85
expenditures, 46, 105, 107, 111, 114, 116, 122, 124, 144
major crop uses, 52–53
number, 36, 56
old, 85
risk reductions in policy scenarios, 105, 107, 108, 111, 112, 114–117, 124
substitutes for, 106, 124, 131
TMRCs for, 60
tolerance revocations under policy scenarios, 105–107, 109, 111, 113–114, 116
volume of use, 46–47, 49, 52–53
worst-case impact of Delaney Clause on, 71
year of first tolerance, 52–53, 85
Hoelon, *see* Diclofop methyl
Hormones, juvenile insect, for pest control, 154, 235, 238

I

Imidazolinone, 144
Innovations in pest control
challenges to, 155–158
economic incentive for, 145
effect of Delaney Clause on, 9–10
indicators of rates and trends in, 142
in insect control, 234–247
for minor crops, 10
nonchemical, 9, 150–155
pesticides, 8–9, 125, 128–129, 131, 137
process, 137–139
prospects for, 145–148, 150–155
role in pesticide regulatory action, 226

trends, 226–247
in weed control, 228–233
see also Research and development in pest control
Insecticides
amidinohydrazones, 237
avermectins, 236–237
bacterial, 239–243
benzoylphenylureas, 237
cancellation of uses of, 51, 56
estimated dietary risk from, 5
fungal, 245–246
historical perspective of R&D in, 142–144
innovation in, 9, 129, 146–147, 234–247
insect hormones, 235
low-application rate, 234
milbemycines, 236–237
number of CFR tolerances for, 19, 35
octopamine agonists, 236
organochlorine, 138, 142, 234
percent oncogenic, 4, 47, 56
plant products as, 235, 238
proinsecticides, 237–238
R&D expenditures, 149–150
trioxabicyclo[2,2,2]octanes, 236–237
viral, 243–245
see also specific active ingredients
Insecticides, oncogenic
acre treatments, 47–48, 122, 124–125
active ingredients affected by policy scenarios, 106–107, 109–111, 113–114, 116
estimated risk from, 5, 69, 74–77, 79, 82, 84, 85
expenditures, 48, 105, 107, 111, 114, 116, 122, 124–125
number, 36, 56
risk reductions in policy scenarios, 105, 107, 108, 111, 112, 114–117, 122
substitutes for, 106, 124
synthetic pyrethroid, 47, 52, 55, 68, 77, 84, 142–143, 234, 237
TMRCs for, 60
tolerance revocations under policy scenarios, 105–107, 109, 111, 113–114, 116
worst-case impact of Delaney Clause on, 71
International Agency for Research on Cancer, 66

K

Kelthane, see Dicofol
Kerb, see Pronamide

L

Lannate, see Methomyl
Larvadex, see Cyromazine
Larvin, see Thiodicarb
Lasso, see Alachlor
Lead arsenate, 52
Liability for minor crop failures or crop
　injury, 10, 155–156
Lindane, 52, 56
Linuron
　crop uses, 52, 68, 76
　dietary oncogenic risk from, 68, 74, 75,
　　82, 83, 84, 98
　herbicide market share, 98
　possible date for tolerance revocation,
　　98
　potential short-term impact of Delaney
　　Clause on, 98
　Q* for, 55, 76
　risk estimate approaches for, 66
　risk reduced through tolerance
　　revocations, 110, 121, 124
　TMRC, 76
　volume of use, 47, 52
　weight-of-the-evidence classification, 67,
　　76
　year of first tolerance, 52, 68
Lorox, see Linuron

M

Maleic hydrazide, 52
Mancozeb
　crop uses, 52, 68, 77
　dietary oncogenic risk from, 68, 77, 83,
　　85, 97, 132
　fungicide market share, 97, 132
　possible date for tolerance revocation,
　　97, 132
　potential short-term impact of Delaney
　　Clause on, 97, 132
　Q* for, 55, 77
　risk reduced through tolerance
　　revocations, 127
　TMRC, 77
　volume of use, 52
　weight-of-the-evidence classification, 67,
　　77

year of first tolerance, 52, 68
Maneb
　crop uses, 53, 68, 77
　dietary oncogenic risk from, 68, 77, 97,
　　132
　fungicide market share, 97, 132
　possible date for tolerance revocation,
　　97, 132
　Q* for, 55, 77
　risk reduced through tolerance
　　revocations, 110, 120–121
　TMRC, 77
　volume of use, 53
　weight-of-the-evidence classification, 67,
　　77
　year of first tolerance, 53, 68
Meat
　estimated oncogenic risk from, 73–74, 94
　red, consumption estimates, 57–58
Metalaxyl
　application of Delaney Clause to, 216
　dietary oncogenic risk from, 215–216
　effectiveness, 127
　potential uses of and alternatives to,
　　216–217
　regulatory status, 215
　tolerances, 215, 216
　volume of use, 214
Methanearsonic acid, 53
Methomyl, 53
Metiram
　crop uses, 53, 68, 77
　dietary oncogenic risk from, 68, 77, 83,
　　85, 97, 132
　fungicide market share, 97, 132
　possible date for tolerance revocation,
　　97, 132
　potential short-term impact of Delaney
　　Clause on, 97, 132
　Q* for, 55, 77
　TMRC, 77
　volume of use, 53
　weight-of-the-evidence classification, 67,
　　77
　year of first tolerance, 53, 68
Metolachlor
　crop uses, 53, 68, 76
　dietary oncogenic risk from, 68, 76
　Q* for, 55, 76
　risk reduced by tolerance revocations,
　　113, 121
　TMRC, 76
　volume of use, 47, 53
　weight-of-the-evidence classification, 67,

76
year of first tolerance, 53, 68
Milk and dairy products
consumption estimates, 57–58
estimated oncogenic risk from, 79, 94
oncogenic risk from, 73–74
Minor crops
challenges to innovation posed by,
155–157
dietary oncogenic risk from, 10
liability problems with, 10, 155–156
pesticide registration fees, 156
tolerances for, 155
USDA InterRegional Project 4 for,
156–157
vulnerability to tolerance revocations,
10, 71
with processed forms, 10
Mutations of biological insecticides, 241

N

National Food Processors Association, 72
Nuclear polyhedrios viruses, pest control
with, 154

O

O-Phenylphenol
crop uses, 53, 68, 77
dietary oncogenic risk from, 68, 77, 85
Q* for, 55, 77
volume of use, 53
weight-of-the-evidence classification, 67,
77
year of first tolerance, 53, 68
Oncogenicity
data necessary to support a finding of,
38
distinction between carcinogenicity and,
3, 30–31
see also Dietary oncogenic risk
Oncogenicity potency factor (Q*)
definition, 64
derivation of, 63–64, 182, 186
for EPA-designated oncogenic active
ingredients, 55
number of active ingredients with and
without, 56
quantification of, 54–55
uncertainty in, 64, 194–195
variables in, 3, 49–50
Oncogens, definition, 30
Orthene, *see* Acephate

Oryzalin
crop uses, 53, 68, 76
dietary oncogenic risk from, 68, 76, 84
Q* for, 55, 76
TMRC, 76
volume of use, 47, 53
weight-of-the-evidence classification, 67,
76
year of first tolerance, 53, 68
Oxadiazon
crop uses, 53, 68, 76
dietary oncogenic risk from, 68, 76, 83,
84
Q* for, 55, 76
TMRC, 76
volume of use, 53
weight-of-the-evidence classification, 67,
76
year of first tolerance, 53, 68

P

Paraquat
dietary oncogenic risk from, 98
herbicide market share, 98
major crop uses, 53
possible date for tolerance revocation,
98
potential short-term impact of Delaney
Clause on, 98
volume of use, 47, 53
year of first tolerance, 53
Parathion
crop uses, 53, 68, 77
dietary oncogenic risk from, 68, 77, 84
market life, 137
Q* for, 55, 77
risk reduced through tolerance
revocations, 121
volume of use, 53
weight-of-the-evidence classification, 67,
77
year of first tolerance, 53, 68
PCNB, 53
Peanuts
dietary oncogenic risk from pesticide
residues, 133
effect of policy scenarios on, 105, 107,
110–111, 114, 116–117, 128–129
pesticide use levels on, 48, 52–53
risk reduced by tolerance revocations,
122
Permethrin
application of Delaney Clause to, 88, 90,

92–93, 218–220
application rates, 47, 53
crop uses, 53, 68, 77, 92–93
dietary oncogenic risk from, 68, 74, 76, 77, 83, 84, 85, 88, 217–218
Q* for, 55, 77
risk estimate approaches for, 66
risk reduced through tolerance revocations, 121
weight-of-the-evidence classification, 67, 77
year of first tolerance, 53, 68
Pest resistance
to bacterial insecticides, 239–240
Delaney Clause and, 10–11
effect of pesticide use patterns on, 49
to fungal insecticides, 246
to fungicides, 10, 130, 198
management of, 10–11, 157–158
to non-oncogenic pesticides, 10–11, 130
to synthetic pyrethroids, 144
to viral insecticides, 243
Pesticide active ingredients
Acceptable Daily Intake of, 31–32
analyzed in this study, 4
availability, 20
contact with nontarget crops and organisms, 17–18
degradation products of, 29, 31, 37
dietary exposure to, 32, 59; *see also* Dietary exposure to pesticides
expenditures on, 49, 184
exposure to, *see* Dietary exposure to pesticides
field trials for, 29
historical perspective on R&D on, 141–145
impurities, 31, 37, 88, 90
legal basis for regulation of, 11–12
levels in foods, 61
metabolites, 29, 31, 37, 41, 42, 54, 88, 90, 93–94
patent life, 139
prior-sanctioned, 91–92
registration under FIFRA, 23–24, *see* Registration of pesticides; Reregistration process
with retracted or unpursued tolerance applications, 90
suspected oncogens, EPA policy on, 50–51
synthetic chemical, 9
toxicological data on, 182
use cancellations, 56

see also Crop-level scenario analyses; Fungicides; Herbicides; Insecticides; specific active ingredients
Pesticide active ingredients, new
application of Delaney Clause to, 2, 36, 41, 86–96
prospects for, 146–150
recommended safety criteria for, 11–12
simultaneously used with old pesticides, 10
Pesticide active ingredients, non-oncogenic
innovations in, 8–9, 125, 128–129, 131, 137, 148–149
tolerance setting under section 408, 31–33
tolerance setting under section 409, 35
Pesticide active ingredients, old (registered before 1978)
application of Delaney Clause to, 2, 35, 41, 95–96
benefits of, 7–8, 43
dietary oncogenic risk from, 11, 85
EPA application of Delaney Clause to, 95–96
oncogenicity data on, 41, 51
recommended safety criteria for, 11–12
simultaneously used with new pesticides, 10
Pesticide active ingredients, oncogenic
affected by policy scenarios, 106–107, 109–111, 113–114, 116
in animal feeds, 71–74
dichotomous risk standards of sections 408 and 409, 40, 161–170
estimated dietary risk by, 75–77, 83–84
highest risks ever calculated for, 65
low-risk, 7
projections of, 36
Q* for, 55
registered for processed foods, 4–5
with section 409 tolerances, 4–5, 36, 63
substitutes for, 43, 105–106, 149, 200–201, 205
theoretical policy scenarios for regulating, *see* Scenarios for regulating oncogenic pesticides
TMRCs, 60
Waxman list, 50–51
weak, 10, 13–14, 42–43, 95
Pesticide use
benefits associated with, 14, 32–33, 43, 103, 123
cancellation/suspension of, 24, 51, 56; *see also* Tolerance revocation/denial

data on, 184
factors affecting, 48–49
label specifications for, 24, 93
patterns in U.S., 46–49
regional variation in, 17, 61
Pest management programs, integrated, 153–155, 231
Plant breeding, innovation prospects in, 9, 150–151
Policy recommendations
analytical framework, 15–16
coordination between EPA and FDA, 11–12
high-risk pesticide/crop uses, 14–15
negligible-risk standard, 12–14
Potatoes
consumption estimates, 57–59
effect of policy scenarios on, 105, 107, 111, 114, 115–116, 126–127
estimated oncogenic risk from, 78–80, 83, 84, 134
pesticide use levels on, 48, 52
risk reduced by tolerance revocations, 122
vulnerability to tolerance revocations, 10
Pounce, *see* Permethrin
Processed commodities, *see* Commodities, processed
Pronamide
crop uses, 53, 68, 76
dietary oncogenic risk from, 68, 76, 98
herbicide market share, 98
possible date for tolerance revocation, 98
potential short-term impact of Delaney Clause on, 98
Q* for, 55, 76
TMRC, 76
volume of use, 53
weight-of-the-evidence classification, 67, 76
year of first tolerance, 53, 68
Pseudomonas syringae, 154

Q

Q*, *see* Oncogenicity potency (Q*)
Quantitative risk assessment
conservatisms in, 50, 54, 60
constituents policy on, 39, 88, 90, 94, 207–208
EPA's current methodology, 3, 33–34, 50, 59–60
limitations of, 33–34

qualitative factors in, 3
risk/benefit balancing, 18, 19, 24, 25, 32–35, 42–43, 226–227
sensitivity-of-the-method approach, 38, 40, 73, 88, 90, 93–94, 120, 223–224
uncertainties in, 33–34, 51, 54
weight-of-the-evidence approach, 3, 54–55, 66, 101
see also EPA policy, current dietary oncogenic risk estimation

R

Registration of pesticides
burden on registrant after, 24
cancellation/suspension, 24, 51, 56
data required to support, 20, 24, 36, 51
label specifications, 24, 93
minor-use, 156
relation to tolerance-setting process, 23
standards for, under FIFRA, 24
Registration standard, 97
Reregistration process
application of Delaney Clause in, 2, 12
Data Call-In Program, 36–37, 96–97
residue chemistry data supporting, 20
Research and development in pest control
in chemical pest control, prospects for, 145–148
effect of Delaney Clause implementation on, 9–10, 137, 140, 249–255
expenditures on pesticides, 129, 139–141, 149–150
historical perspective of, 141–145
in nonchemical pest control, 9, 150–155
studies of regulatory effects on, 139–140, 249–255
see also Innovations in pest control
Residue chemistry data
gathering and interpretation of, 29, 36–37
required to support registration, 20, 24, 36, 51
required to support tolerance petitions, 27–29
Ridomyl, *see* Metalaxyl
Risk
definition, 65
see also Dietary oncogenic risk; Dietary oncogenic risk estimation; Quantitative risk assessment
Ronilan, *see* Vinclozolin
Ronstar, *see* Oxadiazon
Roundup, *see* Glyphosate

S

Scenarios for regulating oncogenic
    pesticides
  analytical methods, 102–103, 187–190
  criteria for, 104
  crop-level analyses, 7, 102–103, 117,
    123–129, 190
  crop-pesticide combinations used for,
    102
  crops losing tolerances under, 106,
    109–110, 113–116
  cropwide tolerance reduction, 131–134
  impacts analyzed in, 101–102
  impacts by pesticide type, 118–120
  impacts on benefits and risks, 123–129
  impacts on individual active ingredient
    risk, 120–123
  negligible-risk, processed foods (scenario
    4), 6, 7, 103–104, 114–117
  negligible-risk, raw and processed foods
    (scenario 3), 6, 7, 104, 110–114
  zero-risk, processed foods (scenario 2),
    6–7, 104, 107–110
  zero-risk, raw and processed foods
    (scenario 1), 6, 103–107
Sodium arsenate, 53
Sodium arsenite, 53, 56
Sonalan, *see* Ethalfluralin
Soybeans
  effect of policy scenarios on, 107, 111,
    114, 116–117, 124
  estimated oncogenic risk from, 15, 78,
    79
  pesticide use levels on, 52–53, 89
  risk reduced by tolerance revocations,
    122
  tolerances for processed forms, 64,
    219–220
Sulfonylureas, 144
Sulfur, effectiveness as potato fungicide,
    127
Surflan, *see* Oryzalin

T

Terbutryn
  crop uses, 53, 68, 76
  dietary oncogenic risk from, 68, 76, 84,
    98
  herbicide market share, 98
  possible date for tolerance revocation,
    98
  potential short-term impact of Delaney

Clause on, 98
  Q* for, 55, 76
  TMRC, 76
  volume of use, 53
  weight-of-the-evidence classification, 67,
    76
  year of first tolerance, 53, 68
Tetrachlorvinphos, 53
Theoretical Maximum Residue
    Contribution (TMRC)
  calculation of, 32, 181–182
  conservatisms in, 60
  distribution of, by pesticide type, 60
  reduction of, 33
Thiodicarb
  application of Delaney Clause to, 88, 90,
    93–94, 222–224
  degradation to methomyl, 222
  dietary oncogenic risk from, 88, 93–94,
    221–222
  major crop uses, 53
  metabolite, 222–223
  volume of use, 53
  year of first tolerance, 53
Thiophanate-methyl, 53
Tobacco mosaic virus, 152
Tolerance Assessment System (TAS)
  conversion factors for concentration of
    residues, 62
  data base, 59, 174–175
  limitations and improvements in, 57–59,
    175
  number of processed foods in, 64
  treatment of residues in processed
    foods, 61–63
  use in this study, 51
Tolerance revocation/denial
  dietary oncogenic risk increased by, 8,
    14–15, 41–42, 126, 127, 128, 131–134
  EPA policy, 34
  under policy scenarios, 105–117
  possible dates for, on selected fungicides
    and herbicides, 97–98
  regional impacts, 125–126, 128
  vulnerability of minor crops to, 10
Tolerance setting
  actions for which Delaney Clause was
    cited, 88
  benefit consideration in, 18, 19, 24, 25,
    32–35
  dichotomy in statutory standards for, 2,
    11, 40–41, 161–170
  EPA policy for, 2, 27–36, 41, 196–224
  EPA responsibility for, 18–19

under FDC Act, 19, 24–36
for new active ingredients, case studies of, 91–95
for non-oncogenic pesticides, 31–33
for old active ingredients, case studies of, 95–96
for oncogenic pesticides under section 408, 33–35
process, 27–36
relationship to registration process, 23–24
on suspect oncogens, 51
zero-risk vs. negligible-risk, 2, 6–7, 12–14
Tolerances
affected by negligible-risk scenario 3, 112–114
affected by negligible-risk scenario 4, 115–116
affected by zero-risk scenario 1, 106–107
affected by zero-risk scenario 2, 109–111
conversion into dietary intake estimate, 59
cropwide reduction of, 131–134
data sources on, 178–179
data required to support requests for, 27–29
definition, 18, 23
dietary oncogenic risk by type of, 67–71, 85–86
fees for, 90, 156
incentives for lowering, 220
influence of Delaney Clause on content of, 90
level-of-detection, 131
levels, 29
minor-use, 155
notice and comment in *Federal Register*, 27
number in CFR by pesticide type, 19, 35
oncogenic risk associated with date of, 85–86
opposition to, 29
petitions for, 27
processed by-products needing, 72
regulatory status data, 182–183
risk by date of, 85–87
Tolerances, processed commodity (section 409)
basis for determining need for, 28
number, 19, 64
for oncogenic pesticides, 4–5, 36, 63, 69
risk from, 67–71
standard for, 1, 25–27, 35–36

Tolerances, raw commodity (section 408)
basis for, 28
benefits considered in determining, 32–33
for oncogenic pesticides, 36, 69
risk from, 67–71
standard for, 1, 25
Tomatoes
concentration of residues during processing of, 81–82, 218–219
consumption estimates, 57–59
effect of policy scenarios on, 107, 111, 114–116, 127–128
estimated oncogenic risk from, 78–83, 85, 134
pesticide use levels on, 48, 52
risk reduced by tolerance revocations, 122
tolerance limited to raw form, 88, 90
tolerances for processed forms, 64, 81
vulnerability to tolerance revocations, 10
Toxaphene, 53, 56
Toxicity data/studies
no observable effect level, 31–32
required for tolerance petitions, 29
safety factor in, 32
Treflan, *see* Trifluralin
Trifluralin
estimated dietary oncogenic risk from, 98
herbicide market share, 98
major crop uses, 53
possible date for tolerance revocation, 98
potential short-term impact of Delaney Clause on, 98
volume of use, 47, 53
year of first tolerance, 53

U

U.S. Department of Agriculture
food consumption surveys, 57
InterRegional Project 4, 156–157

V

Vegetables
consumption estimates, 57–58
dependency on pesticides, 49
importance of fungicides in production of, 8
pesticide use levels on, 48, 52–53, 89

regional variation in pesticide use on, 17
Vinclozolin, 90

W

Waxman list, 50–51

Z

Zineb
  crop uses, 53, 68, 77
  dietary oncogenic risk from, 68, 77, 85,
    97, 132
  fungicide market share, 97, 132
  possible date for tolerance revocation,
    97, 132
  potential short-term impact of Delaney
    Clause on, 97, 132
  Q* for, 55, 77
  TMRC, 77
  volume of use, 53
  weight-of-the-evidence classification, 67,
    77
  year of first tolerance, 53, 68